Saving Lives in Wartime China

China Studies

Edited by

Glen Dudbridge
Frank Pieke

VOLUME 26

The titles published in this series are listed at brill.com/chs

Saving Lives in Wartime China

How Medical Reformers Built Modern Healthcare
Systems Amid War and Epidemics, 1928–1945

By

John R. Watt

BRILL

LEIDEN • BOSTON
2016

This paperback was originally published in hardback as Volume 26 in the series *ChS*.

Cover illustration: The ABMAC Blood Bank saved combat soldiers in west China in 1944. Source: ABMAC Archive.

Library of Congress Cataloging-in-Publication Data

Watt, John R. (John Robertson), 1934–
   Saving lives in wartime China : how medical reformers built modern healthcare systems amid war and epidemics, 1928–1945 / by John R. Watt.
      pages cm. — (China studies ; volume 26)
   Includes bibliographical references and index.
   ISBN 978-90-04-25645-3 (hardback : alk. paper) — ISBN 978-90-04-25646-0 (e-book)
1. Public health—China—History—20th century. 2. Medical care—China—History—20th century. 3. China—History—20th century. 4. Health care reform—China—History.
I. Title.

   RA527.W38 2013
   362.10951—dc23

                                                                                             2013027832

This publication has been typeset in the multilingual "Brill" typeface. With over 5,100 characters covering Latin, IPA, Greek, and Cyrillic, this typeface is especially suitable for use in the humanities. For more information, please see www.brill.com/brill-typeface.

ISSN 1570-1344
ISBN 978-90-04-31076-6 (paperback, 2016)
ISBN 978-90-04-25645-3 (hardback, 2014)
ISBN 978-90-04-25646-0 (e-book, 2014)

For Anne

CONTENTS

LIST OF PHOTOGRAPHS, GRAPHS, MAPS, AND TABLES

Photographs

Graphs

Maps

Tables

FOREWORD

Throughout the late 19th and the 20th centuries health care for urban and national populations was highly variable. Western European nations and the United States led the way in recognizing that public health necessitated providing clean water, sewage control and isolation of patients to control the spread of infections.

These practical public health measures were lacking in China, with devastating consequences for the Chinese people, especially the peasants. Superimposed on the existing health problems in that era were the devastating civil and Sino-Japanese wars, which greatly magnified the problems of survival in a population already near starvation.

This volume chronicles how China faced the urgent need to find solutions to the problem of mass suffering of the Chinese people. In time a few leaders emerged. These health reformers, in the words of the author, faced five severe problems: 1) communicable disease, 2) superstition and illiteracy, 3) patriarchal oppression, 4) warfare, and 5) deep seated disregard for the peasant population except as a source of labor, rent and taxes.

This magnificently detailed history clarifies the role of specific physicians and scientists who rose to prominence in that era and who found these conditions unacceptable. These individuals emerged from the more forward looking medical institutions in China, the Peking Union Medical College, a number of Chinese medical colleges and the Chinese Red Cross.

Ultimately, this volume demonstrates how the personal resolve and dedication of a small number of physicians and scientists and a unique set of political, social and economic conditions met in a remarkable confluence to mitigate appalling suffering and initiate the promise of an improved health care system in China for the future.

John Watt, a specialist in Chinese history, has had 36 years of participation in the progress of the American Bureau for Medical Advancement in China (ABMAC). This organization had its beginnings in 1937 during the Japanese invasion and supported Chinese medical agencies throughout that war. In 1949 it moved to Taiwan. The ABMAC organization has played a significant role in the development of the national system of

health care and medical education in Taiwan and, more recently, in Mainland China.

Gerard M. Turino, M.D.
John H. Keating Sr. Professor of Medicine (emeritus)
Columbia University College of Physicians & Surgeons
President of the ABMAC Foundation

Kung-ming Jan, M.D., Ph.D.
Associate Professor of Clinical Medicine
Columbia University College of Physicians & Surgeons
Executive Director of the ABMAC Foundation

PREFACE

This study has grown out of my thirty-six year association with the American Bureau for Medical Aid to China (ABMAC, later Medical Advancement in China), as consultant, executive director, historian, and then as Board Director of ABMAC and its successor the ABMAC Foundation. During this time I published a booklet on ABMAC's history (A Friend Indeed: ABMAC and the Republic of China 1937–1987) and a larger edited volume, tracking ABMAC's commitment to healthcare in mainland China and later Taiwan from 1937 to 2000 (Healthcare and National Development in Taiwan).

When Japan invaded China in August 1937, the founders of ABMAC determined to do something to help save Chinese lives threatened by the furious military onslaught. During the war that mission expanded into helping China's medical leaders build a modern army medical service and a public health structure for what they saw as a newborn nation. After 1945 the decline of U.S. financial support and the collapse of the Nationalist regime took the wind out of these goals; but they remained intrinsic to the mission of ABMAC and are embedded in its archive at Columbia University. Saving lives and advancing healthcare mattered then and matters now.

The Japanese invasion was part of a more complex problem. China at that time was bombarded by infectious diseases and by malpractice in birthing as well as maternal-child health. For millions of rural people starvation and famine were never far away. China in the 1940s was a dangerously high fertility and high mortality society, however the Nationalist government did not see this as the major threat to its mandate. But during the War against Japan the social contract by which the government extracted resources from its people and in return ensured conditions of at least minimal peace and livelihood reached near breakdown. Only the medical reformers understood the vital importance of curtailing disease and saving lives in an impoverished, war-torn and starving country.

After considering this situation for over 20 years, I am convinced that more research into modernization of developing countries with large populations will affirm that managing basic public health issues is a precursor to economic advancement, even during war time. This study spells out the challenges to health in China in the 1930s and 1940s, showing how both the Nationalists and the Communists recognized the need for biomedicine and basic public health as they struggled to save lives despite horrifying losses during this period. It looks at public health, military health, maternal-child health, initiatives in some of the Communist base areas, health education, and the impact on health of a brutal war. Although there is little vital statistical data for that era, a good deal of information was gathered from documents in the ABMAC Archive and from policies undertaken by bold innovators. The resulting study is designed to make the results of this research accessible to people concerned about healthcare in China. I've learned that if given a chance Chinese healthcare innovators were second to none in achieving advances in public healthcare, even during this chaotic war period. In short, this is a story worth telling.

ACKNOWLEDGEMENTS

This work has been a long time in the making, set aside repeatedly in the interest of making a living, and yet something that I could not ultimately let drop. To begin with, I could not forget the people I knew who took part in this story, so I should start by acknowledging their claim on my conscience. All of them, not incidentally, are Chinese.

Among those who supplied me with essential documentary material are Drs. Yang Wen-tah, Pan Shu-jen, Fan Rixin and Robert McClure, Nurse Chu Pao-tien (Zhu Baotian), Prof. Sa Benwang of the former Beijing Institute of International Strategic Studies, retired Public Health Vice Minister Yang Chun and officers of the Chinese Red Cross in Beijing, Mr. John Ma (former China librarian at the New York Public Library), Christina and Peter Gilmartin, Caroline Reeves, Priscilla Armstrong, Nicole Barnes, Lingling Zhang, Wang Yintong of the Shanghai Academy of Social Sciences, Michael Gasster, Suzanne Pearce, Hope Phillips, and Yanfang Su. I could not have completed this study without their help.

I was also fortunate to receive some very helpful financial and technical support. Financial support came initially from the Pacific Cultural Foundation and later from the China Medical Board and the ABMAC Foundation. I am indebted to Dr. Lincoln Chen and the directors of the CMB and to Drs. Gerard Turino, Kung-ming Jan and Richard N. Pierson of the ABMAC Foundation for stepping in to help this study at times when I really needed some assistance. Operating from retirement is not the ideal perch from which to launch a complicated, research-driven project.

For technical assistance of various kinds I am indebted to Yanfang Su, Chelsea Lei, Bill Schneider, Alison Watt, and Ethan Kuo. I am particularly grateful to Dana Bille, who made the photographs and maps clear and readable and solved computer problems, and Bao Truong, who prepared the exemplary graphs, drawing meaning out of tables of indigestible numbers. The photographs, graphs, and maps are all essential elements in making this story come alive.

Among those with whom I was able to have interviews and consultations I am happy to acknowledge Professor Chang Peng-yuan of Academic Sinica, Drs. Wang Kaixi, Yang Wen-tah, and Mr. Liu Yung-mao (all former members of the Chinese Red Cross Medical Relief Corps), Dr. Fan Rixin and Nurse Chu Pao-tien (former public health agents in

China during the 1940s), a group of senior officials at the Chinese Red Cross offices in Beijing, Mrs. S. C. Wang (a graduate of the PUMC Nursing School) who for years guided me on everything to do with nursing in China, Dr. Chai Tso-yung, and Dr. Xie Xide, with whom I was able to meet several times in Shanghai and who was among those who knew Dr. Lin Kesheng personally.

Among many friends and colleagues who helped to point me and/or the text generally in the right direction I should mention Bridie Andrews, Yanfang Su, Christina Gilmartin, Nicole Barnes, Jane Knowles, Bob Ross, and Mike Liu of Academia Sinica. Special thanks are due to Caroline Reeves for prodding me into action in so many ways and to Ronald Suleski, who sponsored publication of my essay on medical education in China and introduced me to a representative of E. J. Brill. At Brill I was fortunate to receive outstanding service on many fronts from Qin Higley, Karen Cullen, and Tom Begley. Last but not least, Ezra Vogel not only provided useful connections but has been an inspiring example of how to get busy when retired.

Readers who know what editing is all about will hopefully recognize that this work has been edited and reedited to remove the padding, sharpen the argument, and make the text more readable. For those services I am hugely indebted to my lifetime partner Anne. During the last two years she has spent countless weeks and months tracking down every weakness in the text and making me rethink every chapter and most paragraphs at least twice. In addition, she worked generously over the technical aspects of organizing photographs, and particularly preparing the maps: making sure that they were accurately drawn, labeled, captioned with relevant 'stories', and placed appropriately in the text. For this plus numerous phone calls and emails, her reward is a dedication, justly earned, and from time to time breakfast in bed. I also want to acknowledge several friends and my daughters for keeping my spirits high during many long years.

I could not complete these acknowledgements without expressing my thanks to the Chinese people for creating and preserving a civilization that has been a constant source of enrichment. My goal in this work has been to recognize the contributions of China's people to that civilization, and to pay my respects to those individuals who sought to take care of their health and wellbeing in a time of crisis.

LIST OF ABBREVIATIONS

ABMAC	American Bureau for Medical Aid to China (美国医药援华会)
AMA	Army Medical Administration (junyishu 军医暑)
AMC	Army Medical College
ARC	American Red Cross
CEF	Chinese expeditionary force
CFHS	Central Field Health Station (*Zhongyang Weisheng Sheshi Shi-yanchu* 中央卫生设施实验处)
CRC	Chinese Red Cross
CRCHQ	Chinese Red Cross Headquarters
CRCMRC	Chinese Red Cross Medical Relief Corps
DBS	delousing, bathing and scabies
EMSTS	Emergency Medical Service Training Schools
MCH	Maternal Child health
MRC	Medical Relief Corps
NAC	Nursing Association of the Republic of China (中华民国护理学会)
NHA	National Health Administration (*weishengshu* 卫生署)
NIH	National Institute of Health (*Zhongyang weisheng shiyanyuan* 中央卫生实验院)
NMJC	National Medical Journal of China
NMPPS	North Manchurian Plague Prevention Service (北满防疫处, later 东北防疫事务总处)
PUMC	Peking Union Medical College
SOS	services of supply
UCR	United China Relief
UNRRA	United Nations Relief and Rehabilitation Agency
WAMC	War Area Medical Centers
WHO	World Health Organization

INTRODUCTION

SAVING LIVES IN THE CONTEXT OF DISEASE, POVERTY AND WAR

A guaranteed cure!
Don't cough like that, Little Shuan!
A guaranteed cure!
　　　　　　　　　　　—From "Medicine," by Lu Xun, 1919[1]

The field of public health and medical services is ... closely involved in
people's lives, and essential for societies to grow and develop.
　　　　　　—Japan International Cooperation Agency, 2005[2]

In 1919, a former Chinese medical student published a story about a boy,
who died from tuberculosis because of a radically improper treatment.
At that time there was no public health in China beyond street cleaning
in a few big cities, and the vast majority of rural people depended on
temples, priests and quacks for medical services. Modernity in the form of
biomedical healthcare existed in a few mission settlements, where curative services were available, but the majority of Chinese people still lived,
epidemiologically, in a pre-modern world characterized by poverty, illiteracy, high fertility and high mortality. The boy was expensively treated
with bread dipped in the blood of an executed "criminal." The author used
this notion of healthcare to emphasize the harsh realities of life for most
Chinese people.

　　Such a story presents in microcosm dilemmas facing China in the early
twentieth century. After half a century of peasant rebellions, imperialist
encroachment, shameful defeats and infection with opium, the great traditional civilization of China was falling apart. In 1905 Confucianism was
officially abandoned, and in 1911, after executing many martyrs, the imperial regime collapsed, leaving the intelligentsia with no clear leadership
function. Warlord armies crisscrossed the country, opium smoking continued, Japan replaced China as East Asia's leading power, and foreigners

---

[1] From Yang Hsien-yi and Gladys Yang (1972), 31. The Chinese text is *"Bao hao, Xiao*
Shuan, nibuyao zheme ke, bao hao" (包好小栓你不要这么咳包好). The family name of
father and son was Hua 华, meaning "China."
　[2] From foreword to Japan International Cooperation Agency (March 2005).

controlled significant areas of China's public life. China's great literary tradition was also was scarred by these upheavals. In *Diary of a Madman*, one of the most celebrated texts of early twentieth century Chinese litera-ture, Lu Xun depicts a scholar who becomes obsessed by the dark aspects of human existence. Between the lines of historical texts he keeps seeing the words "eat people." Shaken by this vision he fears for his own life. The 'diary' ends with a pathetic appeal to "save the children."

In early twentieth century China the idea of saving children had little traction. China's children were targets of human oppression, devastating diseases and dangerous malpractice. Circulation of infectious diseases— e.g. cholera and plague—had been greatly increased by nineteenth century imperialism and trade. In "Medicine," however, Lu Xun chose tuberculosis, a disease long embedded in the Chinese population, as the symbol of early death. As we shall see, this disease was believed to kill a million or more Chinese people a year, many of them children. The public authorities were seemingly indifferent to the problem, as they did nothing about it.

But while China sank into the status of "sick man of East Asia" (东亚病夫 *dongya bingfu*),[3] huge changes were going on across the world, precipitated by industrialization, World War I and the Soviet Revolution. A few Chinese patriots trained in modern clinical and laboratory-based medicine thought that doing nothing in China was unacceptable. Living outside of China these medical scientists already knew a good deal about agents of infectious disease and were teaching such knowledge in bio-medical schools. If Japan could get infectious disease under control, surely Chinese medical reformers could do as much.

Yet the challenges to transforming healthcare in China were immense. Internationally public health discourse and legislation was still in its early days. Although public health reforms began in Britain in the middle of the 19th century, a British Ministry of Health was not established until 1919, by which time fundamental reforms of urban sewage and water systems were in place and most dangerous infectious diseases were under con-trol. Up to that time no such changes had taken place in China and no public understanding of the need for public health existed. A statement such as that of the Japan International Cooperation Agency cited above,

---

[3] The idea of China as "sick man" apparently originated with the philosopher Yan Fu (严复) in the aftermath of China's defeat by Japan in 1895. See "Dongya bingfu" (东亚 病夫) in http://baike.baidu.com/view/582724.htm.

which today reads like a truism, could not even have been formulated in China in 1919.

This book highlights the work of a small but dedicated group of medical reformers who took on the challenge to deal with China's high rates of sickness and death. These reformers were individuals who obtained professional education in colleges that taught clinical and laboratory-based medicine, hereafter referred to as biomedicine, that is, study based on careful examination of patients, laboratory data collection and microscopic analysis, along with the principles of modern nursing, midwifery and public health. Initially they obtained their education in China, Hong Kong or Japan, or farther away in Germany, France, Britain, Canada, and the United States, and in some cases with advanced study in public health or tropical medicine.

After the dedication of the Rockefeller-sponsored Peking Union Medical College (PUMC) in 1921, this college became a fertile source of medical reformers. Some learned about public health by working at urban and rural health centers cosponsored by PUMC. In the 1930s and 1940s the Nationalist government's National Health Administration (NHA), several national medical colleges and provincial health administrations, and the Chinese Red Cross Medical Relief Corps (CRCMRC) and Emergency Medical Service Training Schools, educated or hired individuals who would play significant roles as healthcare reformers.

A few missionary agencies also were a source of new leadership. Qilu (齐鲁 Cheloo) Christian University Medical College cosponsored a rural health service in Shandong; and several physicians who served the Chinese Red Army and Chinese Communist base areas during the 1930s and 1940s were educated at missionary institutions. Practitioners of Chinese medicine also took on leadership roles in the Chinese Communist medical services of this era. Even the experience of healthcare reform in East Europe and the Soviet Union after World War One came into play in China. In short, different pathways existed in China for promoting modernity through healthcare.

The most active reformers were interested in following the path of "public healthcare" (公医 *gongyi*) as a strategy for dealing with widespread illness and premature death common among uneducated people. Many reformers chose to work specifically in the fields of public health and military medicine. They emphasized preventive medicine (防疫 *fangyi*), hygiene and sanitation, or more broadly public health (卫生 *weisheng*, literally meaning "guard health"). *Weisheng* had sufficient importance for Nationalist China's Ministry of Health to call itself in 1928 the "*weisheng* ministry," suggesting that the state was now interested in guarding the health of the people. In the early 1930s the Red Army changed the names of its military healthcare units to *weisheng* units to emphasize their preventive health role.[4]

What, then, were the specific challenges that the reformers faced? From an epidemiological perspective, China was still locked into a pre-modern, pre-transitional state dominated by five severe problems: communicable disease, superstition and illiteracy, patriarchal oppression, warfare, and disregard for the peasantry except as a source of rent and taxes. We will briefly review these five problems before proceeding on with the work of the reformers.

Communicable Disease

In 1945, a professor of agricultural biology at Qilu University calculated that around a quarter of the annual average death rate estimated at 15 million people resulted from fecal-borne diseases.[5] During the eight year War of Resistance against Japan (1937–45) some thirty to thirty-five million people may have died of fecal-borne diseases, while "probably five to ten million" died as a direct result of the war.[6] In a more cautiously worded survey of prevalent communicable diseases, Dr. Fan Rixin (范日新, J. H. Fan) estimated that bacillary dysentery (杆菌痢疾) formed ninety percent of reported hospital cases during 1940–44 and that the available data was only a small fraction of incidence. He wrote that during the war dysentery was probably more present and widespread than ever before.[7] In China there was then little statistical data available to researchers. But information of this nature indicates that war helped to spread infectious

---

[4] The meanings of *weisheng* in both Japanese and Chinese culture, and its association with the emergence of a modern health-oriented Japanese nation, are explored in detail in Ruth Rogaski, *Hygienic Modernity: Meanings of Health and Disease in Treaty Port China* (Berkeley: University of California Press, 2004). Chapters 4 and 5 provide interesting comparisons of the treatment of *weisheng* in China and Japan.

[5] Gerald F. Winfield, 1948.

[6] Winfield (1948), 112–113. 'Fecal-borne' diseases include bacterial diseases such as cholera, typhoid, bacillary and amoebic dysentery and diarrhea, and parasitic diseases such as hookworm, schistosomiasis and ascaris.

[7] J. H. Fan (1945): 495–536. Dr. Fan was a PUMC graduate and had a Ph.D. in public Health from Johns Hopkins. The writer interviewed him on several occasions. Fan's emphasis on dysentery is supported by data collected by Zhang Taishan and presented in tables 1–10 and 1–11 in Zhang Taishan (张泰山) (2008), 60–62.

disease and that bacterial and parasitic infection in China destroyed considerably more human life than did military conflict.[8]

Other diseases contributed significantly to China's chronically high rates of disease and death. Due to poverty and malnutrition tuberculosis was endemic in China and caused an annual mortality estimated at 900,000 to 1.2 million people, many of whom were students. Smallpox was also endemic and caused an annual mortality also estimated at 900,000, much of it occurring in early childhood.[9] Other directly transmitted diseases included measles, diphtheria, scarlet fever; childbirth diseases and complications for mothers and infants resulting from unhygienic midwifery; insect-borne diseases such as malaria, typhus, bubonic plague, and relapsing fever; parasitic diseases, e.g. hookworm and schistosomiasis; and venereal diseases, principally syphilis and gonorrhea.[10] As this study will illustrate, whole regions could be depleted by onslaughts of cholera, malaria and syphilis.

The oppressive rates of disease and death found in China in the 1930s and 1940s expressed not only the public health and war-induced problems of that time but also more underlying cultural patterns, such as pervasive superstition, conducive to social and physical pathology. As the reformers noticed, these underlying cultural patterns made it hard to deal with the destructive impact of epidemics and inadequate medical practice. Ghastly as the destruction of Nanjing was, the main dangers to human life were disease, malpractice, ignorance, poverty and starvation. Because of such circumstances China had to fight an eight-year war against the modernized Japanese military with a population whose health and wellbeing were compromised from the outset.

---

[8] This is the basic argument underlying the path-breaking book by William H. McNeill (1976). The Japanese discerned the dominance of disease in creating wartime casualties during the Sino-Japanese war of 1894–1895. See Rogaski (2004), 157–160.

[9] Tsefang F. Huang (1927), reported in Lamson, *Social Pathology in China* (1935), 270, 280, and chapter 11.

[10] Winfield (1948), 105. Based on various studies, Winfield calculated the mortality rate at approximately 30/1,000. The National Health Administration had used the same ratio in 1937; so did Herbert D. Lamson in *Social Pathology in China*. Public health specialists of the time considered a death rate over 15/1,000 as excessive.

Superstition

Superstition was a special curse for the Reformers. Wu Liande (伍连德), the noted public health reformer, captured the sentiments of his colleagues when he wrote:

> As long as there is ignorance of the laws of physiological and sanitary righteousness and it is commonly believed that all forms of disease are traceable to the action or influence of innumerable spirits and demons over whom there can be no permanent human influence or control, there will be little real progress in public health.[11]

One can understand the frustration of the reformers. They were dealing with a belief system lasting for 2,000 years or more and deeply rooted in literary and oral traditions.[12] For the vast majority of the Chinese population temples, shrines, images, and beliefs handed down through generations were the main agencies for helping individuals, families and small communities to fend off demonic assaults.

A large assortment of healthcare gods catered to individuals living in the oral tradition, chief among them the god of pestilence (瘟神, *wenshen*) and the king of the underworld (阎王, *yan wang*/Yama).

When angered by human misconduct *Wenshen* unleashed multitudes of *wen* spirits, which spread disease. Supplication to higher deity was necessary to persuade *Wenshen* to recall the *wen* spirits. Other gods arbitrated over afflictions caused by cold and heat, wind diseases, eye diseases, dysentery, convulsions, smallpox, measles, and plague. A study published in 1924 found that out of 500 prayer slips 484 requested healing from disease.[13]

It was the dense population of lower-order demons that caused the most trouble. Demons who died unnatural deaths tried to trap people into similar deaths. Demons who died in childbirth tried to cause other women to die in childbirth. If a child was sick, a demonic attack might be the cause. Buddhist and Daoist priests made a living exorcising such demonic activities. These notions now seem farfetched, but D. C. Graham,

---

[11] Wu Lien-teh (1924), 44, 45, cited in Lamson (1935), 455. Note his use of the Confucian term "righteousness" (义 *yi*) in this English language essay.

[12] Among many studies of Chinese religion J. J. M. De Groot (1972 reprint), provides detailed and heavily documented accounts of religious management of psychosomatic disorder, particularly in volumes 5 and 6. The account in this chapter draws on De Groot's treatment.

[13] Clarence Burton Day, *Chinese Peasant Cults* (1969), 13, 39–40. This valuable account of peasant cults has several passages dealing with demonic disorder.

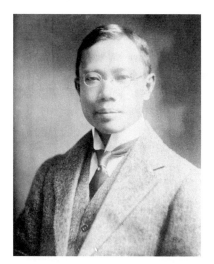 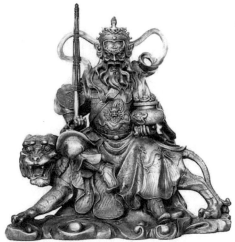

Photographs I.1 and I.2: *Dr. Wu Liande* and *Wenshen*

1. Dr. Wu Liande. Overseas Chinese, pioneer public health advocate, he brought a major plague epidemic under control and co-founded the National Medical Association and the National Medical Journal of China. (*Source*: George Grantham Bain Collection, Library of Congress, website: http://www.loc.gov/pictures/item/ggb2005014227/.)
2. Wenshen. Disease deity, arbiter of health in many rural Chinese communities. (*Source*: http://www.baike.com/wiki/%E7%98%9F%E7%A5%9E&prd=so_auto_doc_list.)

writing in the 1950s, insisted that: "the fear of demons in West China can hardly be exaggerated."[14]

Much of the problem with superstition had to do with pervasive illiteracy as much as with spirits and demons. But in the 1930s and 40s the tradition was still strong enough to persuade educated individuals who obtained vaccinations against epidemic diseases to continue to support temple cults that responded to epidemics with rituals. The question for the reformers, including Mao Zedong, was: why should so many people be left to combat bacteria and parasites with animism and chicanery, when modern science could do better?

Yet the question for the people was, why abandon a cult such as that of *Wenshen* that was rooted in popular culture and that seemed to have its own way of controlling disease?[15] Its rituals promoted fasting, interrupted social commerce, and required people to stay at home and keep their

---

[14] David Crockett Graham (1961), 123–29. Dr. Graham was for ten years professor at West China Union University in Chengdu.
[15] See "Wenshen" in baike.baidu.com/view/145335.htm.

doors fastened against entry by evil spirits. As indicated by Francis Hsu, such practices were still flourishing in Yunnan in the 1940s, at a time when a cholera epidemic spread by Japanese military bacterial warfare was devastating southwest China.[16] So entrenched were these beliefs that they could cause rural people to flee with their children rather than allow them to receive vaccinations from unfamiliar, white coated people (white was associated with death).[17] Short of the direct assault on the demonic world favored by Mao Zedong, the influence of gods and demons would not be easily dislodged.[18]

Patriarchal Oppression

Following the collapse of the empire in 1911 the Chinese people entered a period of government characterized by incompetence, military violence, and rapacity. In his study of the peasant movement in Hunan Mao Zedong described political authority, from the center down to townships, as a "thick rope" binding the Chinese people in several key ways.[19] The strongest part of the "rope" was the brutal squeeze accompanying rural tax collection. The replacement of China's Imperial system by warlord regimes led to infliction of nightmarish tax levies as well as predatory scavenging, burning and killing by warlord armies.[20]

The worst famine in the period under study was that which occurred in and around Henan province during 1942–1943. In their well-known diatribe *Thunder Out of China*, White and Jacoby charged that two years of poor harvests were followed by a year in which harvests failed while taxes and rent collection continued. They concluded that of the thirty million people of Henan, probably two to three million fled the province as refugees and a similar number died of disease, while the loyalty of the people had been "hollowed out by the extortion of their government."[21]

---

[16] Francis L. K. Hsu (1983) provides a fascinating insight into this question from an anthropological perspective.

[17] "Guomin zhengfu shiqi gongyizhidu shouxiao shenwei yuanyin tanxi," (2011).

[18] Mao Zedong (1927).

[19] Mao Zedong (1927), section on "Fourteen Great Achievements."

[20] One particularly obscene example of this phenomenon is discussed by Edward A. McCord (2001), 18–47.

[21] Theodore H. White and Annalee Jacoby (1946), 176–177. A more comprehensive but much less well-known analysis, written by an American missionary who lived through it all, concluded that the famine was "largely man-made"; it "would not have occurred

Another aspect of Mao's thick rope critique was the system of clan authority embodied in landlord-tenant relationships. A characteristic method by which landlords deployed squeeze was to get their land withdrawn from government tax rolls, leaving less powerful and more vulnerable people to cover the cost of the tax levies.[22] The direct method was through coercion of rent and seizure of peasant assets in times of distress. A third of Mao's "thick ropes", masculine authority, ensured that women and children would be the first to suffer in times of stress through such methods as being starved, denied healthcare, or sold into slavery or marital subservience. Among the many healthcare hazards related to this oppression of women, one must include the old-style midwifery and the social context in which it operated, which prevailed in China during the first half of the twentieth century. These conditions produced very high rates of death among infants and young mothers. During wartime rape also flourished, as described in chapter 7.

Conduct of Warfare

A "thick rope" not discussed by Mao involved the prevailing systems of authority governing rank-and-file soldiers and recruitment of conscripts.[23] We will see how these systems functioned and their impact on the health of soldiers and conscripts. Here it is sufficient to point out that anemia, malnutrition and starvation were characteristic problems affecting Chinese soldiers and conscripts, especially in the later years of the War of Resistance against Japan. These afflictions also had a seriously negative impact on the Chinese Communist resistance in Jiangxi province in 1934. The starvation that occurred during the War of Resistance resulted not only from corruption at higher levels but also from a systemic incompetence in management of services of supply that dogged Nationalist China's armed forces and conscription systems. These problems were the

---

had not war, selfishness and greed been raging near that area." See Ernest M. Wampler (1945), 274.

[22] An aerial survey of one Jiangxi district, carried out from May 1932–June 1934, found that 300,000 mu of arable land, constituting twenty-three percent of the district's arable land, had not paid taxes in "hundreds of years." See American Board of Commissioners for Foreign Missions, Shaowu archive, volume II, Reports, #37, section on land tenure.

[23] In 1926 Chinese Communist soldiers had fought in the Northern Expedition under the overall command of Chiang Kaishek. The Red army was officially launched on August 1, 1927.

product of pre-modern military attitudes that saw soldiers and conscripts as expendable commodities, who could survive on pillage.

The book also considers ways the belligerents conducted warfare during this period and their effect on Chinese lives. All modern warfare is brutal, but the Chinese civil war and the war between China and Japan were fought with unusual ferocity.[24] To root out Communism the Nationalist forces used scorched earth tactics and generally executed identifiable Communists. The Communist forces took military prisoners to make use of their skills but had no tolerance for enemies such as landlords and landlord militias. The Japanese military, in the belief that they were punishing an upstart government, made use of many methods for destroying opposition. These included massive bombing of urban centers, extended scorched earth tactics, chemical warfare, bacterial warfare, aerial machine-gunning of refugees, slaughter of prisoners on the battlefield or in bacterial warfare laboratories, widespread rape, and indiscriminate use of the bayonet. A particular feature of the Japanese military assault, especially during the Shanghai campaign in 1937 and Operation Ichigo in 1944 was to undermine civilian morale by setting off massive drives of panic-stricken refugees. Tens to hundreds of thousands of these front line victims succumbed to cholera, dysentery, malaria, typhus, starvation, and freezing cold, in the process blocking roads and pathways, destroying marginal sanitary systems, spreading infection, and straining healthcare services to the utmost.[25] Due to lack of records, the loss of life caused by these chilling strategies is not accurately measurable.[26]

Disregard for the Peasantry

Underlying these oppressive forces lay the intense poverty and marginalization of living conditions for millions of the poor and illiterate in urban and rural China in the early 20th century. In some regions, such as

---

[24] In Chinese writings the war is called the War of Resistance Against Japan (抗日战争 *kangrizhanzheng*); in Japan it was known as the China Incident.

[25] For an account of the Japanese military strategy towards refugees, see McClure, (November 1941), 640–645.

[26] The methodology of Drew Faust's remarkable study of death during the American Civil War could not yet be applied to the subject of death in China during the War of Resistance with Japan because of the lack of relevant statistical and personal data. See Faust (2008).

northwest China, villagers were generally worse off than others; those living in areas subject to flood and/or drought were especially vulnerable.

The Nationalist government's extraordinary decision to blow up the Yellow River dyke at Huayuankou on June 9, 1938, provides a graphic example of this kind of crisis. Intended to block the Japanese military advance into central China, the breach of the dyke unleashed a massive volume of water, which swept without warning into the Huai river basin. The flood submerged a reported 9.36 million *mou* (equivalent to 1.38 million acres or 624,000 hectares) of Henan's arable land, and reportedly drowned 470,000 people in Henan alone (about 1.5 percent of Henan's population), leaving another 1.4 million people homeless and destitute. Altogether 890,000 is widely used as an estimate of deaths in the three provinces of Henan, Anhui and Jiangsu due to drowning or starvation.[27] Although inflicting an appalling calamity on well over two million Chinese people, the stratagem only temporarily delayed the Japanese capture of Wuhan.[28] Despite various efforts to downplay—or not even mention—this disaster, a detailed eyewitness report to the International Red Cross leaves little doubt about its impact.[29]

Historians and social scientists, including the present writer, are still a long way from understanding the full effect of this sustained and overwhelming trauma on the Chinese people.[30] A recent Chinese film assesses how the trauma played out during the Japanese military assault on the capital city of Nanjing from late 1937 to early 1938.[31] The film graphically reconstructs the assault on the city and its inhabitants from the perspectives of various Chinese, Japanese and Western participants and provides shocking enactments of how they were made to suffer for what

---

[27] Wang Tianjiang 王天将, September 1990), 349, entry for June 9, 1938. The text does not indicate how these numbers were calculated. The broad implications of the flooding are discussed in Odoric Y. K. Wou (1994), chapter 6. A major contemporary account is Louis Calame (November 1938), 967–1016. Online sources generally estimate population loss at 890,000 in forty-four affected counties in Henan, Anhui and Jiangsu.

[28] This event is considered one of the 'three great calamities' (san da can'an 三大惨案). The other two in this category are the great burning of Changsha in November 1938 and the relentless bombing of Chongqing. The Japanese air force was responsible for the third calamity, but Chinese military forces were responsible for the Yellow River and Changsha calamities. An account with map of how the Japanese military circumvented the flood is in Stephen R. MacKinnon, *Wuhan, 1938* (Berkeley, CA: University of California Press, 2008), chapter 3.

[29] Calame (1938).

[30] Diana Lary (2010) is a welcome exception to this observation, as is Diana Lary and Stephen MacKinnon (2001).

[31] "City of Life and Death," directed by Lu Chuan, (2009).

happened. Some of these enactments are based on contemporary photographs. The Nanjing war museum constitutes another impressive effort to visualize the broad physical and psychic impact of the destruction of Nanjing and its people.[32] *Red Sorghum*, by Nobel prizewinner Mo Yan, offers a vivid reconstruction of Japanese military brutality in the North China countryside.

To understand the challenges to saving lives we have to take into account the overall vulnerability of mothers and infants in childbirth, young undernourished children, young men and boys conscripted into military service against a much better armed and trained invader, girls sold into slavery and concubinage, men and women taken down by opium, large populations hit by drought, flood and famine, tens of thousands of soldiers left to die on battlefields, conscripts marching to death from starvation or disease, innumerable refugees scattered to the winds by enemy armies on the march, millions of victims of epidemics, millions more victims of bombing and invasion, and still more victims of pervasive poverty and malnutrition. All such categories have to be reviewed in order to come up with viable estimates of morbidity and mortality before and during the War of Resistance against Japan.

Pervasive poverty is an especially intractable problem, and one with a ruthless impact on human immune systems, especially of people living on the edge. "The misery and misfortune of China!" exclaimed Agnes Smedley, writing in 1937. "Floods, famines, droughts, wars! Poverty indescribable, and the people always on the verge of starvation. Can you conceive of the disasters of a war when even in peacetime the Chinese people live on the verge of starvation?" After another such outburst, set off by Smedley's effort to treat a young peasant suffering from blood poisoning, an intellectual from Beijing informed her that: "sympathy with the people is utterly useless. There are too many of them." "Do you mean," Smedley responded, "that I should not help that boy with blood poisoning?" "It is useless," he replied—echoing a long-standing official sentiment that saw the "foolish people" (*yumin* 愚民) as ignorant and expendable.[33]

Ironically the British Raj began counting military deaths in India in the 1850s and 1860s, discriminating them by location, ethnicity, rank and disease.[34] In 1869 the Indian Sanitary Commissioner called it indispensable

---

[32] See Yang Daqing (2001), 76–96.
[33] Smedley (1938), 9, 17.
[34] David Arnold (1993), 67–71.

to ascertain community death rates and their preventable causes, in order to apply remedies. In 1852 the Massachusetts Sanitary Commission noted a disturbing discrepancy between the life expectancies of farmers and mechanics and urged physicians to find out the causes.[35] These were early stirrings of a fundamental premise of public health research, namely collection of vital statistics as a guide to policy. Until the 1930s China lacked such information.[36]

The Argument

It is the thesis of this book that several important initiatives took place during the era under study that did address the waste of life apparent to reformers of that era, and that these efforts were significantly extended during wartime conditions. We will find that many thousands of country people were trained in basic methods of triage and disease prevention, and that a strong focus on advancement of hygiene and prevention of epidemic disease emerged as the healthcare reformers took stock of what their options were. This book names and discusses the work of people who made a difference in all these respects, and whose achievements are attracting recognition in contemporary China.

It is also argued that political leadership was an indispensable ingredient in promoting and validating these initiatives. Most healthcare reformers lacked the political skills to build the support required for their initiatives to gain traction as political priorities. The troublesome fact is that despite the urgent need for advances in public healthcare, the subject never became a top political priority in Nationalist China. In Nationalist leadership circles healthcare had to compete with military and ideological priorities enjoying a much greater level of political support; and sadly, during the Nationalist era healthcare became the object of an internecine struggle between biomedical and Chinese medicine practitioners. By contrast Communist forces, short in numbers and struggling for survival, were more apt to see health work as an essential ingredient of overall policy, one which by saving lives and embracing modernity contributed to advancement of policy goals rather than acting as a financial and bureaucratic

---

[35] Prabhat Jha (2012).
[36] In June 1925 Dr. Tsefang F. Huang urged provinces to send monthly reports of prevalence of notifiable diseases, but returns came only in three categories with no exact numbers. *American Journal of Public Health* (October 1926), 16/10, 1030.

drag. For the medical reformers, many of whom had seen modern society at work in Britain, France, Germany and the U.S., complacency towards loss of life was no longer acceptable.

This study aims to pull healthcare, death and lifesaving into mainstream analysis of 1) the bitter conflicts characterizing the history of Nationalist China, 2) the will to promote better care of vulnerable people despite the forces resisting this goal. Just as the mind-numbing destruction of huge conscript armies during World War One forced a century-long reappraisal of European culture and politics,[37] so too the huge loss of life in China during the 1930s and 1940s calls for sustained evaluation. It urges us to investigate how reformers were able to find ways to protect so many lives at risk and to assess how far the value of lifesaving rose because of their efforts or because of the impact of war.

Discussions of these issues are organized as follows. Chapter 1 considers how the health reformers assessed the problems they faced up to the outbreak of civil war between the Nationalist and Communists in 1928. How concerned were they with disease and death rates on the one hand and with national strength on the other; and given their limited personnel and financial resources, along what lines did they organize their priorities? Who supported the strategy expressed in English as 'state medicine' and in Chinese as 'public healthcare system' (*gongyi zhidu* 公医制度), and what were its objectives and results?

Chapter 2 deals with organizers of national governmental civilian health services and their work in promoting public healthcare strategies. The chapter discusses the political as well as public health problems that the civilian health administrators encountered, how they mobilized resources and prioritized goals, and how senior leaders exploited them to advance national political priorities. It deals with basic weaknesses in national health administration during the 1930s. It discusses work in model counties as an example of how medical reformers were able to creatively address the substantial problems of providing rural and school healthcare.

Chapter 3 takes up the radically different experience of the Red Army and civilian leadership in developing health services in the Jiangxi base area and sustaining them during the Long March. Particular attention is given to the civilian health campaign mobilized during 1933–1934, what

---

[37] Hochschild (2012), while weighted towards British participation, provides gripping descriptions of battles such as at the Somme and Passchendaele and the ghastly casualty tolls inflicted.

its goals were and what it accomplished even during times when a brutal civil war was going on. The chapter discusses how the Red Army was able to maintain a viable healthcare service during the critical Long March from southeast to northwest China during 1934–1936.

Chapter 4 deals with the army medical services available to Nationalist China to meet the Japanese military invasion in 1937 and the agencies developed by healthcare reformers to strengthen the army medical services. The CRCMRC and the Emergency Medical Service Training Schools are the key agencies discussed. It features the leadership and political fall from grace of a remarkable medical scientist, Dr. Lin Kesheng. The chapter illustrates how far the reformers were able to go in strengthening what were marginal army medical services; it reviews the opposition and setbacks that they experienced while carrying out this work.

Chapter 5 goes further into the hostility towards Dr. Lin Kesheng expressed by senior generals and American civilian relief agencies and its negative impact on military medical morale. Cooperation with US military medical services helped to validate the work of the Emergency Medical Service Schools at a time when the pressures of Japanese military campaigning and financial inflation were at their worst. The general indifference of the top Nationalist leaders towards army nutrition and conscript health continued throughout the war. The crisis caused by the Ichigo campaign enabled Dr. Lin to come back into office, but by then the health of soldiers in Nationalist armies had been seriously compromised.

Chapter 6 covers the work of the civilian National Health Administration (NHA) during the War of Resistance against Japan (1937–1945). Despite the chaos that that war precipitated, the NHA was able to reorganize in West China and push the case for preventive health care. Two epidemic prevention bureaus produced large amounts of vaccines that mitigated the spread of epidemic diseases and showed what Chinese healthcare reformers could do to get that curse under control. Despite war and inflation, NHA agencies focused on public and preventive health and demonstrated in modest ways the importance of that work in protecting public order. But they continued to suffer from lack of political influence, which worsened during the late 1940s.

Chapter 7 focuses on the military and civilian health work undertaken by Mao Zedong and the Yan'an government and its armed forces in north China during the War of Resistance against Japan. Chinese sources emphasize the interest of communist party leaders in healthcare and the contributions of international physicians in upgrading the quality of front line military healthcare. At the same time civilian healthcare focused on improving management of communicable diseases, maternal child health and public hygiene in what was one of the poorest and most vulnerable regions in all of China. Military healthcare made much faster progress than civilian, primarily because it was less encumbered by superstition and chicanery, and also because of its strategic significance.

Chapter 8 sums up the achievements of the health reformers and the costs incurred. The healthcare world of 1948 was very different from that of 1928. By 1948 public health was established as a state responsibility; communicable diseases were on the defensive; and paramedics had emerged as significant players in the modern healthcare world. But the question of the overall importance of lifesaving as a national priority remained ominously unresolved.

CHAPTER ONE

EPIDEMICS, WARS AND PUBLIC HEALTHCARE ADVOCACY
IN REPUBLICAN CHINA, 1911–1928

*In any effort to understand what lies ahead, as much as what lies behind,
the role of infectious disease cannot properly be left out of consideration.*
—William H. McNeill[1]

*It would be better for the little girl to die. What's the point in saving a
little girl?*
—Comment about Lu Lihua, reported by Wang Zheng[2]

Epidemics have played an ominous part in human history. In Europe both
the sixth century Justinian plague and the fourteenth century Black Death
killed tens of millions of people, fundamentally affecting the course of
European history. Smallpox has ravaged humanity, especially children, for
at least 3,000 years. In the nineteenth and early twentieth centuries cholera epidemics swept across Asia and Europe, flourishing because of public ignorance of how the disease was spread. Infections have also hugely
affected military conflicts. The influenza pandemic of 1918–1919 struck
down combatants on the Western front and helped bring World War I
to a close. Estimates of its worldwide death toll range from 20 million to
as high as 70 million.[3] Smallpox and measles enabled Cortez and Pizarro
to overwhelm the Aztec and Inca populations in the sixteenth century;
and as the noted bacteriologist Hans Zinsser pointed out in 1934, lice and
typhus have repeatedly struck down armies on the warpath.[4]

Written history of the Chinese Republic (1911–1949) has focused on
the ideological and military struggles in China to throw off internal and
foreign oppression and reestablish strong government. And yet most of
the lives lost during these years were due not to combat but to infection,

---

[1] William H. McNeill (1976), 257.
[2] Wang Zheng (1999), 147.
[3] There are numerous articles on this subject on the internet. Almost all emphasize its
crushing impact, especially in India, and the lack of attention by historians to its effect
during the closing weeks of the war.
[4] Hans Zinsser (1935). For history buffs, this well-researched and witty book is a 'must
read'.

prejudice and malpractice, and if due to combat were more often struck down by disease than by wounds. As one Indian army medical manual put it, "it was early realized, as it is universally agreed today, that losses of men in war from sickness far exceed the losses from even the bloodiest of campaigns." Frederick of Prussia said: "fevers cost me as many men as seven battles."[5] A Chinese Red Cross manual, published in 1937, included a chart of British army casualties over the previous thirty years, showing that casualties due to diseases were four times as many as casualties due to wounds, and deaths due to disease 4.6 times as many as deaths due to enemy action.[6] These ratios do not include all the other causes of mortality noted in the introduction.

Such overwhelming disease trauma did not go unnoticed by Chinese graduates of national and internationally recognized medical schools. As early as 1915 Dr. Wu Liande published an article in the missionary-sponsored Chinese Medical Journal pleading with his foreign medical colleagues to set up a public health service in China and end its reputation as "the most insanitary nation on earth."[7] During that year he joined with several other Chinese medical reformers to establish the National Medical Association and set up their own medical journal—the *National Medical Journal of China* (*NMJC*).[8] These reformers grappled with a succession of epidemics and with key problems in health diagnostics and treatment, publishing their results and proposals in the *NMJC* and other publications. Unfortunately little of their research has made its way into standard histories.

It was the people's vulnerability to disease that first concerned this small group of patriotic medical reformers. They treated and studied infectious diseases during the time leading up to the establishment of the Nationalist Government's Ministry of Health in 1928. Aided by international health advisers, they advocated low cost ideas for dealing with China's immense problems of disease and healthcare. These ideas and strategies, grouped under the rubric of "state medicine" (in Chinese *gongyi zhidu* 公医制度 public healthcare system), became the principle guide for practitioners of publically managed healthcare in Nationalist China. Until war and inflation became dominant in the early 1940s, application of publicly managed

---

[5] *Field Service Hygiene Notes* (1945), 2.
[6] *Jiuhu Shouce* (1937), 298.
[7] Wu Lian-teh (1915).
[8] Wong and Wu (1936), 603–605.

healthcare helped spur significant progress in public health, saving many thousands of lives in the process.

Virulent infections were the most obvious problem confronting human health in early twentieth century China. Pneumonic plague traveled from Siberia along railroads into northeast China, and cholera spread inland from coastal cities, where it was delivered by trading vessels. These diseases were aided by the spread of imperialism and its communications systems into China and by the superstitions of local people and authorities that prevented them from responding effectively. As one medical journal put it, attribution of epidemics to annual visitations of gods and difficulties concerning wind and water were still rampant in the minds of most officials.[9] New kinds of technical medical capability, themselves the product of an imperialist era, were needed to deal with such contagions.

Other infectious diseases, such as smallpox, tuberculosis and malaria, were more deeply rooted in China; the word for malaria or ague (疟 *nue* originally 瘧) was in use over three thousand years ago.[10] Symptoms of smallpox were described in a fourth century text and a method of inoculation was successfully employed in the early eleventh century. Syphilis, however, appears to have entered China through the port of Guangzhou in the early sixteenth century.[11] Diseases favored by wartime conditions, such as dysentery, typhus and scabies, have long histories of occurrence in China, but the wartime conditions of the early twentieth century facilitated epidemic outbreaks.[12] It was these epidemics, plus the widespread incidence of tuberculosis, smallpox and malaria, which galvanized the medical reformers into seeking effective responses.

Another major pathology of this era involved the health of women and children. Childbirth was a major cause of disease and death, affecting both infants and mothers. Children's lives were at great risk through the age of five and at continuing risk through the age of ten. The dangers to the health of women have to be seen in the context of a fundamentally patriarchal culture, in which women in the early twentieth century were still binding the feet of their young daughters, and in which unknown tens of

---

[9] Editorial (1923): 154–157.

[10] *Xin Zhongguo Yufang Yixue Lishi Jingyan* (1988), 286.

[11] K. Chimin Wong and Wu Lien-teh (1936), 215–219, 273–275. A virulent outbreak occurred in Naples in 1495. Vasco Da Gama carried the disease to Calcutta in 1498 and it is said to have reached China by 1520.

[12] *Xin Zhongguo Yufang Yixue Lishi Jingyan* (1988) 68, 145. (This volume does not include a chapter on scabies (疥疮), but there is plenty of information about this disease on the Chinese internet.)

thousands of girls were still being forced into marriage or bondage, especially in times of economic crisis.[13] In such a patriarchy, the health of girls and women mattered considerably less than that of boys and men. During the early 1920s a very active and passionate women's movement burst into flower in urban China, spurred on by the writings of men. It focused initially on women's rights but before long its advocates were linking the awakening of women to the improvement of China's tenuous national strength.[14] At that time childbirth was still considered the responsibility of the birthing mother; if the child was not a healthy boy, both the gender and the health status were the fault of the mother.[15] Thus urban women were slowly freed from one set of fetters (foot-binding, concubinage and slavery) only to be locked more firmly into another (boy-preference).[16] It would be hard, for men especially, to imagine the trauma that this caused birthing mothers of girl children.[17]

The conditions of childbirth among the masses living outside of urban China remained dependent on hygienically untrained traditional midwives or on the birth mother herself. Thanks to the prevalence of infectious diseases the rates of morbidity and mortality in rural China were believed by reformers in the absence of hard data to be far in excess of those occurring in modernized countries. Military diseases were equally lethal, as treatment lay in the hands of marginal military medical systems staffed predominantly by untrained personnel.

Thus the questions raised in this chapter are, how did China's twentieth century healthcare reformers respond to these realities? What resources did reformers have at their disposal? How effective were they in dealing with opposition, especially if it was of foreign origin? What was meant by "public healthcare system," and how far were these patriotic reformers able to make it a reality?

---

[13] Lillian Li, (2007), 303, provides sales prices of boys, girls, and young women during the North China famine of 1928–1930. Boys, at 10 yuan a head, were cheapest. Girls fetched a higher price—10–30 yuan.

[14] This is the subject of Wang Zheng's study on Women in the Chinese Enlightenment (1999).

[15] Ye Shaojun's story, "A Posthumous Son," provides a gripping insight into this mentality. See Joseph S. M. Lau and Howard Goldblatt (1995), 35–43.

[16] Tina Phillips Johnson (2011), chapter 2, provides a groundbreaking treatment of this subject.

[17] An appalling example is the case of Wang Yiwei, cited by Wang Zheng. Wang was accused as an infant of having a hard fate that 'ate up' (killed) her four-year old brother. This had a permanently negative impact on her life and the life of her family. See Wang Zheng (1999), 222–223.

Epidemic Disease and Public Healthcare up to 1928

Not long after the 1911 revolution a handful of Chinese health care reformers, most of them educated overseas, began to articulate a modern, science-based, healthcare policy for China. At the time biomedicine in China was mostly practiced by missionaries. It was curative in nature and focused on individual patients treated in clinics or hospitals. In the mission world, curing bodies was a metaphor for curing souls and was the pathway to better life. Thus medical care was an important aspect of missionary work, but less so than directly saving souls.[18]

The Chinese medical reformers were concerned with the people's vulnerability to epidemic diseases and the absence of an effective science-based public health service to counteract these scourges. They winced at unfavorable comparisons between health services in China and Japan. They pointed to the need to inject science-based thinking and health management into China's schools and colleges, and further to the need to reduce the political upheavals that impeded social progress. One cannot read far in the *NMJC* before coming across reports on epidemic and contagious diseases, particularly plague (鼠疫), cholera (霍乱) and tuberculosis (结核). A famous pneumonic plague epidemic occurred in northeast and north China from 1910–1911 and reportedly took 60,000 lives. Its successful control by the pioneer public health physician Dr. Wu Liande led to an international conference on plague in Shenyang (Mukden) and in 1912 to the establishment of a North Manchurian Plague Prevention Service (北满防疫处, later 东北防疫事务总处) in Harbin. This was a watershed event in the emergence of modern, science-based public healthcare in China. During this epidemic, central government response was considered quite effective and local officials appeared indifferent but as a rule friendly.[19]

---

[18] Liping Bu (2009) provides a broader cultural context from which to assess the problems of health and modernization facing China in the early 20th century and the steps taken by various individuals, including the eminent missionary physician Dr. W. W. Peter, to provide public education about healthcare. The account in this chapter focuses more on the views of China's medical reformers who faced the long-range responsibility to develop a public health service for China's people.

[19] There is a good deal of discussion of this event on the Chinese internet. Although Dr. Wu came from what is now Malaysia (but was in his time a British colony) and was trained at the University of Cambridge and the London School of Tropical Medicine, his contributions to plague control have given him a well-deserved reputation as a Chinese hero and patriot.

Another outbreak of pneumonic plague in Shanxi province and elsewhere in north China in 1917–1918 reportedly cost 16,000 deaths but led
to the establishment of a Central Epidemic Prevention Bureau (*Zhongyang Fangyichu* 中央防疫处) in Beijing's Tiantan Park in 1919. During the
War of Resistance against Japan this Bureau, relocated in Kunming, would
assume a substantial role in manufacturing vaccines to aid delivery of
public healthcare. The Army Medical School, led by its director, Dr. Quan
Shaoqing (全绍清), played an important part in bringing this later plague
epidemic under control. But compared with the activist North Manchurian Plague Prevention Service (NMPPS), the Bureau was reportedly ham-
pered by insufficient funds and a "superabundant staff of non-workers."[20]
In addition, local officials appeared "indifferent, even hostile," and the
local populace "ignorant and often uncontrollable."[21] Another outbreak of
pneumonic plague occurred in northeast China in 1920–1921 resulting in
a reported 9,300 deaths. The *NMJC* charged that the epidemic was spread
by ignorant soldiers, who interfered with the work of sanitary officers.
An editorial complained that high officials and educated people—not to
mention ordinary people—still lacked knowledge of the simplest rules of
hygiene. As a result, physicians had to fight prejudice and ignorance as
well as the plague.[22]

In pre-1930 China, cholera was generally reported in coastal or river
cities handling commerce, where reporting mechanisms were more available than in the interior. In 1919 a cholera epidemic occurred in major
cities, including several inland in Henan, Anhui, Hubei and Hunan provinces. The number of dead due to cholera during the summer months
was said to be at least 300,000. It is likely that cholera would have spread
into the countryside of a populous province such as Henan, but no estimate of rural fatalities was available.[23] The disease was spread by rail, the

---

[20] This unfavorable comment comes from Dr. Wu Liande, who was the mover and
shaker of both the NMPPS and the NMJC. See Wu Lien-teh (1923), 1–6.

[21] Editorials, (March 1918), 37–39, and (September 1918), 88–94. See also Wong and Wu
(1936), 592–594, 602 and other writings by Dr. Wu, who rose to prominence as a result of
his work on the 1910–1911 epidemic. The Central Epidemic Prevention Bureau became part
of the National Health Administration (at that time still Ministry of Health) in 1929. After
the Japanese military invasion of North China in 1937, its buildings were secretly taken
over by the Japanese military bacterial warfare program.

[22] Editorial, (June 1921), 38. An editorial in NMJC (March 1921), 2–4, reports that two
noted physicians lost their lives during this epidemic.

[23] Under August 1919 the Henan chronology reports laconically that cholera spread from
Fuzhou to Kaifeng, Anyang and Xinyang, and that there were very many deaths. It also
reports epidemics of plague and cerebrospinal meningitis (*naojisuimoyan* 脑脊髓膜炎)

number of flies was unusually great, and the poor reportedly defecated everywhere. Because of the hot weather people ate melons and drank unboiled water. In Harbin, where the authors of this report had first hand knowledge, 4,500 deaths occurred in just over six weeks. Rogers' hypertonic saline solution was available to treat cholera victims lucky enough to reach the right urban hospital in a matter of hours, otherwise the death rate would have been higher.[24]

Even a relatively modernized city such as Shanghai was vulnerable to cholera. In the summer of 1925 at least 3,000 cases occurred with over 1,000 fatalities. In 1926 16,000 cases were reported with a death rate of about thirty percent. The city's foreign authorities were displeased because of the discovery of live vibrios (cholera bacteria) in samples taken at Shanghai's Chapei (zhabei 閘北) waterworks. In return, an NMJC editorial writer criticized the foreign authorities for not acting fast enough to enforce quarantines in various ports. In 1919 approximately 20,000 cases of cholera occurred in Fuzhou (capital of Fujian province). The authorities there responded in 1920 by mounting a big anti-cholera campaign. The campaign enlisted 2,380 volunteers. Two hundred and twenty thousand people saw its displays, and it distributed at no expense to the public over 300,000 pieces of literature. In Changsha (capital of Hunan province) during August 1920 over 48,000 people were said to have attended sixty-six lectures on cholera.[25] A study published in 1928 of a cholera epidemic in the much smaller Fujian town of Hsinghua (Putian) (population 40,000) stressed the connection between overflowing cesspools and wells in spreading cholera and noted that "the large number of leaking latrines and their close proximity to the wells is staggering." But use of Roger's

---

for that year. See Wang Tianjiang, (September 1990), Introduction, note 28. In 1917, however, Huang County (黃县), on the northern coast of Shandong and in the prefecture of Yantai, recorded that 16,000 of its population of 270,000 died of cholera. See Zhang Taishan (2008), 93.

[24] Wu Lien-teh and J. W. H. Chun (December 1919), 182–198; Wu and Chun (1920), 4–16. "*The Cholera Epidemic*" (September 1919) estimated the number of deaths at 400,000.

[25] W. W. Peter (1920), 24–236. *The Caduceus* reported an estimated 19,000 deaths in Fuzhou in 1919. "Review of Journals" (1926). Dr. William W. Peter (1882–1958?) was a missionary surgeon in central China who turned his attention to public health because of the need for new thinking about health care priorities. He served for a year with the Chinese volunteer battalion in World War I, obtained degrees in public health from Harvard-MIT and later Yale, then returned to Shanghai and lived there until 1926, returning again for several months in 1929. (information from http://www.grc/nia/nih.gov/branches/bisa/founders.pdf).

saline treatment, rapid disinfection of wells and vigorous propaganda at well sites kept the death toll down to around 150.[26]

At this time a few larger cities had departments of public health, but managing urban public health was very challenging. Dr. Li Tingan (李廷安) pointed out that in Guangzhou notifiable infectious diseases were not reported because many physicians did not realize the need, while many Chinese medicine practitioners did not know the diagnostic terminology of Western medicine. Public nuisances included public cesspools, stagnant water, rats, flies, mosquitoes, waste matter in rivers, defective plumbing, public spitting, dead animals, and human defecation into rivers. The city water supply came from sources contaminated with sewage. Dr. Jin Baoshan (金宝善 P. Z. King), describing problems in Beijing, noted that each year, out of a population of 800,000, thirty thousand became sick and three thousand died because of gastrointestinal diseases. In the south of the city many people depended on river water, which was subject to numerous infectious diseases. Dr. Jin wanted regulations to prohibit sale of melons and all impure drinking materials during the summer. Many of the sick, he noted, were women and children.[27] As for lesser-sized cities, they had negligible public health services, if any.[28]

Tuberculosis (结核病) was also a major source of sickness and death. The missionary physician J. L. Maxwell described it as "rampant throughout China."[29] Spitting was the worst way of spreading the disease; serving food with infected chopsticks was another means of infection. Tuberculosis was prevalent around Suzhou; in Zunhua it was the greatest single source of death. In Guangzhou (Canton) there was no organization to counteract it. In Harbin it was responsible for twenty-five percent of reported sickness, more than the next four diseases combined. The degree of frequency of tuberculosis in Harbin was attributed to overcrowding and

---

[26] M. K. Yue (1928), 151–153. Dr. Yue obtained a DPH from Cambridge University.

[27] Li Tingan (李廷安) (October 1925), 324–375; Jin Baoshan (金宝善) (1926), 253–261. A graduate of PUMC, Dr. Li received a doctorate from the Harvard School of Public Health. Dr. Jin's degrees were from Chiba University and Johns Hopkins School of Public Health. Both were active advocates of public health.

[28] See, for example, Chia K'uei (Jia Kui), "A Sanitary Survey of Tsunhwa (Zunhua)." NMJC, 11, 5 (1925): 313–323. In this city of at least 50,000 people around 150 km. east north east of Beijing, no municipal or other organization was responsible for public health. Whatever little was done was under the control of the police, whose chief knew nothing about public health. Not surprisingly, a bad cholera outbreak occurred in the summer of 1923. There is much more information along these lines in this article.

[29] J. L. Maxwell, *The Diseases of China Including Formosa and Korea,* second edition (Shanghai: 1929) 23, cited by Lamson, *op. cit.,* 326.

ill-ventilated rooms.[30] Exasperated by the ease with which this disease could spread, Dr. Feng Zhongen (酆仲恩) published an article in 1928 on what physicians could do to get rid of it.[31] He pointed out that since people continued spitting after catching the disease, physicians must teach preventive measures. They must look for early signs of symptoms and teach people how the disease is transmitted. Sick people should be isolated and kept away from family members. Physicians should promote the anti-tuberculosis movement. Cities should establish tuberculosis hospitals, sanitariums and prevention stations. Since a national anti-tuberculosis conference held in Shanghai in 1933 noted that China's annual death rate due to tuberculosis could be as high as 1.2 million, there was certainly good reason for recognizing the high economic and social cost that tuberculosis exacted.[32]

Childhood disease and mortality constituted a problem for which only improvement of maternal, child and school health offered a way forward. Writing in 1923 Dr. P. Y. Chang charged that "negligence of the health of children is a fault practiced everywhere throughout China."[33] Eleven years later Dr. Yang Chongrui (杨崇瑞) reported that "some people" estimated that around half the children born in China were unwanted and were therefore carelessly brought up.[34] For such children infectious diseases, especially diarrhea and dysentery, were lying in wait; but data on mortality was difficult to pin down because in police censuses, data on children less than fifteen years of age were liable to be left out.[35] Dr. W. P. Ling (林文秉 Lin Wenbing) estimated that there were between sixteen and twenty million blind people in China and that trachoma (typically a childhood infectious disease) was the most prevalent eye disease and the

---

[30] Information from i) P. Y. Chang (1923), 297–304; ii) Li Guangxun (1923): 122–131; iii) Chia K'uei (1925): 313–323; iv) Li Ting-an (1925), 324–375; v) Lin Chia-swee (林家瑞) and Wu Lien-teh (February 1927), 24–82. Dr. Lin was a graduate of the Army Medical College and a close colleague of Dr. Wu. See http:/news.china.com.cn/rollnews/2011-01/19/content_6143208.htm.

[31] Feng Zhongen (酆仲恩), (1928) 149–153.

[32] Wong and Wu (1936), 758. Winfield, writing in the immediate aftermath of World War II, put annual deaths from tuberculosis at "approximately" 1.5 million. He described its prevalence among students as "particularly distressing." See Winfield (1948), 107–108.

[33] P. Y. Chang (1923), 297–304.

[34] Marian Yang (杨崇瑞) (1934), 786–791.

[35] Lin Chia-swee (林家瑞 Lin Jiarui) and Wu Lien-teh (February 1927), 24–82. In this survey, scarlet fever was fourth in order of mortality after tuberculosis, smallpox and dysentery.

most common cause of blindness.[36] Epidemics of scarlet fever in children were reported in another article, and the disease was found to be prevalent in northwest China, while a "large number of cases" were reported every year in Beijing.[37] Given such deficiencies, one author called school hygiene "the most promising field of endeavor in public health;" another called for promotion of public health practice especially for children.[38]

Lack of Scientific Rigor

Reformers with biomedical training writing in the 1920s were acutely concerned with what they saw as lack of scientific rigor in the practice of medicine in China. This was probably the single most important factor leading to the creation of the Chinese Medical Association and the NMJC. The reformers sought to transform medicine into a research-based and examination-tested profession, which would make study and prevention of disease a national priority.

At that time gods, ghosts, unqualified practitioners and harmful concoctions dominated health care, in their view, as did foreign religious and secular missionaries. China's intelligentsia lacked control over an increasingly troubled area of China's public life. People had no conception of preventive health: washing hands, brushing teeth, not spitting etc., or of the importance of sanitation. China's intelligentsia had to find new ways forward, responsive to the urgent problems facing their country. Those reformers who chose the new field of biomedicine believed it could contribute significantly to the revival of China, especially if built on a

---

[36] W. P. Ling (林文秉 Lin Wenbing) (February 1924), 20–24. Dr. Lin (1893–1969) was a graduate of Harvard (Shanghai) and Cambridge, MA, medical schools and a faculty member of Peking Union Medical College, National Central, and National Shanghai Medical Colleges. His paper was first delivered at the 1922 National Medical Association Conference. See Wong and Wu (1936), 666–667, and http://www.hudong.com/wiki/林文秉. After 1949 he joined the faculty of the Number Two Army Medical College. He is noted for his publications on eye pathology and dissection and for establishing the impact of a variety of infectious diseases on eye health.

[37] Yang Ting-kuang and W. H. Shih (1924): 153–170. (No information was found on either of these authors).

[38] S. M. Wu (胡宣明 Hu Xuanming) (1924), 98–100; Zhao Shifa (赵士法) (February 1925), 4–17. A noted public health specialist, Dr. Hu was a graduate of the Johns Hopkins University Medical School and author and translator of a number of books on public health. Zhao was the author of books and articles on student health, emergency healthcare and military health.

foundation of ethics and science. They believed that as physicians they could play a significant public role in post imperial China.[39]

Government Indifference

A major problem facing the medical reformers during the 1920s was the ignorance and indifference of governing authorities towards public health. While Japanese medical researchers were scoring one breakthrough after another and Japanese officials were laying the groundwork for medical education and public health in their colonies, Chinese governments and educated classes seemed impervious to the importance of public health.[40] Enforcement of sanitary methods lay in the hands of poorly educated and paid police and marginal "scholars," who were oblivious to such matters as preventing overcrowding, supervising food and water, and collecting vital statistics. In China, said one angry writer, the sanitary assistant was often "a mere Chinese scholar, with no knowledge of medicine or modern health work." A frustrated eulogist of Dr. Sun Yat-sen claimed that those who held government positions "were no better than idiots;" the idea of sacrificing themselves in order to make China prosperous and strong was "entirely foreign to them." Adopting a more businesslike stance, Dr. Lee Shufen (李树芬 Li Shufan), who held leadership positions in Guangzhou and Hong Kong, defined three responsibilities of Chinese physicians: 1) produce as many teachers and practitioners as possible to meet the present emergency of having only one physician worthy of the name per 100,000 people; 2) cultivate the scientific spirit by doing sound work and research and get China onto the map of medical science; 3) translate international medical research and teach in Chinese so that physicians in less densely urban areas could learn what was being accomplished. Another task was to create public health centers to reduce the appalling

---

[39] Cf. i) E. S. Tyau (刁信德, born 刁庆湘, Edward Sintak Tiao/Diao Xinde) (November 1915), 1–6; ii) "The National Association of China," ibid., 22–25; iii) Minutes of the First Meeting of the National Medical Association of China, February 5, 1915, ibid., 9–31. Dr. Diao received his M.D. from St. John's University in Shanghai and a D.P.H. from the University of Pennsylvania. His chosen name signals a commitment to ethics.

[40] What distinguished Dr. Sun Yat-sen from such people is that he attended high school in Hawaii and medical school at the University of Hong Kong, where he studied with several distinguished parasitologists.

death rates in China.[41] All these responsibilities would increase in urgency as war with Japan approached and took hold.

Injecting Science-based Thinking into Chinese Education and Public Policy

The medical reformers knew that little progress would be made in improving public health until science-based thinking entered the mainstream of Chinese education. Here is how Chen Sibang (陈祀邦), a thirty-two year old Singapore-born physician with medical credentials from Cambridge University and St. Thomas's Hospital in London saw the problem:

> In the struggle for existence the chances of a nation depend entirely on progress, and the country that is contented with remaining stationary and does not endeavor to seek the path of progress is certain to go under. The progress of a nation is measured chiefly, nay entirely, by its achievements in science... What is the present situation in this country? China's achievements in the realm of modern science can be summed up practically in one small word—nil.[42]

Western countries were long free of smallpox (天花), typhus (斑疹伤寒) and plague (鼠疫), but not China. Much existing medical education was still controlled by foreigners. Each medical school set its own curriculum and examinations and conferred its own degrees.

In 1918, after a second major plague epidemic had shaken the medical world, Dr. Wu Liande published an article with views close to those of Dr. Chen. The authorities, he wrote, were not yet alive to the urgent needs of scientific and technical education. "Our nation is backward... Only a

---

[41] Information from i) Wu Lien-teh (1922), 286–290; ii) I. K. Wong (1925), 193–195; iii) Lee Shu-fan (1926), 57–61. Dr. Li was a graduate of Hong Kong University Medical School and the University of Edinburgh Medical School, where he passed the examination to enter the Royal College of Surgeons. He served in many capacities in Hong Kong and Guangzhou, including as medical adviser to Dr. Sun Yat-sen. His memoir, *Hong Kong Surgeon*, was published in New York by E. P. Dutton in 1964. Although educated in medicine in English, he learned how to teach it in Chinese.

[42] S. P. Chen (Chen Sibang 陈祀邦) (June 1916), 4–19. Dr. Chen was born in Singapore in 1884. After study at Cambridge University and St. Thomas's Hospital in London he obtained his M.B.B.Ch. degree in 1907. He was at one time medical officer of the NMPPS in Harbin and later director of the small government isolation hospital that opened in Beijing in 1915. From January till May 20, 1918 he served as one of three commissioners on the Shanxi Plague Commission, with responsibility for investigating plague conditions in Shanxi around Datong and the Beijing-Suiyuan railroad. By 1919 he was medical director of Beijing's Central Hospital and a lecturer in medicine at the Peking Union Medical College. See i) China Weekly Review (1936); ii) Alex. Ramsay (1922); iii) "Pneumonic Plague" (1918), 88–94.

proper understanding of scientific thought as exemplified in the practice of modern hygiene can alleviate it."[43] At that time the Yale-educated Dr. Yan Fuqing (颜福庆) was publishing appalling findings regarding hookworm (钩虫) infection in a colliery in Hunan.[44] During October-November 1918 the influenza pandemic (流行性感冒) struck China. In southern Manchuria the epidemic reportedly "victimized" around 15,000 Chinese and Japanese people between late 1918 and spring 1919.[45] In summer 1919 cholera rampaged through coastal and northeast China. Year after year scarlet fever (猩红热) threatened young children living in central and north China.[46] At that time internationally trained scientists such as Ding Wenjiang (丁文江) were still struggling to inject scientific perspective into public discourse about China's future.[47]

By 1928 the reformers knew that China's health leaders would have to focus attention on preventive medicine and that medical schools and public health agencies would have to take on that task. Unfortunately the culture, from their perspective, was still stuck in a pre-scientific mentality and the country still in political chaos, barring any hope of progressive social legislation. Whereas in Japan the "old-style quacks and herbalists" had been gradually weeded out, the masses encouraged through schools and newspapers to rely upon the new medicine, and Japanese physicians provided with government aid to visit Europe and the US, no such initiatives had occurred in China. In China, the spirit of help and an understanding of science were still rarely present among officials and wealthy classes.[48] And doctors themselves were not oriented to public health concerns such as investigation of housing, drinking water, food, or family customs. Nor did they see the importance of their work to national health.[49] To be sure, in June 1925 the Central Epidemic Prevention Bureau made a start on collecting routine information on occurrence of the more important communicable diseases. But China still had no quarantine service, noted Dr. Ludwik Rajchman, the Polish Head of the League of Nations

---

[43] Wu Lien-teh (1918), 132–139.

[44] See articles by Dr. Yan on this subject in NMJC, 4, 3 (1918): 81–87; 4, 4 (1918): 140–145; 5, 1 (1919,): 57ff; 6, 2 (1920): 71–92.

[45] Chun, J. W. H. (1919), 34–44. Dr. Chun studied medicine at Cambridge University.

[46] Yang Ting-kuang and W. H. Shih (1924), 153–170; Lin Chia-swee and H. M. Jettmar (December 1925), 399–412.

[47] D. W. Y. Kwok (1965).

[48] Editorial (1926), 253–257.

[49] Gao Wei (高维) (1926), 563–568.

Health Organization, while on a visit to China in 1926. Not surprisingly he concluded that: "modern medicine in China is practically non-existent."[50]

Ill Health and National Weakness

While Rajchman was concerned about epidemics; Chinese medical reformers such as Yan Fuqing and Chen Wenda were troubled by the relationship in China of poor health and poverty to national weakness.[51] A sure sign of this weakness was the resurgence of opium after 1917, attributable to the decline of civil authority and the growth of militarism. An endless supply of foreign opium and opium derivatives (morphine, heroin, and morphine pills) was flooding into China, much of it from Persia, and foreign concessions were havens for drug traffickers. The National Anti-Opium Association, founded in 1924, felt its hands tied. "A feeling of loneliness is possessing us," wrote the acting general secretary Huang Jiahui (黄嘉惠 Garfield Huang), "as we are doing our utmost to cope with the opium evil and find that we are without strong allies." The Hague anti-opium convention of 1912, to which China was a signatory, was still not operative in China, and the new Nationalist government depended on income from the opium trade to support its military force.[52]

An unnamed correspondent bleakly summed up the health environment as follows. The defunct Peking government had merely codified sanitary laws, most of which had never been put into operation. China's death rate was probably "not under 30 per 1,000," double that of the West. In a population of 400 million, this meant six million unnecessary deaths per annum (i.e. twelve million deaths instead of six million). Struck by this terrible waste of life, the writer blasted the medical profession as being full of half-trained doctors, many graduated from incompetent provincial medical schools. The army medical service, he charged, was a dumping ground for untrained, incompetent and in some cases corrupt doctors and nurses, unworthy of wounded soldiers fighting for a revolutionary cause.[53]

---

[50] L. Rajchman (1927), 288–292.

[51] i) Yan Fuqing (1927), 229–240; ii) Chen Wenda (陈闻达) (1928), 105–107.

[52] Correspondence (1929), 520–524; Leonard P. Adams (1972). See further discussion on opium in chapter 2.

[53] Letter to the Editor, *NMJC*, 15 (February 1929): 114–116. Even the more cautious John Grant had calculated that there were at least 4 million unnecessary deaths per year. See John B. Grant (1928), 65–80.

As it happened, the revolutionary cause had just been championed by the Northern Expedition of Nationalist and Communist forces led by Generalissimo Chiang Kaishek, which swept up from Guangzhou to central China during the summer and autumn of 1926. The establishment of the Nationalist government in Nanjing in 1927, and the formation of a national Ministry of Health a year later, appeared to the medical reformers as a gift from Heaven. At last there would be an opportunity for their ideas to take shape within a favorable policy setting.

State Medicine and Gongyi Zhidu (公医制度)

The rationale adopted by the medical reformers is known in Chinese as Public Healthcare System (*gongyi zhidu*) and in English as State Medicine. Due to the brief and conflict-ridden history of the Nationalist era (1928–49), the idea that its medical reformers might have had a rational policy for dealing with China's health problems seems surprising. When vast amounts of blood were being shed over ideology and military aggression, how much importance could be attached to well-meaning policies pursued by a handful of medical reformers? But realization that even in wartime more lives are lost due to communicable diseases than to wound casualties should have caused military healthcare to take on added meaning.

The concept of state medicine as a strategy for promoting public healthcare had its origins in public health reforms launched in the early 19th century in West European countries. It was articulated in publications by the middle of the 19th century,[54] and in the later 19th century it became a guiding factor in the development of the British colonial medical system in India.[55] A more immediate stimulus for Chinese reformers came from reforms in East European health services following the destruction caused by World War One. These reforms focused on the socio-economic contexts in which epidemic diseases such as cholera, typhus and malaria occurred, the adoption of preventive health services, and a recognition that public healthcare must bring rural communities into the orbit of healthcare delivery. These initiatives were strongly advocated by healthcare reformers in Poland and Yugoslavia and actively supported by the League of Nations Health Organization and the Rockefeller Foundation's

---

[54] See, for example, Henry Wyldbore Rumsey (1856).
[55] See David Arnold (1993).

International Health Board. Representatives of all these agencies would play an important part advising the Chinese reformers shaping the practice of state medicine and public healthcare in Nationalist China.[56]

The idea of state medicine was advocated in China in January 1928 by Dr. John Grant while he was chair of the PUMC's Department of Public Health.[57] The establishment of the Ministry of Health in Nanjing in November 1928 provided an institutional framework for promotion of state medicine. In 1935 the government's Commission on Medical Education adopted state medicine as a guiding philosophy and began to introduce it into medical education. Several important papers on state medicine were published in June 1937 in the Chinese Medical Journal by Drs. Wu Liande, Chen Zhiqian (陈志潜) and Lin Kesheng (林可胜, Robert K. S. Lim), just before the war with Japan broke out.

During the War of Resistance to Japan (1937–1945) state medicine became a significant formula for programs of the National Health Administration (*weishengshu* 卫生署 NHA), the Army's Emergency Medical Service Training Schools, and a number of provincial health organizations. It became the guiding philosophy of several national medical colleges formed or reorganized in the 1930s to increase and diversify China's national medical manpower.[58] The strategy recognized China's need for a publicly sponsored preventive health program and the inability of private, uncoordinated medical systems, including missionary clinics and hospitals, to handle constant epidemic outbreaks in a time of nation-wide political upheaval.

Before going further we should distinguish between the general sense of "state medicine" and the general sense of "*gongyi zhidu*." "State medicine" is generally taken to mean areas of sanitary care for which the state assumes responsibility. This can include everything from vital statistics, food sanitation, water and sewage management, to prevention of infection, registration of practitioners, care of the elderly, incapacitated,

---

[56] The subject is treated extensively in chapter 2 of AnElissa Lucas (1982). See also Mary Brown Bullock (1980), chapter 6 (on John Grant). For studies of post World War One epidemics in East Europe see M. A. Balinksa (accepted 1999); Gabriel Gachelin and Annick Opinel, (April/June 2011).

[57] Ka-che Yip points out that Chen Zhiqian and other students at PUMC were discussing state medicine in the mid 1920s; Grant's article appears to be the first statement by a public health leader. See Ka-che Yip (1995), 39–40; see also C. C. Chen (1989), 46–56, especially 53, where he uses the term "state-supported medicine."

[58] They included National Xiangya, Guiyang and Zhongzheng medical colleges. Aspects of medical college commitment to state medicine are discussed in Watt (2012).

and poor, and more recently national insurance. *"Gongyi zhidu"* (public healthcare system) focuses on the wellbeing of the population, which in the case of China in the 1930s meant addressing the high rates of death and disease, the perceived backwardness of the people's health, and the dangers resulting from uncontrolled epidemics and high rates of mortality of mothers and infants. It represents a coordinated means for addressing these problems and a cost-effective delivery system through public channels. 'Public healthcare,' advocates in China in the 1930s visited the Soviet Union and Croatia to learn more about their state medical initiatives.[59] [60] Further, public healthcare in China included experimental programs introduced at the county level mainly by medical colleges for the benefit of local people, with the support of local administrations but without management by national government authority.

It is necessary to make these distinctions since Chinese medical reformers are liable to use the term *"gongyi zhidu"* in Chinese language texts and the term "state medicine" in English language texts and to be drawing on both definitions (especially since many of them were trained in English medium schools) even while discussing the needs of 1930s Chinese people and country. The discussion of public healthcare in the late 1920s and 30s is superimposed onto a public health system largely limited to a few urban centers, featuring street cleaning, and managed by police departments. The reformers were eager to get the discussion of public healthcare well beyond this primitive context.

It should also be noted that state medicine in Japan is represented in the concept of *weisheng*. *Weisheng* came to mean "hygienic modernity" and was the means by which the Japanese state achieved a modern, scientific health system. *Weisheng* was also the term used to represent the national health authority (*weishengbu/weishengshu*) in Nationalist China; but the Nationalist Chinese political and military elite did not recognize *weisheng* as a pathway to national political and physical strength with

---

[59] Among the principles of Soviet medicine that drew attention in China were 1) Health care is the responsibility of the state; 2) health care should be cost-free; 3) preventive care is paramount; 4) popular support is a necessary ingredient. See Mark G. Field (1967) especially chapters 3 and 4.

[60] Chen Zhiqian notes in his memoirs that he and Dr. Lin Kesheng traveled to the Soviet Union in 1935 to attend a conference on physiology and visited several health institutions while they were there. Dr. Chen subsequently visited Croatia, where Dr. Berislav Borcic hosted him. Certain aspects of the rural health program, e.g. construction of wells, impressed him; he was also favorably impressed by the skills represented at the Institute of Hygiene in Zagreb. See C. C. Chen, (1989), 100–104.

anything like the same level of commitment shown by the Japanese political elite.[61]

To return now to the discourse in late 1920s China: In his article "State Medicine—A Logical Policy for China," Dr. John Grant (*Lan Ansheng*) argued that medical work should fit into overall community goals, particularly protection against disease. China had two immediate problems: first, to control excessive loss of life; secondly, to find ways to treat around sixteen million daily illnesses. The solution to this huge logistical problem would depend on both medical and non-medical factors. Grant suggested a structure of simple dispensaries and first aid facilities in rural health stations, backed by a hierarchy of local and base hospitals for dealing with more complicated cases. Personal hygiene should be emphasized, particularly in schools, to develop a citizenry trained to avoid infection. Such goals depended on the emergence of a centralized and diversified medical authority pursuing a policy of state medicine. The scheme was very much that of the East European and League of Nations reformers and was in line with strategies developed in Beijing and Dingxian with Grant's guidance.[62]

Dr. Grant's ideas were part of a stream of advice from public health reformers, among them Drs. Yan Fuqing, Chen Wenda, Wu Liande, and Ludwik Rajchman, emphasizing the importance of public health to national reconstruction and urging the newly established Nanjing government to set up a national public health authority. After the Ministry of Public Health (卫生部 *weishengbu*) was launched, with Dr. Liu Ruiheng (刘瑞恒) of PUMC as its first technical vice minister, Dr. Rajchman was invited to China to conduct a public health survey.[63] This set the stage for the involvement of League of Nations advisors in the development and monitoring of Nationalist China's public health policy. This policy and its enactment before 1938 is the subject of the next chapter.

---

[61] Rogaski (2004), chapter 5, is particularly helpful in clarifying the degree of Japanese elite commitment to a policy of national strength through *weisheng*.

[62] John B. Grant (1928): 65–80. See also Bullock (1980), 151–152.

[63] When Rajchman first visited China in April 1926 he concluded that China needed a system of public preventive medicine based on a national effort and assisted from abroad. His second visit, as Ministry advisor, was in November 1929. See Wong and Wu, (1936), 726–727; Rajchman (1927), 288–292; League of Nations Health Organization (1930).

CHAPTER TWO

ADVANCES AND SETBACKS IN NATIONALIST CHINA'S PUBLIC HEALTH MANAGEMENT, 1928–1937

There is nothing more difficult to carry out, nor more doubtful of success, nor more dangerous to handle, than to initiate a new order of things.[1]
—Machiavelli

This chapter discusses the public healthcare policies initiated by the leaders of the new health ministry and the problems they ran into. It asks what were these problems, what mistakes did the reformers make, how did they pay for them, and how were they able to persevere within a regime that had bitter fights with warlords and ideological opponents on its hands? In a decade of continuing civil war and mounting conflict with Japan, it assesses what chance the public health reformers had of making any significant progress, let alone paving the way to a new social order in which China could control infection, save lives and demonstrate modernity. While science and public health were seen as progressive values characteristic of modernity, World War One, the Bolshevik Revolution, the Great Depression, and the rise of Fascism and Militarism unleashed more strident and destructive values. In the 1920s and 30s rising tides of revolution and class war made their way to China, and China's health reformers could not escape them. It would take perseverance of a very high order for the reformers to find their way forward.

Rise and Fall of the Ministry of Health, 1928–1931

The organization of the Ministry of Health illustrates the maze of problems into which the healthcare reformers stumbled. Initially health policy was situated in the Ministry of the Interior, management of which was turned over to the Christian warlord Marshal Feng Yuxiang (冯玉祥). Feng chose as minister Xue Dubi (薛笃弼), a young but close associate,

---

[1] Machiavelli, *The Prince and the Discourses* (New York: Random House, Modern Library, 1950), chapter 6, 21.

who had served as Mayor of Beijing and governor of Gansu province. Then it transpired that direction of the Interior Ministry was needed for Zhao Daiwen (赵戴文), an early follower of Dr. Sun Yat-sen and senior associate of Yan Xishan (阎锡山), another major northern warlord whom the Nationalist leaders wanted to bring into the new government. To solve this problem the Nationalist central leadership took the health department out of the Interior Ministry and set it up under Xue as a separate Health Ministry. Xue brought with him two associates as secretary general and political vice minister. The position of technical vice-minister went to Dr. Liu Ruiheng (刘瑞恒), a prominent physician and Director of the Peking Union Medical College. Dr. Liu was a graduate of Harvard College and Harvard Medical School, who had a relationship with the influential finance minister Song Ziwen (宋子文 T. V. Soong, also a Harvard graduate).[2]

Installing a public healthcare system was not a reason for establishing the Health Ministry until Dr. Liu came in as technical vice-minister. Even then enacting such a policy depended on the patronage of Marshal Feng and Mr. Xue. But in early spring of 1930 a falling out occurred between the Nationalist military leaders and the two northern warlords. As a result Xue had to resign abruptly, leaving Dr. Liu in an awkward position as acting minister without a clearly designated patron. The weakness of his status can be seen in the subsequent ebb and flow that beset the health administration. In November 1930 the central leadership abolished the Ministry and in April 1931 reconstituted it as a National Health Administration (*weishengshu* 卫生署 NHA) under the Interior Ministry. In 1935 it was raised to sub-cabinet status under the Executive Yuan. After the outbreak of the War of Resistance in 1937 it was combined with the Army Medical Administration to form a Combined Health Services Ministry (*qinwubu* 勤务部). Early in 1938 the Combined Ministry was dissolved and the NHA relegated to a department of the Interior Ministry. In April 1940 it was promoted back to sub-cabinet status, at which level it remained until the end of the war. During the government reorganization of 1947 it was restored to ministerial status, only to be once more

---

[2] Fu and Deng (1989). Xue was at the time only 36 whereas Yan's associate Zhao Daiwen who displaced him was 61 and had been a member of the Tongmenghui. Dr. Liu was even younger at only 31; his association with Song Ziwen developed during the time when both were students at Harvard University. The part played by Dr. Grant and Feng's wife Li Dequan (李德全) in these negotiations is reported in Bullock (1980), 152–155.

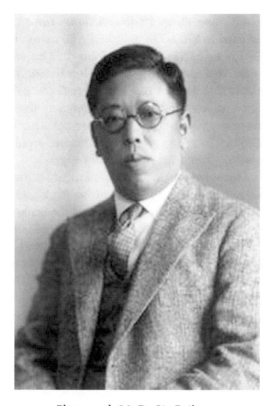

Photograph 2.1: *Dr. Liu Ruiheng*
Director Peking Union Medical College, Deputy Minister of Health, Director General, National Health Administration, wartime medical director of China Lend Lease, medical director, ABMAC. Strong advocate for Anglo-American biomedicine. (*Source*: ABMAC archive)

consigned to the Interior Ministry as the Nationalist government retreated to Taiwan.[3]

The new Ministry set up an impressive organization that included five departments, a secretariat, two offices for counselors and technical experts, an editorial committee, a National Board of Health, and an International Advisory Council. Several separately administered health

---

[3] Zhu Chao (1988), 95; Wong and Wu (1936), 719–721, 734; Fu and Deng (1989); ABMAC Archive, box 21, "The Chinese NHA . . .," rev. October 1941. I am indebted to Dr. J. H. Fan (Fan Rixin 范日新) for providing a copy of the article by Fu and Deng. A larger study, not seen, is Fu Hui and Deng Zongyu, *Jiu Weishengbu Zuzhi de Bianqian* (旧卫生部组织的变迁) (Beijing: Zhongguo Wenshi Chubanshe, 1996).

agencies gradually came under its jurisdiction.[4] The annual operating budget was restricted to $700,000, only $200,000 more than the amount allocated to health management by the city of Canton (Guangzhou) in 1926–27. As pointed out by Ka-che Yip, the Health Ministry budget accounted for only 0.11 percent of the total national government 1929 budget. These comparisons indicate the perfunctory level of interest of Nationalist government leaders in public health.[5] This attitude would change only in 1934 when the government launched a public health program in the politically contested province of Jiangxi.

The Ministry's seventeen-member National Board of Health had some predictable names along with others requiring explanation. The leader, Dr. Chu Minyi (褚民谊 Ts'u Ming-yi), studied medicine in France and became an associate of the Guomindang (Nationalist Party) leader Wang Jingwei (汪精卫). After returning to China he was head of the medical corps in the Northern Expedition and became a member of the Guomindang (Nationalist Party) Central Executive Committee. During the early 1930s relations between Wang and Chiang Kaishek frayed; as a result Dr. Chu resigned from the Central Executive Committee in November 1935. After war with Japan erupted, he joined Wang's puppet government and became its foreign minister. After the war Chu was captured and executed. In short, his power in the Guomindang leadership depended on Mr. Wang's, and he could not provide the independent weight that the ministry needed.

The other members of the Board were all physicians holding government or collegiate positions or in private practice in Shanghai.[6] An interesting exception was Dr. Yu Yan (余岩, also known as Yu Yunxiu 余云岫, 1879–1954), President of the Shanghai branch of the Medical

---

[4] Fu and Deng (1989); Wong and Wu (1936), 720–21; Tyau, (1930), 262.

[5] Editorial (1929), 49–52; Ka-che Yip (1995), 62–65. Yip describes expedients adopted by Dr. Liu to raise additional funds.

[6] The other members were: Drs. Yan Fuqing, Wu Liande, Hu Xuanming (胡宣明 S. M. Woo, Chief Medical Officer, Ministry of Railways), Yang Mao (杨懋 briefly nominated as President, Army Medical College), and Chen Fangzhi (陈方之 Chen Fang-tse, director of the National Hygiene Laboratory, Shanghai); five urban Commissioners of Health: Hu Hongji (胡鸿基 also Hu Hou-ki, Greater Shanghai), Huang Zifang (黄子方 Tsefang F. Huang, Greater Beijing), Quan Shaoqing (全绍清, Greater Tianjin, former president, Army Medical School), Hu Ping (Nanjing; this must be Hu Dingan 胡定安, who was Nanjing's Commissioner of Health at that time), and He Jichang (Ho Tchi Tcheong, Guangzhou); four Shanghai physicians—Drs. Niu Huisheng (牛惠生 Waysung New), Yu Fengbin (俞凤宾 Yui Voonping), Y. H. Zhou and Sung Wei-seng; and Dr. Fang Shishan (方擎石珊 S. C. Fang, Director Beijing Health Demonstration Station). From "National Board of Health Conference (1929), 203–204. For Dr. Chu see Boorman 1967), volume 1, 467a–469a.

and Pharmaceutical Association of China. Like many modern trained physicians Dr. Yu was eager to rescue China from foreign oppression and humiliation. After graduating in medicine at the University of Osaka and seeing how medical science had contributed to Japan's modernization, he felt that science was the key to China's revival. Although trained in Chinese medicine, he concluded that it lacked scientific validity and could not address China's public health problems. Dealing with that issue was one of his agendas.[7]

Assignment to leadership of the Ministry's departments depended on whether the candidate had received training from Anglo-American or German-Japanese medical schools. As a Harvard graduate and PUMC director Dr. Liu Ruiheng headed the former group. To balance his influence direction of the department of medical administration went to Dr. Yan Zhizhong (严智钟) a grandson of the late Qing intellectual reformer Yan Fu (严复) and a graduate of Tokyo Imperial University. Dr. Yan held senior medical agency and university positions in Beijing.[8] The head of the department of preventive health, Dr. Cai Hong (蔡鸿), had studied in France and was not a member of either group.[9] The head of the department of health and sanitation, Dr. Jin Baoshan (金宝善), had an MD from Chiba University but advanced training in public health from Johns Hopkins. He was already an associate of Dr. Liu Ruiheng. The head of the department of general administration, Yang Tianshou (杨天受), was a Tianjin banker with an American degree in economics.[10]

This parceling of top positions reflected a split amongst China's biomedical physicians, which hinged on differences in curriculum studied and disagreement over medical qualifications, particularly the dual track of junior and senior medical degrees in Japanese medical education. The

---

[7] i) Wong and Wu (1936), 161–166; ii) Yu Yunxiu biography, http://baike.bidu.com/view/857802.htm#sub857802; iii) www.jstcm.com/zyxs/detail.asp?newsid=84; Jstcm.com is the website for Jiangsu Traditional Chinese Medicine. A vigorous writer and editor, Dr. Yu was the author of *Yixue geming lunji* (医学革命论集 Essays on Medical Revolution). He had trained in Chinese medicine, but abandoned it in Japan.

[8] Dr. Yan was born in 1889 and was 8 years senior to Dr. Liu. He was apparently in Japan from 1904 to 1917. After returning to China he held positions as director of the government isolation hospital in Beijing, professor of bacteriology and hygiene at the National Medical College of Beijing and technical director of the National Epidemic Prevention Bureau. *China Weekly Review* (1936), 277.

[9] Dr. Cai was a native of Nanchang (Jiangxi). He trained in surgery at the University of Bordeaux. Although associated at one point with Dr. Wu Liande, his influence over preventive health policy appears to have been marginal. See *China Weekly Review* (1936), 231.

[10] Fu and Deng (1989); biographical data from *China Weekly Review* (1936).

split embodied differences over the aims of public health, which in the Japanese model was subject to state surveillance, whereas in the Anglo-American model it was a central plank of late nineteenth century urban social reform. Members of each group regarded members of the other group as sympathetic to the interests and cultural values of the countries where they had trained and in certain instances as publicly or secretly representing them in China.[11] Thus the division of power within the Health Ministry represented a balancing of these contending forces. In 1932 Dr. Liu informed the Chinese Medical Association that the continued existence of several different medical associations and "sects of modern doctors" (e.g. Anglo-American and German-Japanese) was "most deplorable;" he himself was firmly planted in the former and regarded the latter with ill-concealed disdain.[12]

The head of the department of statistics, Jin Songpan (金诵盘 1894–1958), was an exception to this categorization. Dr. Jin was a respected clinician who learned Chinese medicine from his father Jin Cangbai (金沧柏) but also graduated from the German Tongji medical school in Shanghai. He developed strong ties with both Dr. Sun Yat-sen (孙中山 Sun Zhongshan), whom he served as personal physician, and Chiang Kaishek. He became a sworn brother with Chiang and Dai Jitao (戴季陶 a leading Guomindang intellectual and official). He was for several years Chiang's personal physician and director of medical affairs at Chiang's Whampoa Military Academy. He was Headquarters medical officer during Chiang's critical second campaign against the Guangdong warlord Chen Jiongming (陈炯明) and medical director of field operations during the Northern Expedition. He was passionate about saving lives and so was shocked by Chiang's decision to kill Chinese Communists (The White Terror) in April 1927, and abruptly withdrew from military service. He agreed to take a position in the Ministry but preferred working as a clinician and left office after two years.[13]

One of the first acts of the Ministry of Health was to publish a general outline for development of public health work at provincial, municipal and

---

[11] Grant's views on this are reported in note 50 below.

[12] J. Heng Liu (1932).

[13] There are two major texts online about Dr. Jin. 1) baike.baidu.com/view/1630666 .htm; 2) a longer and more interesting text, at club.china.com/data/thread/5688158/2717/ 38/80/4_1.html. Dr. Jin was also upset by the ongoing warlord feuding. His career exemplifies the tensions between political struggle and the commitment of physicians to save lives. He is regarded as an exemplary person who "rescues the times and relieves the people" (*jiushijimin* 救世济民), an attribute associated with China's greatest Confucian sages: Yao, Shun, Yu, Tang, the Duke of Zhou and Confucius himself.

county levels. At the time, professionally directed health agencies existed only in a few major municipalities. In response to this problem the Ministry held a conference in Nanjing in February 1929 attended by twenty to twenty-five mostly non-medical heads of health agencies. The conference was reportedly a "great success,"[14] yet not long after it the Mayor of Beijing appointed his Chief of Police as concurrent Commissioner of Health. A chagrined local branch of the National Medical Association telegrammed the Ministry urging it (ineffectively) to prevent similar incidents occurring elsewhere.[15] Dr. Liu reported that the Ministry was "studying" the idea of state medicine.[16]

Registration of medical practitioners was another concern of the health reformers. Regulations were issued in December 1928, followed by a meeting in February 1929 of the Ministry's National Board of Health, at which it was resolved not to relicense Chinese medicine practitioners after December 1930. A further blow to Chinese medicine practitioners occurred when the Ministry of Education, in April 1929, announced that since instruction in Chinese medicine was not based on scientific practice, its recently organized schools (*xuexiao* 学校) should be renamed apprentice institutes (*chuanxisuo* 传习所), thus depriving them of educational standing. The Ministry of Health forbade Chinese medicine practitioners to use western medicines or equipment and downgraded their hospitals to clinics.[17]

The practitioners quickly organized to protect their profession and block the Ministry's initiatives. By positioning Chinese medicine as a pillar of Chinese national identity they were able to enlist the support of key Guomindang leaders such as Tan Yankai (谭延闿) and Chen Guofu (陈果夫).[18] In March 1931 the Chinese medicine practitioners strengthened their position by organizing the Central Bureau of National Medicine (*Zhongyang Guoyi Guan* 中央国医馆) to represent their interests. They set up branch offices at provincial, city and county levels. The first national director, Jiao Yitang (焦易堂), was a member of the Guomindang's Central

---

[14] Zhu Chao (1988), 96; Wong and Wu (1936), 722.

[15] Peiping Branch, National Medical Association (1929), 469–470.

[16] J. Heng Liu (1929), 135–148.

[17] Shaanxi Zhongyi Xueyuan (1988), 127; Zhu Chao (1988), 114–115; Wong and Wu (1936), 161–165.

[18] i) Wong and Wu (1936), 161–162, 722; ii) *NMJC*, XV, 5: (October 1929), 700; iii) Ralph C. Crozier (1968), chapter 7; iv) Shaanxi Zhongyi Xueyuan (1988), 125–128. The latter source notes that both Yu Yan and Dr. Chu Minyi, were leading opponents of Chinese medicine. Both Crozier and the Shaanxi Zhongyi Xueyuan study describe in detail the methods used by the practitioners and their supporters to frustrate the Ministry's proposal.

Executive Committee with a senior position in the Legislative Yuan (立法院); its Board was joined by the formidable Chen brothers (Chen Guofu 陈果夫 and Chen Lifu 陈立夫). As strong believers in building national strength, and with a powerful patronage system in place, they attacked the Ministry of Health modernizers, accusing them of excessive worship of foreign things and disparagement of the national medical tradition.[19] As Minister of Education, Chen Lifu took on representatives of the Rockefeller Foundation and the China Medical Board, advocating strongly for Chinese medicine and setting up strict regulations for students seeking to study abroad.[20]

While this struggle was going on, the Ministries of Health and Education convened a Joint Committee on School Health in April 1929 to discuss curriculum and training criteria.[21] School health was then a novel idea, although in 1924 a missionary conference had drawn limited attention to the topic. The Health Demonstration center in Beijing studied the health of 3,573 students from kindergarten through middle school, and similar studies existed of small numbers of students in Suzhou, Hangzhou and Changsha. The Beijing study uncovered problems with trachoma, tooth decay and tonsillitis; it showed that at a cost of $2.74 per head significant progress could be made providing children with effective treatment of minor health problems. The other studies discovered significant numbers of students with anemia and skin, glandular and orthopedic problems.[22] Meanwhile medical students such as Chen Zhiqian (陈志潜) and his friends concluded that health education was a critical priority for reformers focusing healthcare on scientific and preventive treatment.[23] Dr. Liu wrote that school health work would be established "as soon as feasible" and would include smallpox vaccination and health education.[24]

---

[19] Wong and Wu (1936), 165–168; Crozier (1968), chapter 5; Fu Weikang (1989), 519–521.

[20] 1) In 1938 (May 6) Chen Lifu subjected Drs. Grant and Yan Fuqing (then director of the demoted National Health Administration) to a twenty minute discussion on Chinese medicine, coming across, in Grant's view, as "extremely aggressive." Rockefeller Foundation, RG12, Grant diaries 1937–1939. 2) In November 1943 the Ministry of Education put in place regulations requiring private students seeking to study abroad to pass a Ministry exam, after which they would be sent for training at the Guomindang's Central Institute of Party and Political Training before being permitted to leave the country. A private China Medical Board response, in a letter dated April 6, 1944, was that Mr. Chen "ought to be stopped in his tracks." CMB archive, box 22, folder 156, Ministry of Education 1934–1950.

[21] The Minister of Education at that time was the educational reformer Jiang Menglin (蔣夢麟 also Chiang Monlin); he resigned in December 1930.

[22] Herbert Day Lamson (1935), 475–478, section on school health.

[23] C. C. Chen (1989), 44–46.

[24] J. Heng Liu (1929).

The Ministry of Health organized early in 1929 an International Advisory Council, to which Dr. Ludwik Rajchman and Dr. Victor Heiser (a member of the Rockefeller Foundation's International Health Board) accepted appointments. In November 1929 Drs. Rajchman and Frank G. Boudreau arrived in Shanghai to review the public health situation in China.[25] As well as surveying medical education, Rajchman and Boudreau agreed to provide advice and training in setting up specialized health agencies. Following this delegation, experts were sent from the League of Nations to study the occurrence of cholera in Shanghai and to develop quarantine regulations. In the summer of 1930 Dr. Berislav Borcic (鮑謙熙), director of the School of Hygiene of Zagreb University, arrived in China to develop a plan for long range collaboration between the Ministry and the League of Nations Health Organization.[26]

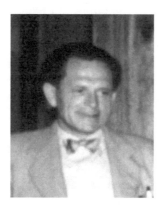

Photograph 2.2: *Dr. Berislav Borcic*
A colleague of Dr. Andrija Stampar, Dr. Borcic was director of the School of Public Health in Zagreb, a leading public health innovator in post World War One East Europe, and a League of Nations consultant to China's National Health Administration. (*Source*: ABMAC Archive)

[25] i) Rajchman (1881–1965) was a bacteriologist and epidemiologist. He studied medicine in Cracow and epidemiology at the Pasteur Institute in Paris. He founded the Polish Central Institute of Epidemiology in 1918 and from 1921 to 1939 served as Director of the League of Nations Health Organization. He extended its scope to include disease prevention, protection of children and invalids, and anti-narcotic work. His Jewish ancestry and support of Republican Spain led him to resign from the League of Nations. He later was associated with UNRRA and the founding of UNICEF. See www.pasteur.fr/infosci/archives/e_raj0.html; ii) Boudreau (b. Quebec 1886) studied medicine at McGill University. In 1925 he became chief of epidemiological intelligence and public health statistics at the League of Nations. He later became Executive Director of the Millbank Memorial Fund. See Journal of the American Medical Association (January 30, 1937), 402.
[26] League of Nations Health Organization (1930); Tyau (1930), 274–282; Wong and Wu (1936), 726–730.

In February 1930 the Ministry's Board of Health held a second meeting, at which it approved a draft Chinese pharmacopoeia for publication.
This work offered a nod to its predecessors in the Chinese medical tradition but concluded that: "today they are nothing but waste paper." The
new pharmacopoeia was based on those of the USA (1921), Japan (1921),
Great Britain (1914), and Germany (1926) and took the Nuremberg code
of 1542 as a direct ancestor. It made no concession to drugs in Chinese
medical practice unless already recognized in Western pharmacy. As Paul
Unschuld points out, the code was inaccessible to practitioners of Chinese
medicine and represented a "complete turn towards Western therapeutic
methods." It was a next step in the Ministry's campaign to downgrade
Chinese medicine. The code was enacted in August 1931 and republished
unchanged in 1937.[27]

It is surprising that a small group of healthcare reformers felt they
could take on hundreds of thousands of Chinese medicine practitioners
and undermine their system of healthcare. Even though Dr. Chu was still
a member of the Guomindang's central executive committee, the reformers lacked the clout to overcome a large constituency whose work was
deeply embedded in China's long cultural tradition. The pharmacopoeia
was intended to set a scientific basis for healthcare in China and throw
practitioners of Chinese medicine on the defensive. In this respect the
reformers were quite successful. Where they fell short was in the political
skills and numbers to back up their technical initiatives.

Consequently at a party conference in November 1930 the powerful,
conservative army general and Minister of War He Yingqin (何应钦)
proposed the dissolution of the weakened Health Ministry. The Guomindang Central Executive Committee approved this initiative.[28] In January
1931 the Health Ministry was demoted and put back under the Interior
Ministry. The number of personnel was diminished by about one-third
and their official ranks and salaries were reduced.[29] The NHA budget was
also greatly decreased.[30]

---

[27] Paul U. Unschuld (1986), 261–267; Wong and Wu (1936), 724–725.

[28] Zhu Chao (1988), 95; H. D. Lamson (1935), 463. The lead taken by General He reflects
the influence exerted by the military in the Nationalist government and almost certainly
was intended in part to snub Marshal Feng Yuxiang.

[29] Zhu Chao (1988), Fu and Deng (1989).

[30] Fu and Deng (1989). In this passage the operative words are "*renyuan jingfei dawei
jianshao*" (人员经费大为减少 personnel and funds were greatly cut back).

This reorganization required a demotion in rank for Dr. Liu. To avoid this embarrassment he was appointed head of the government's Opium Suppression Commission (*Jinyan Weiyuanhui* 禁烟委员会), a position that enabled him to continue to attend cabinet meetings, but entangled him in Nationalist government opium policy.[31] Initially the military-dominated government pursued a policy of overtly suppressing opium cultivation and trade while covertly taxing the lucrative trade to help finance the government's military expenditures. It did so with the aid of the underground Shanghai Green Gang and its powerful leader Du Yuesheng (杜月笙). This policy put both Dr. Liu and Dr. Wu Liande (a Commission member) at the center of bitter attacks by opium opponents. In 1932 and again in 1934 members of the Control Yuan (government supervisory agency) attempted to impeach Dr. Liu on charges of embezzlement and neglect of human life. No doubt because he had assisted Du Yuesheng in overcoming opium addiction at the request of finance minister Song Ziwen (宋子文), Dr. Liu was vulnerable to political criticism. In 1935 the Commission was disbanded, but the attacks on Dr. Liu continued.[32]

Progress under the National Health Administration, 1931–1937

The demotion of the NHA was intended to shrink its agendas and rein in its staff. More broadly it signaled a hardening conservative and military disdain for science and internationalism as pathways to restore national strength. The Ministry of the Interior was in charge of local administration and police work, and public sanitation was a police function and a low level domestic operation. The Interior Minister, Liu Shangqing (刘尚清, 1868–1946), was a northeasterner from Liaoning province with experience in banking and commerce but none in public health; he was not at the center of the Nationalist party hierarchy. Fortunately for public health, Dr. Liu received continued support from Song Ziwen and his sister Mme. Chiang (Song Meiling 宋美龄 Wellesley 1917), as well as the Rockefeller Foundation officials who worked with him when he was director of the PUMC.

---

[31] Fu and Deng (1989).
[32] This paragraph follows evidence assembled in Edward R. Slack, Jr. (2001). This aspect of Dr. Liu's career does not normally arise in accounts of his life or health policy, but it is part of the problematic in which he found himself as the Nationalist government's chief health officer and therefore warrants further study.

Thus the government's public health program, despite its damaged status, continued to edge forward.[33]

One important step during this period of shifting fortunes was to consolidate existing health agencies under NHA control. The Central Epidemic Prevention Bureau (*Zhongyang Fangyichu* 中央防疫处), founded in Beijing in 1919, was brought under NHA control in 1929. In 1934 a branch laboratory was opened in Lanzhou, and in 1935 the Central Bureau moved to Nanjing. The Bureau was responsible for producing sera, vaccines and antitoxins. Its production of biologicals increased rapidly between 1927 and 1935, indicating the value attached to preventive health, but was disrupted by the move to Nanjing.[34]

Another important step taken by the NHA was to centralize the quarantine service (*Shanghai Haigang Jianyisuo* 上海海港检疫所). Before 1928 individual ports had their own services under non-medical Customs officers. This system did not prevent the spread of epidemic outbreaks and led to harsh penalties on Chinese vessels traveling to other countries. A central quarantine service was established in 1930 under the direction of Dr. Wu Liande. It took over management of ten coastal ports, published manuals on cholera and plague, carried out a survey of rats and fleas, and assisted with refugee relief during the Shanghai hostilities triggered by the Japanese military in January 1932. In 1935 the service came under direct management of the NHA. After the outbreak of war in 1937 it was seized by the Japanese military.[35]

---

[33] Fu and Deng (1989); Zhu Chao (1988), 95; Wong and Wu (1936), 734, which reports that Dr. Liu finessed the situation by informing a League of Nations Health Organization meeting in Geneva that: "Recent developments in China have resulted in the amalgamation of the Ministry of Health with the Ministry of the Interior. I have, in consequence, been appointed Director of the new National Health Administration." As Yip points out, Dr. Rajchman was aware of, and worried about, the transition. See Yip (1995), 51. For data on Liu Shangqing, see baike.baidu.com/view/1126192.htm#sub1126192.

[34] Fu and Deng (1989); Wong and Wu (1936), 602, 734, 738. Production of serums rose from 29,373 c.c. in 1927 to 1.39 million in 1935, dropping back to 579,000 in 1936 and 363,000 in 1937. Production of anti-toxins was 16.7 million c.c. in 1927, rose to 133.9 million in 1932, dropped to 85.2 million in 1933 and to 296,000 in 1934. Production of other items continued rising through 1935, fluctuating thereafter. Figures are from ABMAC, Box 21, "The Chinese NHA during the Sino-Japanese Hostilities," by Dr. P. Z. King (Jin Baoshan), Section II, part 5. Its leader at this time was Dr. Chen Zongxian (陈宗贤), a graduate of St. John's Medical College in Shanghai, who had obtained three years' advanced study at Harvard and Columbia Medical Schools. See http://blog.sina.com .cn/s/blog_676014580100o263.html.

[35] Wu Lienteh (1959); Wong and Wu (1936), 729–733.

Two other agencies initiated early on were the Central Hospital (*Guoli Zhongyang Yiyuan* 国立中央医院) in Nanjing and the Central Hygienic Laboratory (*Zhongyang Weisheng Shiyansuo* 中央卫生实验所) in Shanghai. The Central Hospital opened in January 1930 in a temporary structure for treating wounded soldiers. In 1933 a substantial building in Nanjing was completed with financial assistance from a Singapore philanthropist. The purpose of this hospital was to provide clinical treatment, serve as a model Chinese-managed facility, and act as an advanced medical training center. Dr. Liu took was appointed Superintendent to ensure his personal control over the hospital. Two ambitious American-trained physicians, Drs. Shen Kefei (沈克非 James K. Shen) and Qi Shounan (戚寿南 Sheonan Cheer), became heads of the departments of surgery and medicine. Dr. Shen soon rose to vice superintendent and superintendent. Dr. Qi became president of the National Central University Medical School, for which the Central Hospital served as a clinical teaching facility. The training program provided a six-month course in public health and eighteen months of clinical training. Dr. Shen actively promoted it, traveling to medical schools in Beijing, Nanjing and Shanghai to attract graduating medical students. Between 1931 and 1937 the hospital trained over 200 health workers.[36]

The Central Hygienic Laboratory in Shanghai had the job of testing drugs, food articles, drinking materials and pathological specimens. A division of bacteriology prepared vaccines and sera and carried out examinations of air, dust, water, and beverages. During the Japanese attack on Shanghai in 1932 its building and equipment were badly damaged. The director resigned and the facilities were transferred to Nanjing for use by the Central Field Health Station. The Laboratory continued in name and a nominal director was appointed.[37]

For outreach to rural China, the Central Field Health Station (CFHS: *Zhongyang Weisheng Sheshi Shiyanchu* 中央卫生设施实验处) was the most important health agency founded during the Nanjing era. The Yugoslav League of Nations health consultant Dr. Berislav Borcic (鲍谦熙) advised on its planning. The station opened in May 1931 with four departments of Health Education, Sanitary Engineering, Bacteriology and Epidemic Disease Control, and Chemistry and Pharmacology. Later in the

---

[36] Shi Yuquan and He Liangjia (1985), 115–116; Zhu Chao (1988), 112–113; Wong and Wu (1936), 810.
[37] Fu and Deng (1989); Lamson (1935), 465; Wong and Wu (1936), 742.

year it was placed under the influential National Economic Council (*Quan-guo Jingji Weiyuanhui* 全国经济委员会) and provided with an advisory board. During the next two years it added departments of Parasitology, Medical Relief and Social Medicine, Epidemiology and Vital Statistics, Maternal and Child Health, and Industrial Health, making nine departments in all. The director of the Maternal and Child Health department was Dr. Yang Chongrui (杨崇瑞 Marian Yang), a pioneer in modern midwifery education.

During 1931–32 the CFHS participated in flood relief and epidemic control as well as relief work during the Japanese attack on Shanghai. In Spring 1933 it opened up a highway health service, which by 1934 was providing clinical and preventive services in seven provinces. A subsidy from a cotton and wheat loan obtained in August 1933 by Song Ziwen brought the Station's budget for that year up to $514,640, making it the largest financial operation of all central government health services. Later that year Drs. Liu Ruiheng and Jin Baoshan (金宝善) obtained joint appointments as Director and Vice-Director.[38]

An important function of the CFHS was to be a public health demonstration field and training center. During 1935 six hundred students graduated from a variety of courses, the largest number being schoolteachers graduating from a health education course, along with sanitary inspectors, interns and residents. The NHA set up with Rockefeller Foundation assistance a Health Personnel Training Class (later Institute: *Weisheng Renyuan Xunlian ban* 卫生人员训练班, later *suo* 所) to promote training of rural health workers. The grant was the result of a shift by the Rockefeller Foundation away from its earlier focus in China on advanced medical education and towards a strategy favoring rural economic and social development. The Health Personnel Training Institute was one of three governmental and five other university and independent agencies funded for this purpose. Staff for the Institute came from the NHA and the CFHS.[39]

---

[38] Wong and Wu (1936), 738–739; Fu and Deng (1989). The Chinese name for Borcic is from "卫生行政系统的确立" at http://www.cintcm.com/lanmu/zhongyi_lishi/jindaijuan/xiyi/mulu/dierzhang1.htm.

[39] Thomson (1969), 130–148. Thomson's account focuses on the role of Selskar M. Gunn in persuading the Foundation to move funds into rural health development in China.

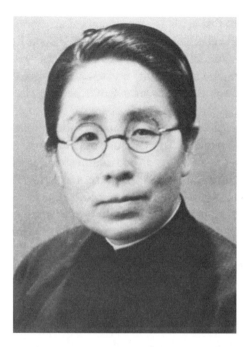

Photograph 2.3: *Dr. Yang Chongrui*
A leading advocate for modern midwifery, member of the Ministry of Health's National Midwifery Board, Professor of Obstetrics and Gynecology at the PUMC, and director of East Beijing Health Demonstration Station. (Source: ABMAC Archive)

Other work by NHA leaders during the Nanjing era (1927–1937) included the establishment of a National Bureau for Control of Narcotic Drugs (*Mazui Yaopin Jinglichu* 麻醉药品经理处) in 1934 and the organization of famine relief during floods in central China in 1931 and in the Yellow River region of eastern China in 1933. Floods have occurred throughout Chinese history, but the Yangtze and Huai River floods of July 1931 were particularly severe. An estimated 34–35,000 square miles were flooded, much of it arable land planted with rice. Nanjing itself became an island surrounded by flooding. "The memory of the season of 1931 still remains with us," wrote one foreign observer, "when thousands of square miles of fertile lands were inundated, peasants and livestock drowned, (and) property destroyed."[40]

---

[40] T. R. Tregear (1965), 108, 241; the quotation is from Lamson (1935), 94ff. (On-line estimates of deaths from these floods range from 140,000 to several million).

In response to this crisis Dr. Liu organized an emergency and preventive health flood relief corps for the National Flood Relief Commission, staffed with one hundred and thirty physicians, eighty-six sanitary inspectors and one hundred and seventy nurses and dressers, as well as auxiliary health workers amounting to over 2,000 people. He put his key aide, Dr. Jin Baoshan (photograph 6.1), in charge of this work. Hospitals, clinics, sanitary and burial teams and a temporary quarantine service provided relief for 150,000 refugees. Through June 1932 the flood relief corps treated over 97,000 cases of skin disease and administered over 200,000 cholera-typhoid inoculations and 246,000 smallpox vaccinations. They buried 13,693 corpses, disinfected 2,000 wells, and provided sanitary services for refugee camps.[41] Dr. Wu Liande noted that though the toll from epidemics including cholera was heavy, "infection remained limited and many lives were saved."[42] It was one of the NHA's most impressive accomplishments.

Getting Preventive Health into Rural and Urban Health Agencies

During the Nanjing era (1927–1937) provincial and municipal health services, except those of key cities, were outside the direct control of the NHA. In two respects the central authorities were able to make an impact: through development of model rural health units and through rural welfare centers, such as those sponsored in Jiangxi province by the National Economic Council and the New Life Movement.

In the 1930s the Shanghai Commissioner of Health Dr. Li Tingan estimated that rural people formed eighty-five percent of China's population. Consequently the state of rural health was of great importance to the health of China as a whole.[43]

---

[41] Fu and Deng (1989); Flood Relief (1932), 233; "Health Work in the Central China Flood" (1933), 75–76.

[42] Wong and Wu (1936), 764.

[43] Li Tingan (1935), 1. Dr. Li carried out a survey of seventeen rural health care agencies during 1934 and published a summary report of findings (Li Tingan, 1934). His book is a detailed handbook on how to identify rural health care problems and organize and carry out an effective rural health care service.

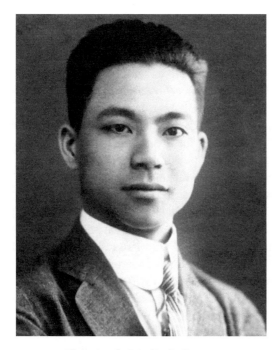

Photograph 2.4: *Dr. Li Tingan*
Received Ph.D. in public health from Harvard School of Public Health, Commissioner of Health, Shanghai in 1930s, expert on vital statistics, author of study on rural health in China. (*Source*: http://show.sysu.edu.cn/?action-imagedetail-pid-3781-uid-124)

Until the 1930s rural health was still the domain of Chinese medical practitioners, gods and demons, temple cults, and sellers of quack medicines. Childbirths were handled by medically untrained midwives viewed by health reformers as *jiushi chanpo* (旧式产婆 old-style birthing women), or by family members if available. In 1930 there were two hundred and twenty-three functioning rural Christian mission hospitals, which recorded over three million outpatient consultations; but it is probable that the majority of the consultations were by townspeople.[44] Rural disorder and the dominance of traditional culture in rural life impeded the diffusion of modern science-based public healthcare, as did the reluctance

---

[44] Lamson (1935), 479–481. Two hundred and five mission hospitals reported having 15,675 hospital beds, 301 foreign physicians, 413 Chinese physicians, 243 foreign nurses, 713 Chinese nurses, 94 nurse-training programs, and 175,217 inpatients during 1930. Lamson (1935).

of trained health specialists to work in rural areas. Under the stimulus of
Dr. John Grant, the PUMC Department of Public Health in 1925 set up an
urban health demonstration center in Beijing, at which several individuals who would become leaders in the public health movement received
their first practical experience.[45] Reform minded students at PUMC published a weekly health supplement in various newspapers, in which they
drew attention to China's health problems. One article published in 1929
stressed the "urgent need for a rural health service practicing scientific
medicine."[46] Beyond the physical definitions of sickness, Yan Yangchu
(晏陽初 James Yen), the education reformer who started the Dingxian
(定县) reform program, saw four great illnesses affecting rural health,
namely poverty, ignorance, physical sickness, and lack of public awareness (贫愚病私). Public health could deal with physical sickness, while
education was needed to deal with ignorance, poverty and lack of public awareness. Public health and education would also help improve the
backward state of the rural economy.[47]

The first incursions of Chinese-led public healthcare into rural China
occurred in 1929 at Dingxian in Hebei province under the guidance of
PUMC's department of public health, and at Xiaozhuang, a short distance
from Nanjing, where the educational reformer Tao Xingzhi (陶行知)
started a rural normal school movement.[48] At Xiaozhuang the Ministry of
Health planned to establish a laboratory to promote village health and a
community hospital. Dr. Chen Zhiqian (陈志潜), recently graduated from
PUMC, was hired to develop a rural health demonstration program at
Xiaozhuang. By that time The Ministry was planning its central field health
station to be "the nucleus of an eventual national field health service,"[49]
and in 1930 the League of Nations dispatched Dr. Borcic to Nanjing to
work with the NHA in surveying municipal and rural health services.[50]

---

[45] They included Fang Shishan (方石珊 Shisan C. Fang), the first director, Hu Hongji
(胡鸿基 Hu Houki) Chief of Vital Statistics, Jin Baoshan (金宝善 P. Z. King) Chief of
Medical Services, Huang Zifang (黄子方 Huang Tsefang), chief of General Sanitation, and
Yang Chongrui (杨崇瑞 Marian Yang), chief of Maternal and Child Health.

[46] Bullock (1980), 144–149; C. C. Chen (1989), 43–56.

[47] Li Tingan (1935), 1.

[48] Bullock (1980), 150 and chapter 7; "Gonggong weisheng shiye de fajan: xiangcun
weisheng" (公共卫生事业的发展: 二乡村卫生 Development of Public Health: Village
Health); Hayford (1990), 132–141, provides a stimulating discussion of Dingxian's rural
health program.

[49] Tyau (1930), 276.

[50] Wong and Wu (1936), 727–728; Bullock (1980), 155. Grant reported in his oral history that the Japanese German physicians regarded both the PUMC and the Rockefeller

A setback to these initiatives occurred when the central government closed the Xiaozhuang program in 1930 for "political" reasons.[51] In its place the CFHS's department of social medicine began a rural demonstration health service at Tangshan (around 25 km. east of Nanjing) to test village health care methods and train village health care workers.[52]

Dr. Chen went on to lead the rural health program at Dingxian.[53] He surveyed the state of Dingxian's rural health and came up with the following disturbing findings. The infant death rate was roughly 164 per 1,000 live births. Thirty percent of children died before the age of five and thirty-four percent before the age of ten. In short, very large numbers of children were dying young.[54] Among preventable deaths the causes, in declining order of magnitude, were tetanus neonatorum, smallpox, diarrhea, dysentery, and diphtheria. Among "partially preventable" deaths the leading causes were "convulsions," measles, scarlet fever, skin infections, and tuberculosis. The sample was taken from children aged 0 to 14 years.[55]

It was unfortunate that the Dingxian reformers had very few years in which to show what they could accomplish. Later in this chapter there is an account of the development of district nursing in Dingxian, led by Nurse Zhou Meiyu (周美玉), one of China's outstanding nursing leaders. But as Charles Hayford recounts in his book on Village China, by 1935 the Japanese military had turned Hebei into a "virtual Japanese puppet province." It was busy promoting the drug trade and undermining Chinese civilian control. Even without this incursion, Dingxian's rural reconstruction movement was unable to overcome local gentry and academic opposition to its work. By summer 1937 the Japanese military were at the

---

Foundation's International Health Division as agents of the U.S. State Department, since some German and French school people were "out and out" agents of their own countries. Borcic was therefore brought out, at Grant's recommendation, to protect the American trained staff in the NHA. John B. Grant, *Oral History*, 311–312, 316.

[51] Hayford (1990), 64; Alitto (1986), 235. In his memoirs Chen notes that he provided Xiaozhuang's teachers with an introduction to the fundamentals of modern medicine. Clinical sessions included a smallpox vaccination program and a treatment for preventing recurrence of ringworm (癣 tinea) of the scalp. Chen (1989), 68–69. The political opposition was almost certainly from local gentry.

[52] Xiangcun Weisheng (Village Health 乡村卫生, as in note 48); Wong and Wu (1936), 749.

[53] For the Tsouping project see chapter 1 and Xiangcun Weisheng/Village Health, as in note 48; Lamley (May 1965), 50–61 (available on-line).

[54] Another source reports an annual China-wide infant death rate of 3.6 million. See Gonggong weisheng shiye de fazhan: fuyou weisheng (妇幼卫生).

[55] C. C. Chen (1933), 680–688.

gates of the county city and the last rural reconstruction workers were rapidly departing.[56]

Zouping County in Shandong province was the site of another model rural program, launched by the Confucian reformer Liang Shuming (梁漱溟). Its health program was developed in collaboration with the Qilu Christian University Medical College. The program was built around a county hospital and thirteen rural district health stations. It ran a one-year training program for health workers and another training class for midwives. It emphasized preventive work to decrease incidence of cholera, diphtheria, typhoid and smallpox, and sent health teams to rural districts to promote hygiene education.[57]

The NHA directly sponsored a rural system of public healthcare at the Nationalist government's Jiangning (江宁) experimental county near Nanjing. The county had a registered population of over 562,000 people. The NHA consultant was Dr. Yao Xunyuan (姚寻源), a PUMC graduate who had previously worked at Dingxian. During the mid 1930s the county developed four health stations and six substations; one of the health stations served as county hospital with fifty beds. The county provided mostly free vaccinations for meningitis, cholera, smallpox and typhoid; it also ran a free maternal child health service. The staff carried out a roving clinical service and a school health program and provided community lectures on topics such as protection against infectious diseases, maternal child health and school health. The health service was guided by the premise that China was an agricultural country, therefore revival of the rural population was the top priority, and preventive health care with cost-free health services was the key to restoring rural public health.[58] As a model experimental county, Jiangning provided the rural teaching field for NHA's Public Health Personnel Training Institute.[59]

It was China's misfortune that all these programs were lost as a result of the Japanese military invasion in 1937. Still, the will to improve rural

---

[56] Hayford (1990), 173–179; understandably Chen Zhiqian does not discuss this painful denouement in his autobiographical account of his work in Dingxian. But he is quoted by Hayford as saying that rural reconstruction would have to wait until liberation from Japan.

[57] Fenxi Guomin Zhengfu Shiqi Gongyi Zhidu Fazhan de Sange Jieduan (2011).

[58] Information from i) Fenxi guomin zhengfu shiqi gongyi zhidu fazhan de sange jieduan (2011); ii) Jiangning gang: minzhong shiqi de mofan shiyan xian.

[59] ABMAC box 21, NHA, 1940–1941, C. K. Chu, Training of Public Health Personnel in 1939–1940."

health through a system of public healthcare would continue during the War of Resistance.

Urban public health had different problems, as indicated by a review of some fifty surveys between 1924 to 1931 of nineteen cities with an average population of 100,000 or above. This study was carried out by Dr. John Grant and Dr. Peng Damou (彭达谋) and published in 1934. The authors found out that with one or two exceptions preventive health programs were not in place. Street cleaning was almost invariably the chief, and in many instances the only, administrative service. In fifteen out of nineteen cities surveyed, 'health administration' was a police function. Apart from Shanghai (not in the survey), only Guangzhou and Nanjing had independent health departments. Health administration in Jinjiang and Zhengzhou was partly under the municipal council and partly under the police department. Except for Guangzhou, Beijing and Nanjing, the budgets were minimal. Personnel were mostly sanitary inspectors and scavengers. Fifteen cities provided no public medical relief. Seven carried out registration of deaths but provided no diagnoses. Practically none of the cities, at the time of the survey, had done anything to control infectious diseases, although five out of nineteen attempted to provide free smallpox vaccinations. Water supplies were not controlled, and food inspection was attempted only in a few cities.[60] In short, the NHA reformers would be starting virtually from scratch.

The Ministry of Health began in 1928 with a nominally supervisory relationship over seven major city health departments: Shanghai, Beijing, Guangzhou, Tianjin, Hankou, Nanjing, and Qingdao. Two other cities later developed departments of health. All other cities were under provincial government management and were not required by statute to establish public health departments. Nine cities had public water supplies, and three others had plans to install public water systems. But in all cases the vast majority of the population used polluted water, and sewerage was restricted to a very small number of cities. The Ministry hoped to get help from the League of Nations Health Organization in collecting data, so that it could develop some activities. But by 1932 all the urban departments of health except those of Shanghai and Guangzhou were back under police departments. According to Dr. Wu Liande, two factors were mainly responsible for "such a retrograde step." One was lack of funds, the other, ineffective management by individuals with general medical

---

[60] J. B. Grant and T. M. Peng (October 1934), 1074–1079.

rather than public health credentials.[61] A third factor could have been skepticism within government bureaucracies about the merits of scientific medicine as sponsored by the NHA.

This situation led the NHA to begin training urban health workers who could promote sanitary and preventive services. Initial steps in that direction were taken by two urban health demonstration centers. The East Beijing health demonstration center was located in a converted temple in a city ward of over 95,000 people. It provided instruction for undergraduates in hygiene and public health administration. Each undergraduate was required to do a community health survey and work as a clerk at the center for a three week period. The center also provided a school health service for 1,800 students and an industrial health service for 1,200 workers.[62] The Wusong Health Demonstration Station in Shanghai opened in 1928. It was sponsored by National Central University's department of health and was used for training of undergraduates in hygiene and public health while carrying on a broad range of urban public health services. The station was destroyed by Japanese warships in 1932 but reopened in 1933.[63] Shanghai also launched a cholera campaign in 1930, inoculating 600,000 individuals. During a severe cholera epidemic in 1932 that affected both coastal cities and provinces in central and northwest China, the cities of Shanghai, Nanjing and Wuhan administered over two million inoculations.[64] In 1933 the Beijing Health Bureau and National Beijing University Medical College set up a Number Two Health station in West Beijing.[65]

But the NHA needed a broader approach to training public health workers. That came with the establishment of the Central Field Health Station and its Public Health Personnel Training Institute. In 1935 the CFHS had one hundred and eighteen people in a 512-hour sanitary inspectors' course and one hundred and nineteen people in a health education course for teachers. It had one hundred and six people in two forty-four hour public health nurses' courses. A one-year course in sanitary engineering provided

[61] League of Nations Health Organization (February 12, 1930); Wong and Wu (1936), 740; Lamson (1935), 456–457; Gonggong weisheng shiye de fazhan: 1. chengshi weisheng gongzuo. This last source adds that people were not clear about the importance of public health.

[62] League of Nations Health Organization (1930); Wong and Wu (1936), 663–664.

[63] League of Nations Health Organization (1930); Wong and Wu (1936), 742–743.

[64] Wu Liande report in *CMJ* 46/9 (September 1932): 931–934; *CMJ* 46/10 (October 1932): 1039–1040; Lamson (1935), 458. Dr. Liu Ruiheng estimated over 100,000 cholera cases and over 30,000 mortalities for 1932.

[65] Gonggong weisheng shiye de fazhan: 1. chengshi weisheng gongzuo.

laboratory training in water, sewage and bacteriology and field practice in operation of water and sewage plants and well and latrine construction. A five hundred hour course for sanitary inspectors provided training in all branches of sanitation, including malaria control and minor drainage.[66] The institute, in short, set in motion a new approach to healthcare training in Nationalist China.

Nationalist Rural Health Initiatives in Jiangxi Province

The most ambitious effort by the Nationalist government to promote rural health during the 1930s occurred in Jiangxi, a semi mountainous and semi forested province in southeast China (see map 3.1). In 1930 Jiangxi had a population estimated at 17.16 million people.[67] It was the scene of violent conflicts between Nationalist and Communist forces, set off by the Nationalist government's efforts to destroy the Communist forces in south central Jiangxi and other rural base areas in central China. These conflicts did not let up until after the Red Army began its historic exodus from the province in October 1934. During the Nationalist government's "fourth extermination campaign" launched in June 1932, efforts began to build a pro-Nationalist government infrastructure within the province.

The Central Field Health Station began by providing healthcare services to the Nationalist armies sent in to destroy the Red Armies. In July 1931, at the outset of the third campaign, Dr. Pan Ji (潘驥), Director of CFHS's Bacteriology and Epidemic Disease Control Department, visited the CFHS field laboratory in Nanchang to investigate outbreaks of dysentery, typhus and malaria among Nationalist army troops. It is possible that the failure of the first two Nationalist campaigns and the difficulties experienced in the third made the government's military leaders recognize that some competent medical assistance for their soldiers might be required. Three years later the Department sent three teams to Jiangxi to help the Nationalist military control a severe outbreak of dysentery. The teams also looked into incidence of malaria and malnutrition. The Sanitary Engineering Department sent four engineers and six sanitary inspectors to Nanchang to install drainage systems and disinfect wells and latrines. The Department of Parasitology investigated malaria cases among

---

[66] Brian R. Dyer (Chinese name Daiya 戴雅) (January 1936), 76–81; Wong and Wu (1936), 802–803.

[67] Tian Xiang Yue and nine other authors (2005): 461–478.

army officers attending a special training course at the Kuling resort on
Lushan Mountain and visited sick soldiers in several military hospitals.[68]
The Bacteriology Department continued its dysentery work until February 1935, reviewing nearly 5,000 cases in base hospitals and examining
2,674 stool specimens. The Sanitary Engineering Department carried out
sanitary work at army camps in Kuling and elsewhere.[69] Dr. Liu Ruiheng
himself visited Nanchang regularly to meet with military health officials
and review military hospitals and provincial and local health service facilities introduced by the Nationalists.[70]

In 1933 the National Economic Council assembled a team of League of
Nations consultants to survey mass education, agriculture and health systems in certain areas of the province. The team consisted of Max Brauer,
a German Jewish social democratic urban administrator in exile from Nazi
Germany, E. Briand-Clausen, a Danish specialist in agricultural cooperation, and Dr. Andrija Stampar, a noted public health leader from Yugoslavia. The team made a thorough review of health conditions. It pointed
out that provincial public health was under the Commissioner for Internal
Affairs and employed only one poorly trained physician, who was away
studying in Nanjing. It harshly criticized a Medical College in Nanchang.
A provincial midwifery school received better treatment; it carried out
1,000 deliveries a year, half of them complicated cases sent in by old-style
midwives, and it had one hundred and seventy students. A nursing school
had just opened with a three-year program. The team recommended closing the Nanchang medical school and a municipal hospital and erecting a
model provincial hospital.[71]

As a result of this report the National Economic Council made a grant
to set up a provincial department of health and finance a provincial hospital and laboratory, the nursing and midwifery schools, a municipal health
station in Nanchang, and ten rural welfare centers. The new administration went into operation in June 1934 and moved rapidly to reorganize
the institutions under its supervision. It undertook health work in areas
formerly managed by the retreating Red Army and Jiangxi Communist

---

[68] Central Field Health Station (1934).

[69] Central Field Health Station (1936). By the time this report was published Dr. Pan
had left the position of acting director of the Department of Bacteriology and presumably
had taken on the new position of Commissioner of Health for Jiangxi province.

[70] Yang Wenda (杨文达) (1989a), 67.

[71] Max Brauer, E. Briand-Clausen and Dr. A. Stampar (January 1934).

government and dispensed free medicine and smallpox vaccines. A new medical college would come in 1937.[72]

The ten rural welfare centers were distributed mainly in the center of the province, with two in the North and two in the reconquered South. Each center operated departments for education, agriculture, health, cooperatives and home industry. The health department of each center was to be supplied by the provincial health service with one doctor and an assistant; late in 1935 a modern, trained midwife was added. The centers each had a hospital-clinic, which offered four to fifteen beds for emergency cases and according to a report by the director of the program were in some cases superior to an average county hospital. Outreach consisted mainly of smallpox vaccination and inoculation against cholera and typhoid.

In 1936 Dr. Stampar made a second visit, during which he toured all the centers and visited the provincial health department. He criticized the program for failing to come to grips with the land tenancy problem, which Stampar regarded (as did the Chinese Communists) as the overriding obstacle to rural reconstruction in Jiangxi. He chided the health departments for focusing too much on treatment and not enough on prevention. Their outreach was too limited; the number of persons vaccinated and the number of deliveries by a trained midwife per year were too low. Very little data had been collected, so that none of his questions on vital statistics, principal local diseases, or care of children could be answered. The provincial health department did not pay enough attention to rural health work; the NHA needed to distribute designs for school buildings, wells and latrines.[73]

A report prepared in May 1936 by Zhang Fuliang (张福良), director of the Jiangxi rural welfare program, pointed out that old customs died hard. Villagers were still willing to spend hundreds or thousands of Chinese dollars pacifying the goddess of smallpox. One center reported that within a radius of 10 Chinese miles (*li*) 50 altars had been built to the goddess in the spring of 1935 costing 500 Chinese dollars per altar. Another reported 700 dollars spent for expenses on an altar for the goddess and much more on eating and amusements.[74] Evidently the pre-modern association of

---

[72] "Health Work in Kiangsi" (1934), 1173.

[73] Houghton Library, Harvard University, American Board of Commissioners for Foreign Missions, Shaowu documents, 1930–39, vol II, Reports, item 41. Dr. Stampar's annex describing the provincial health service is unfortunately missing from the file.

[74] Rural methods for pacifying demons and gods of disease are described in Francis K. L. Hsu (1983), especially 20–23, and Clarence Burton Day (1969).

disease with gods was still flourishing in rural Jiangxi. Healthcare practice was also backward. A local practitioner had collected one dollar per child by collecting material from the nose of a smallpox patient and blowing it into the noses of uninfected children (a not fail-safe pre-vaccination procedure known as variolation). Rural women were reluctant to be attended by a young trained midwife, arguing "how does she know anything about delivery, being both young and unmarried?" Yet they were willing to be treated by old style midwives who made do with old rags, a pair of scissors, and string.[75]

Yet Zhang asserted there had been good results. During much of 1935 only six centers were functioning, yet over 20,000 smallpox vaccinations had been administered. A young trained midwife had achieved "Living Buddha" status by saving the life of a mother with a stillborn child, whom the old-style midwives had been unable to treat. The secretary of the welfare center had been appointed head of the local area, as Stampar recommended. Clinic treatments added up to 42,500, modern vaccinations to nearly 34,000 people and inoculations to nearly 11,000. Student examinations totaled 5,426. Two hundred and four wells and one hundred and sixty-three latrines had been improved. Deliveries by modern trained midwives had risen to 329 and attendance on babies to over 1,000.[76]

Zhang Fuliang's report indicates that most aspects of rural health were handled to some extent. But the figures were modest, and there is no discussion of infectious disease or of security regimes that Nationalist divisions and landlord militias introduced into areas reclaimed from Communist control.[77] A brief report in the Lichuan Center indicates that a visiting nurse carried out home visits three times a week, and a two-month course on the subject of women and the home enrolled sixty women out of a total Lichuan County population of 90,000.[78]

It seems that the health work carried out in rural Jiangxi under Nationalist government auspices lacked the drive and focus found in Dingxian. Yet there were leaders among the reform wing of the Nationalist party

---

[75] "Health Work in Kiangsi" (January 1937), 102–104. The monthly budget for the entire program of each center was $815, except for one that had a budget of $910. See Stampar report, note 73 above.

[76] Shaowu reports (see note 73 above), number 37, "New Life Centers in Rural Kiangsi," May 1936.

[77] For this subject see Benton (1992).

[78] For Lichuan report see Shaowu reports number forty-four, "Brief Report on Lichuan from August 5 1937–September 4, 1939," by Zhang Xiaoliang; for county population see Thomson (1969), 99.

who promoted the modern health movement, among them Song Ziwen, who obtained the financing for the Jiangxi welfare centers, and his sister Mme. Chiang. The latter sent an impassioned appeal to the National Christian Council of China urging it to cooperate with the government health service in bringing 'new life' and specifically modern social services such as smallpox vaccination to China's rural districts. The health authorities, she pointed out in a classic understatement, had "not yet perfected their machinery for reaching all the neglected areas." Until they did, here was one place where the church could still serve the people. From Mme. Chiang's perspective, Zhang Fuliang's program in central Jiangxi was a beacon of light, which others should strive to emulate.[79]

One basic problem, which the NHA could never solve by itself, was how to extend a science-based program, as advocated by reformers such as Drs. Grant, Stampar and Liu Ruiheng. Such a program required the presence in the countryside of science-trained people such as Dr. Chen Zhiqian and Nurse Zhou Meiyu, who could convince local people to put a science-based program into practice. China's educational system of the time, and especially its medical education system, could not produce the numbers or talent needed to do such a job; nearly all graduates that the medical colleges produced preferred to work in urban areas and in private practice. For most such physicians, rural areas were subject to disease, banditry and warfare and were culturally alien territory. Stampar held that mobilization of each local community was needed to enable rural health programs to succeed.[80] The Red Army and Communist Soviet in Jiangxi demonstrated the validity of this point during their public health campaign of 1933–1934 (see next chapter). But the Nationalist provincial leadership was not equipped to mobilize rural people other than those returning to regain control over land expropriated by communist land reform. Nor did they have the means to restore the morale of impoverished villagers in areas trampled by the huge Nationalist invading force of 1934 and still subject to guerilla warfare over the next three years.[81] A modest town-based health system could hardly perform such a task.

[79] Shaowu reports, number 40, "Message to the National Christian Council of China."

[80] Andrija Stampar, "Observations of a Rural Health Worker," New England Journal of Medicine, 218, 24 (1938): 991–997. USSR medical policy made the same point. See Mark G. Field (1967).

[81] Benton (1992). This volume provides a compelling study of a subject still largely passed over in general publications dealing with Nationalist China.

By comparing rural health in China and Yugoslavia one can more easily understand the difficulties that Chinese reformers faced. In 1935 Yugoslavia had over 5,000 physicians, almost as many as China, and most of them were in public service. These physicians were serving a population calculated at 14.534 million in 1931, of whom eighty percent lived in villages. Thus the crude ratio of physicians per head was a little under one per 3,000 people, a ratio unimaginable in 1930s rural China, unless one included Chinese medicine practitioners. But unlike the Communist health leaders, the Nationalist reformers in the 1930s did not include them. Because 1930s data for Yugoslavia indicated that 46.48 percent of all deaths were of children aged ten years or under, the Yugoslav Ministry of Health focused research on diseases responsible for this terrible childhood death rate.[82]

Such conditions could not be replicated in the China of the 1930s, least of all in a mountainous province such as Jiangxi. What China's health reformers did learn from Yugoslavia was that after World War I reform of rural health became a centerpiece of health policy in East Europe. Moreover the Rockefeller Foundation's International Health Board helped to establish schools of public health in Bulgaria, Czechoslovakia, Hungary, Poland, Rumania and Turkey, and it was urging the Johns Hopkins School of Hygiene and Public Health to establish a practical training program for national and international health officials.[83] The importance of rural health, in short, was clear enough to Nationalist China's health leaders.[84] But implementation in the countryside could not brush aside entrenched landed interests and cultural beliefs either in Xiaozhuang or Jiangxi.

---

[82] Stampar, A (1938b). Population data for 1931 is from Institute of Social Sciences, The Demographic Research Center (1974). The influence of East European public health leaders on Chinese social policy of the 1930s is one of the more interesting international phenomena of this period. Osterhammel (1979), 661–680, provides a heavily documented study focused on the role of Dr. Rajchman as the principal technical intermediary between the League and Nationalist China. Although visiting China three times Rajchman was never able to overcome the opposition (for different reasons) of the Japanese and British governments to his work in China. League consultants such as Rajchman, Tawney and Stampar were aware of the primacy of tenancy problems in the Chinese countryside; but finding ways to negotiate the gulf between prevalent rural systems of health care and land ownership was beyond their mandate.

[83] Stampar (1938a); Elizabeth Fee (1987).

[84] For example, in his first report for the Commission on Medical Education, dated June 1936, Dr. Zhu Zhanggeng wrote that the "Peasant University" conducted by the School of Public Health in Zagreb was a model of appropriate training in a backward community. RF, RG1, series 601, box 3, folder 27. The importance of rural health to the Rockefeller Foundation is emphasized in Thomson (1969).

Nursing, Midwifery and Public Health

Nursing and Midwifery were fields in which the NHA and other health agencies made tangible progress. After the establishment of the Ministry of Health in 1928, one of its earliest acts was to organize a Central Midwifery Board. The Board was charged to plan a demonstration school, determine standards for modern midwifery training and investigate public and private midwifery schools.[85] Dr. Liu Ruiheng promised that regular schools of public health nursing would be established when personnel and funds became available.[86]

In 1930 Dr. Liu told a conference of the Nursing Association of the Republic of China (NAC 中华民国护理学会) that he applauded the NAC's interest in training and examination of nurses but suggested that standards should not be set too high. China was estimated to have one nurse per 200,000 people, as compared to the U.S. rate of 140 per 100,000. To get to even 25 nurses per 100,000 people China would have to train 100,000 nurses. "The practical needs," said Dr. Liu, "are such that we cannot afford to be too idealistic." He urged nurses to expand from the sickroom to home visiting, and make the NAC "a really Chinese organization."[87]

To give substance to these views the Ministry of Health took partial responsibility for a midwifery school opened by Dr. Yang Chongrui (杨崇瑞) in Beijing in 1928. The school operated a two-year course for junior high school graduates; it provided training in anatomy, pre- and post-natal examinations, well baby clinics, and performance of at least twenty-five deliveries. Students were expected to become future teachers and supervisors. A six-month course was designed for primary school graduates, with the aim of getting midwives with aseptic training into practice as soon as possible. The school had a seventy-bed hospital, which provided 1,369 deliveries in the first two years of operation.[88] From 1928 to 1930 a Child Health Institute, operated by the school, trained approximately

---

[85] "Law and Legislation: Ministry of Health Organizational Regulation" (February 1929), 75–76. Tina Phillips Johnson (2011) is a heavily documented and persuasively argued study of the development of modern midwifery in Nationalist China, particularly in urban areas.

[86] J. Heng Liu (1929): 135–148, also in Liu Sijin (1989), 287–298.

[87] J. Heng Liu, "Nursing Problems in China," in Liu Sijin (1989), 313–315; for Chinese text see Zhu Baotian (朱宝钿) (c. 1930).

[88] Zhao En-yuan (趙恩源) (c. 1933), in Liu Sijin, op. cit., 170–173; CMJ, 46 (1932), 232; Wong and Wu (1936), 751–753, where it is noted that nursing graduates could take the two year course in a year; Bullock (1980), chapter 7. The authors give different dates as to when the school opened.

two hundred and fifty "old-style" midwives, of whom one hundred and fifty passed a qualifying examination.[89] The NHA organized a National College of Nursing in 1932 and a National Midwifery School in 1933, both in Nanjing.[90]

Dr. Liu's interest in public health nursing grew out of initiatives at PUMC with which he was personally involved. The Beijing health station's Department of Nursing was responsible for family visits, school and factory health services and public health education, as well as for administering courses in public health nursing. School health was particularly emphasized because of its potential for improving personal hygiene as well as reaching families through their children. The station's nursing service began with a supervisor and five staff nurses and by 1930 had grown to 17 nurses.[91]

In PUMC's rural health program at Dingxian nurses focused on school health. Each nurse would provide 1,500 to 2,000 children with physical examinations, immunizations, treatment of minor health problems and instruction in basic hygiene. Heads of families were invited to participate in the examinations so that they could collaborate in maintaining the health of their children. If a problem was identified, there would be a further examination in three months. Nurses were also responsible for supervising the hygienic conditions of schools. Schools that could not provide boiled water were expected to chlorinate their cold water. Children were to use only their own cups. The nurses were expected to provide the children with simple lessons on hygiene, to weigh them as a way to stimulate them to exercise, and to organize cleanup teams. It was their job to provide smallpox vaccinations and inoculations for cholera, typhoid fever and diphtheria. They were to encourage children to bring preschool

---

[89] W. W. Yung, M. D. (1936), 562–572; Bullock (1980), 175. As Bullock points out, nursing and midwifery—the latter as conceived by Dr. Yang Chongrui—were at this time pursuing different and conflicting objectives. The NAC wanted to professionalize the work of women in health care; Dr. Yang wanted to produce midwives who could reduce the very severe infant and maternal sickness and death rates. Bullock (1980), 173, and Marian Yang (杨崇瑞) (1934), 786–791.

[90] Johnson (2011), 135; Wong and Wu (1936), 753–754. The National (Central) Midwifery School set up a two-year program. The first class graduated in 1935, with 12 of 21 students passing the examinations. See *CMJ*, 49/8 (August 1935): 802. In 1935 the course was extended to three years, with fifty-seven students enrolled. Wong and Wu (1936), 753–754. Hunan began a small provincial maternity service in September 1934 with two midwives and four students and four more midwives as volunteers. A description of the program can be found in *CMJ*, 49/8 (August 1935): 803–804.

[91] Wang Xiuying (1987), 224–230. Data for 1930 from League of Nations Health Organization (1930).

siblings for diphtheria inoculations and to inspire school children to act as hygiene scouts and advocates in their villages and homes.

In the community at large nurses were tasked to inspect latrines and wells, encourage personal hygiene, aid local midwives and community health workers, and take community health as their scope of operation. Since female public health nurses had already received modern midwifery training and had handled at least twenty deliveries during their training, it was important for them to keep an eye on local old-style midwives and maternal child health.[92] Community health advice covered basic activities such as food preparation, care of infants, toilet sanitation, dental care, and control of trachoma.[93]

As the Dingxian program developed, the nursing staff rose to nine visiting health nurses, seven clinical nurses and one trained midwife, plus several student nurses. The staff developed two nursing education programs: a three-year course for local women and a six-month course for hospital-trained nurses.[94] With this level of capability on board, Dingxian became a laboratory for testing all the preventive health strategies that the public healthcare reformers were advocating. The visiting nurse served as the point person in delivering the preventive health approach to health care.

In 1928, the Beijing health station was the only place where training in public health nursing could be found. Dr. Liu Ruiheng urged provincial and urban health departments to send graduate nurses there for at least three months training.[95] Shanghai began a school health service in 1928 staffed with a physician and four public health nurses. In 1929 it was serving fourteen schools with 9,000 students and by 1934 fifty schools with around 32,000 students.[96] Two local health stations were opened in the greater Shanghai area in 1929, each with services in public health nursing, school and industrial hygiene and health education. In the Ministry's Xiaozhuang health center a physician with public health training (this was Dr. Chen Zhiqian) carried on health work in schools assisted by two

[92] Zhou Meiyu (1936).
[93] Mamie Kuo Wang, personal communication. Ms. Wang was a graduate of the PUMC School of Nursing.
[94] Zhou Meiyu (1936); C. C. Chen (1989), 96.
[95] Liu, J. Heng (1929), 135–148.
[96] League of Nations Health Organization (1930); Li Ting-an, "A Report on the Bureau of Public Health, City Government of Greater Shanghai," (1934), found in the library of the New York Academy of Medicine.

nurses.[97] It was from this modest base that the country's public health nursing got started.

By 1934 the NHA had developed a rural health service plan designed to position public health nurses in county and market cities and a nurse with training in public health and midwifery in smaller rural towns of 10,000 to 15,000 people. The CFHS began a short course in public health nursing.[98] In 1935 the NHA set up its public health personnel training institute which by 1940 reported having trained five hundred and forty-three public health nurses and midwives.[99]

Another development during this period was the founding of provincial nursing and midwifery schools. In October 1935, the Fujian provincial administration set up a midwifery school in Fuzhou with eighty-four students, over half of whom came from farming families. It had a maternity hospital with twenty beds. A provincial nursing school, also in Fuzhou, enrolled twenty-five students. These city institutions were not reaching country people, but an Anglican mission in Putian (around 90 km south west of Fuzhou) began a rural midwifery service with seven centers, which carried out home visiting.[100] Kunming had a municipal hospital with an attached midwifery school; in 1936 a provincial school of nursing and midwifery was established with fifty-five students.[101] The Attached Number One Hospital of National Zhongshan University Medical College in Guangzhou administered a nursing school and a school of midwifery.[102] Provincial midwifery schools were also founded in Jiangsu, Zhejiang, Anhui, Shandong, Hebei, Gansu and Shaanxi, and a provincial maternity service in Hunan.[103]

---

[97] League of Nations Health Organization (1930). For Dr. Chen's work at Xiaozhuang, see Chen (1989), 61, 66–69.

[98] Brian R. Dyer (1936), 76–81. The course offered 25 hours of lectures and 19 of field-work.

[99] ABMAC archive, Box 21, National Health Administration, "Training of Public Health Personnel in 1939–1940," annual report by Dr. C. K. Chu (Zhu Zhanggeng). A 1936 report noted that the course ought to include more practical experience. Wong and Wu (1936), 803.

[100] A. Stampar, (1937): 1091–1101. Dr. Stampar was troubled that the maternity hospital had only carried out twenty-four deliveries between October 1935 and April 1936. He recommended that the midwifery school open up classes for 'old-style' midwives.

[101] *CMJ*, 50 (1936), 86; Yao Hsun-yuan (1938), 577–583.

[102] Booklet on National Chung-shan University Medical College by Tsou Lu (director) dated January 1, 1935, in ABMAC, Box 18.

[103] Wong and Wu (1936), 754–755; "Gonggong weisheng shiye de fazhan: fuyou weisheng."

The above accounts suggest the extent to which public health practice was still dependent on hospital-based services and training. After inspecting sixty-six nursing schools the Commission on Medical Education's nursing sub-committee reported that the curriculum was made to suit hospital needs; students were brought in to work on the wards. Such schools could not offer basic subjects such as citizenship training, Chinese, personal hygiene, home economics, sociology, psychology, or public health nursing. Students were overburdened with hospital duties and had little time for study.[104] In an attempt to redress this situation the Commission put together ten six to nine month fellowships for teacher training and practical experience, and another thirteen fellowships for a nine-month course in public health visiting at PUMC's School of Nursing.[105]

Surveys of midwifery published in 1936 provided the following information about childbirth practices. In Nanjing old style midwives or family members carried out nearly 14,000 births between July 1934 and June 1935, but over 4,000 were performed by state midwives or in hospitals or clinics. Deliveries by state midwives were only three hundred and twenty-seven in 1931–1932, but this number increased by 1934–1935 to 2,565. The infant mortality rate was recorded as 168.4 and the maternal mortality rate as 15.2. In the Beijing first health station modern midwives and nurses delivered forty-three percent of the 2,836 births recorded during 1934–1935. The station provided clinical and delivery services and home visiting.[106] In the Kaochiao Health Station in Shanghai modern trained midwives delivered two hundred and eighty-two babies in homes, constituting one-third of total recorded births in the county; this service was free to women taking prenatal examinations. In short, modern midwives were beginning to take a modest but noticeable part in childbirths in major cities with modern midwifery training programs and health stations.

To sum up, a major innovation in this era was the development of the visiting public health nurse as the point person in the extension of preventive health care and public medicine into rural China. This was a Chinese-led development of nursing service to meet Chinese health care

---

[104] As Nurse Zhou Meiyu points out in her memoirs, because missionary hospital budgets were limited, students worked to pay for their board and lodging, and in effect received an apprentice style of training. Zhang Pengyuan (张朋园) (1992), 27–28.

[105] Rockefeller archive, RG 1, series 601, box 3, folder 27, "Initial year of the Medical Education Program," by C. K. Chu. According to Nurse Zhou, in the mid 1930s the majority of nursing students were from lower middle schools. Zhang Pengyuan (1992), 28.

[106] H. H. Huang, M. D. and T. H. Wang, M. D. (1936), 554–561; W. W. Yung, M. D. (1936), 562–572.

conditions. Even if nursing education still remained primarily in the hands of mission hospitals, a big future for nursing lay in community settings. This was a breakthrough in China's public health policy. The advancement of midwifery was by contrast a much slower and more arduous process. Thousands of young women and millions more children would continue dying in childbirth or from early childhood diseases before the obstacles to maternal child health could be faced head on.

The National Health Administration's Summary of Public Health Results during the Nanjing Era 1928–1937

On August 3, 1937, while Chinese and Japanese armies mobilized for the battle of Shanghai, a Chinese delegation arrived in Bandung to join a Conference of Far Eastern Countries on Rural Hygiene. The delegation contained most of the country's top public health leaders, but its rural expertise favored the Jiangxi program, not Dingxian's. The delegates brought a Conference report reviewing China's public health work since 1928.[107]

The report acknowledged difficulties due to poverty and illiteracy in rural China, but noted that League of Nations advisors helped introduce rural health services in nine provinces. The most significant developments occurred in Jiangxi, where there were now over two hundred rural health units. The report insisted, without giving details, that these work centers showed how modern medicine was penetrating the masses and taking root. As this claim contrasts with Dr. Stampar's assessment, one

---

[107] Members included 1) Dr. Liu Ruiheng; 2) Dr. Jin Baoshan, Delegation President; 3) Dr. Wu Liande, Director, National Quarantine Service; 4) Dr. Zhu Zhanggeng, Secretary, Commission on Medical Education; 5) Dr. Leonard S. Xu (Xu Shilian 许仕廉), Councilor, Ministry of Industry, Professor, Yanjing University; 6) Professor Wu Xian (吴宪), PUMC; 7) Dr. Zhang Fuliang (张福良), Rural Reconstruction Expert, Director, Jiangxi Rural Health Center; 8) Dr. Xu, head of Rural Health Center, Jiangning county, Jiangsu province; 9) Mr. M. Tao, Sanitary Engineer, CFHS. See League of Nations Health Organization (1937a). (copy seen in Library of New York Academy of Medicine).

Note: Dr. Xu Shilian was a widely published sociologist, at one time Dean of Yanjing University's College of Social Sciences, member of the Executive Yuan's Rural Reconstruction Commission, and Vice Director of the Bureau of Rural Reconstruction of the National Economic Council and co-author with Y. S. Djang (Zhang Yuanshan 章元善) of Rural Reconstruction Experiments in China. Dr. Wu Xian was Professor of Biochemistry at Peking Union Medical College, author of General Treatise on Nutrition (1929), and co-developer of the Folin-Wu method of blood analysis. For Dr. Xu see China Weekly Review (1936), 98; For Dr. Wu see ibid., 261, and John Z. Bowers (1972), 98–99.

must assume that political pressure influenced it. Vital statistics, collected by police, did not include village level data, thus the estimates were the usual: crude birth rate 30/1,000, crude death rate 25/1,000 (but also given as 30/1,000), infant death rate 200/1,000, maternal death rate 10/1,000.[108] Given the government's military and ideological investment in Jiangxi, advocacy of the Jiangxi program is understandable. But in view of Dr. Liu's personal support of the Dingxian program, it is ironic that this project, led by his own former students and colleagues, was not represented and only briefly mentioned.

The standout finding was that forty-five percent of children died before the age of five. This number could not be documented. It is twice as bad as the child mortality rate reported in rural Yugoslavia, although an improvement on a 1930 estimate by Dr. Wu Liande that half of China's children died before the age of one.[109] Even so it signals the precarious child life environment of rural China and the extraordinary problems that the reformers and the Chinese people faced. The report blamed "old style" practitioners and midwives and deplored that farmers were willing to pay heavily for drugs while balking at ten cents for a smallpox vaccination. Since public funds were minimal, the key to any change in rural health had to lie in public education and preventive measures. Home visits on a grand scale were economically unfeasible, but nurses were beginning to penetrate schools. The report blamed natural calamities and local and international politics for lack of progress.

On sanitary improvements the NHA had to rely on surveys done in its model Jiangning County, where seventy-four percent of the county's village population relied on contaminated pond water. Stool examinations of 1,000 primary school children showed 72.5 percent ascaris (蛔虫) infection, 25 percent hookworm (钩虫) infection, and 78 percent total helminth (蠕虫) infestation. Data on diseases in rural areas was limited to those listed by the Conference conveners. The report did not discuss such prevalent diseases in rural China as cholera, dysentery, smallpox, tuberculosis or syphilis. It noted that ninety-five percent of malaria occurred in rural districts, because the anopheles larvae (虐蚊属幼虫) bred well in rice fields. On tuberculosis and pneumonia the authorities lacked comprehensive information. Finally, China had 3.99 million registered opium

---

[108] The 200 per 1,000 infant mortality rate was favored by Dr. Huang Tsefang, who estimated a rate of 100 or less in Western countries. See Lamson (1935), 269.

[109] Cited by Lamson (1935), 272.

smokers, for whom nine hundred and sixty-four anti-opium hospitals and two hundred and ninety-nine other anti-opium institutions offered treatment. But many addicts evaded hospitalization.

The report, drawn up by Dr. Liu Ruiheng, does its best to put a positive spin on a spotty record. Owing to the absence of representatives from Dingxian or Zouping, it did not get into mass education although acknowledging that mass education was an essential platform for rural health reform. Nor is there any significant discussion of the work of visiting nurses. The report does identify the huge problems in rural maternal child health, noting that these included the inferior status of women and that farmers undervalued children. The surprisingly modest discussion of sanitary work tells us that modern management of rural human waste remained outside the scope of what could be accomplished, leaving rural (and urban) people still at the mercy of intestinal epidemics. The central government's insistence on turning Jiangxi into a model of rural health reform deflected attention from other provinces with greater potential for economic output, or other priorities—such as vaccination—with greater potential for saving lives.[110] The work of public health training, which Dr. Liu and his colleagues vigorously pursued, gets little attention, suggesting that the conference conveners (or Nationalist government superiors) were less concerned about this initiative. Thus the report does not reflect some good points in rural health reform in China during the 1930s while it does expose many of its limitations.

Conclusion: How the National Health Administration Made a Difference during the Nanjing Era, 1928–1937

Any attempt at objective appraisal of Nationalist government health policy during the Nanjing decade must begin by recognizing that health policy was the poor cousin among Nationalist government priorities. It lost ministerial status after only two years. Its budget was miniscule and it lacked significant patronage. The Nationalist central leadership's obsession with military and ideological priorities left little room for public health leaders

---

[110] According to the 1937 report to the League of Nations, the number of county health centers in 1936 was as follows: Jiangxi led with 81, then came Shaanxi with 9, Fujian 8, Hunan 6, Gansu 5, Shandong 4, Anhui and Yunnan 3, and Hebei 1 public and 1 private. Jiangsu had 44 county hospitals, Zhejiang 12 and Guangxi 5. No data was listed for Henan, Hubei, Shanxi, Sichuan, Guangdong, or Guizhou.

to do a cost benefit analysis of health initiatives. The alignment of the powerful CC Clique and other Nationalist party leaders with Chinese medicine practitioners left the public healthcare leaders out in left field, while the Central Military Commission's prevarication over opium politics made the public health leaders on the Opium Suppression Commission look like window dressing. Guomindang party priorities required the NHA leaders to focus their rural health initiatives in Jiangxi province, where biomedical practitioners and public awareness of infection were very thin on the ground, even in the provincial capital, and where results would at best be modest.

China's epidemiological status in the 1930s was another problem for the health reformers. The slow but sure transition away from high infection and high mortality—characteristic signs of pre-modernity—had not yet begun in China. Tuberculosis, cholera, plague, smallpox and typhus, which were disappearing rapidly, if not already history, in Europe, North America and Japan, were still rampant or smoldering in China. Malaria, dysentery, syphilis, gonorrhea, hookworm disease, trachoma and neonatal tetanus flourished, compromising the health of millions of children and adults. Even such top administrators as Japan's Goto Shimpei, who saw the relevance of health policy, could well have blanched if confronted with the unrelenting problems that China's public health reformers faced.

A third factor was the lack of institutional groundwork available to the health reformers. How happy they would have been to inherit the palliative institutions, the trained personnel, the data collecting capacity, available in India in the 1930s. While India was developing these capacities in the late 19th and early 20th centuries, China was caught up in revolution, warfare and militarism. To be sure, modernization, including health improvement, was on the agenda of idealists and party political entities in Nationalist China, but through the 1930s militarists held the cards and set the priorities.

Yet Nationalist China's public healthcare reformers did make some significant advances. They established a National Health Administration that stood its ground and stayed in business. Realizing that public health needed personnel who could not be produced by existing medical or teacher colleges, they set up ways of training public health personnel. They established the case for having a public health visiting nurse as rural health point person and started training hundreds of visiting nurses. They set up a functioning national quarantine service. They established experimental model rural health centers and began the process of building a public healthcare system centered on the county as primary managerial unit. They responded to emergencies such as the Yangzi floods of 1931 and did as much as they could to promote and support efforts to train modern midwives.

None of this was enough to demonstrate modernity: the latter would have required a significant retreat by communicable diseases and significant decline in excess mortality. But the NHA did begin to demonstrate what form modernity would take in its health policy aspects. For the first time a visiting nurse, a woman, visited schools, weighed children, vaccinated them against smallpox, checked their eyes for trachoma, checked the latrines for parasites, visited homes and taught some basic health habits. This was a vital development in undermining the world in which disease was determined by gods and demons. That world was still flourishing in the heartland of Nationalist China in the 1930s and would continue to do so in the 1940s. But little though they knew it, the gods and demons were being slowly undermined by an agency more persistent than Chinese or Japanese military forces. That agency, staffed by young women, was the emerging rural public healthcare system. In the next chapter we will see how this process was initiated by the Red Army and in chapters 6 and 7 how it developed during the War of Resistance against Japan.

CHAPTER THREE

RED ARMY HEALTH SERVICES IN JIANGXI
AND ON THE LONG MARCH, 1927–1936

*The way to consolidate these bases is, first, to construct adequate defenses,
second, to store sufficient grain and, third, to set up comparatively good
Red Army hospitals. The Party in the border area must strive to perform
these three tasks effectively.*

—Mao Zedong, October 1928[1]

This chapter examines the Red Army healthcare practices that took shape
in Jiangxi in the largest of the early Chinese Communist base areas, and
during the Long March. Although the Jiangxi base area was tiny compared
with the areas for which the Nationalist government's National Health
Administration was responsible, its problems were comparable to those
of the much larger NHA areas. They included epidemic diseases, malnutrition, lack of hygiene and sanitation, reliance on gods for relief from disease, lack of biomedically trained individuals, and policies often adverse
to the welfare of soldiers and ordinary people.

There were some stark differences however. Red Army commanders and healthcare leaders were forced by their small numbers and
precarious circumstances to learn the importance of preserving lives.
Five campaigns with Nationalist armies put a premium on treating and
returning soldiers to the front, which worked until the fifth Nationalist
encirclement campaign overwhelmed the Communists. The Red Army
mobilized Chinese medicine physicians and pharmacists and enlisted
individuals trained in Christian medical schools and mission hospitals,
and others who had received medical training in Moscow, to develop
highly mobile medical and preventive health delivery systems. It also
managed to organize workshops to supply medical and herbal products,
and created training programs for physicians and health care aides. Under
the guidance of Dr. He Cheng (贺诚) Jiangxi base area leaders even sponsored an ambitious public health drive in 1933–1934. Unfortunately many

---

[1] The original text is: 巩固此根据地的方法: 第一，修筑完备的工事; 第二，储备
充足的粮食; 第三，建设较好的红军医院. 把这三件事切实做好，是边界党应该
努力的. From "Why is it that Red Political Power can Exist in China," Collected Works,
volume 1, (Peking: Foreign Languages Press, 1965), 70.

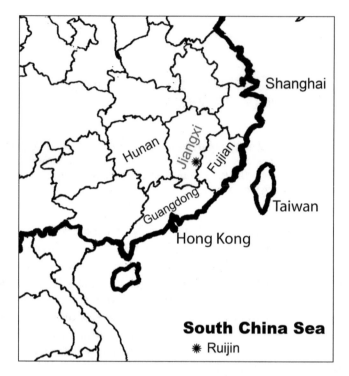

Map 3.1: *Jiangxi Province, Southeast China*
The mountainous and malaria-ridden province of Jiangxi was the main arena in
which the early Chinese Communist revolutionaries learned how to survive and
attract support. They trained military medical aides to help minimize casualties
while improving civilian hygiene to maximize healthcare. Their main base area
was in southeast Jiangxi Province around Ruijin. Chiang Kaishek's huge Fifth
Encirclement Campaign put an end to the Jiangxi Soviet causing the start of the
Long March in October 1934. (*Source*: J.R. and A.S. Watt.)

of these achievements were lost when the Red Army was forced to escape
Jiangxi and undertake the 12 to 24 month Long March starting in October 1934. Thus this chapter will examine the innovations in healthcare
undertaken by Red Army leaders in Jiangxi and the problems that they
encountered.

Creating Healthcare under the Stress of Civil War, 1927–1930

The civil war between China's Nationalist and Communist forces began
with the white terror launched by Chiang Kaishek (蔣介石) in Shanghai
in April 1927. That purge was followed by a campaign of terror through

the Hunan and Jiangxi countryside and as far south as Guangzhou.[2] Communist forces that had just fought with Nationalists on the Northern Expedition under Chiang's leadership were caught unawares. Agnes Smedley reported that Zhu De (朱德) was so staggered by news of the Shanghai massacre that he couldn't even think.[3]

In August Communist leaders responded with an agrarian uprising. It began with the temporary capture of Nanchang (capital of Jiangxi province), but after a few days the Communist forces retreated towards southeast Guangdong and reached Ruijin in southeast Jiangxi, where a four-day battle cost hundreds of dead and around a thousand wounded, including three hundred troops under Zhu De's command.[4] The battered force turned east towards Tingzhou in southwest Fujian, where relief awaited in a formerly British Baptist hospital directed by Dr. Fu Lianzhang (傅连暲 Nelson Fu). Fu turned his hospital into a temporary military medical center and took in around three hundred wounded soldiers. Among his patients were the later military leader Chen Geng (陈赓), who had a severe leg wound, and Xu Teli (徐特立), Mao's teacher.[5]

The Red Army then crossed into eastern Guangdong province and attacked the port city of Shantou, where its main force was shattered. Zhu De's rearguard troops suffered 1,500 casualties, while "hundreds" of peasants were killed or wounded.[6] Autumn harvest uprisings met with no better fate, and this led Mao Zedong to retreat to a base area in

---

[2] In an attempt to quantify the slaughter, Su Kaiming (1985), 129, states that: "As many as 380,000 Communists and their supporters were massacred." Many accounts of the terror rely on orders of magnitude or euphemisms, such as "many" or "thousands." A more detailed analysis of incomplete data, published on-line in 2011, concludes that between April 1927 and the first half of 1928, up to 310,000 people, consisting of CCP and left wing Guomindang party members, democratic scholars and innocent masses caught in the maelstrom, were eliminated. See 1927 *nian dageming shibai hou de da tusha he zhanshou*, 年大革命失败后的大屠杀和斩首 (1927 massacres and decapitations following the failure of the great revolution in 1927). That this involved "massacres" is indicated by the decapitations, which judging from photographs were gruesome. See www.360doc.com/content/11/1108/22/1241083_162918954.shtml.

[3] Smedley (1956), 192.

[4] The figures are from Smedley (1956), 205. A Chinese source states that the losses were "very numerous" (shen zhong 甚众). See Zhang Ruguang, Guo Fangfu, He Manqiu (1989), 3.

[5] Feng Caizhang, Li Baoding (1991), 71, biography of Fu Lianzhang. See also Howard L. Borman (1967), vol. I, 190–192, biography of Chen Geng. It was Chen's good fortune that Dr. Fu decided against amputation. The figure of three hundred patients comes from Zhang Ruguang (1989), 9.

[6] Smedley (1956), 208–209. C. Martin Wilbur (1983), 149.

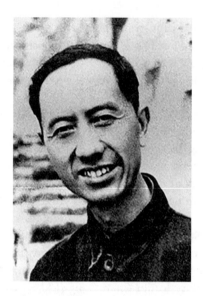

Photograph 3.1: *Dr. Fu Lianzhang*
Trained in a British missionary hospital, he provided hospital care for Zhu De's
wounded soldiers in 1928 and was an early Red Army medical leader. He treated
Mao Zedong for malaria, enabling him to travel on the Long March. (*Source*: Syndey
Today, http://www.sydneytoday.com/content/143380)

the Jinggangshan Mountain region of southwest Jiangxi. An uprising in
Guangzhou in December 1927 was another disaster, but a positive outcome was to bring Dr. He Cheng into the world of Red Army healthcare.
By then, according to Smedley, Zhu De was convinced that his forces
would be "destroyed by further fighting."[7]

In those days Red Army health units could only do simple remedial
work, and medical aides were liable to abscond. Because of lack of medical staff, provisions and clothing, as well as the harried campaigning,
troops suffered from malaria, dysentery, and leg ulcers (a consequence of
poor nutrition) as well as war wounds. They were often icy cold and had
to be bedded in peasant dwellings or left to die on the road. Mao Zedong,
Zhu De and Chen Yi (陈毅) were very concerned about these conditions.[8]
Mao's forces arrived in Jinggangshan with thirty soldiers badly wounded

---

[7] Smedley (1956), 216–225; Rue (1966), 73–90, differs in several respects from the
Smedley account. Zhang Ruguang (1989), 4–5, lists uprisings in Hunan, Hubei, Guangdong,
Jiangxi, Shaanxi and Guangxi and counts over one hundred uprisings in all.
[8] Zhang (1989), 5–10.

and one hundred or more with malaria. They needed hospitalization. At the time, according to a participant, the region possessed one Chinese medicine doctor and one pharmacist. Consequently several soldiers died who might have been cured, including a trusted commander.[9]

After forming a base area in Ninggang, Mao's forces set up a hospital-clinic in October 1927 in an old Confucian academy building. This became the Red Army's first hospital. The hospital had four doctors, twelve trained nurses and ten or more bearers and could accommodate forty to fifty patients. As equipment and medicines were marginal, the hospital relied on local herbs and home remedies.[10]

When Zhu De's depleted forces arrived in Jinggangshan in April 1928, he and Mao began to develop strategies for more quickly removing the wounded from battlefields so that less lives would be lost. They decided to create a rear base hospital in the central Jinggangshan region. Its second director, Dr. Duan Zhizhong (段治忠), had served in a Nationalist army division but was wounded and captured and threw in his lot with the Red Army. This hospital, set up in summer 1928, had four administrative divisions, two for lightly wounded, one for cadres under Dr. Wu Huiguo (伍辉国, a woman doctor), and one for severe cases directly under Dr. Duan and two other physicians. The hospital had a clinic, pharmacy and wards for patients, and a staff of over ten physicians and twenty or more nurses. In autumn 1928 Mao proposed the addition of a "comparatively good hospital" (*tiaojian jiaohao de yiyuan* 条件较好的医院) for sick and wounded civilians. The plan called for four buildings capable of housing 1,000 patients. One building was ready by January 1929 and was named "Red Shining Hospital."[11] The hospital used Chinese herbs to treat internal diseases.[12]

Unfortunately Red Army health units lacked medications and medical equipment, and several party agents seeking drugs were captured and killed. For example, for lack of saline solutions, wounds were cleansed with liquids from Coptis root (黄连 *huanglian* Chinese goldthread, an anti-inflammatory drug) or Honeysuckle flower (金银花 *jinyinhua*, an

---

[9] Feng and Li (1991), 43 (biography of Zhang Lingbin 张令彬); Whitson states that Mao arrived in Sanwan, (Yongxin County) with around seven hundred survivors, most of them with malaria. Whitson (1973), 28.

[10] "Jinggangshan Hongjun Yiyuan Yiwen" (2008) Mao's living quarters are reported in Zhang (1989), 10.

[11] "Jinggangshan Hongjun Yiyuan Yiwen," (2008); more detailed sources as in note 13.

[12] Fan Pu (樊圃) (1988), 134. This source notes that Western trained doctors handled surgical cases.

antibacterial drug). Pig lard was used in place of Vaseline, boric acid in place
of disinfectants, and opium in place of anesthetics. As herbs flourished on
Jinggangshan, Chinese medicine doctors organized teams of local people
to help collect them.[13] Simple items of equipment (e.g. tweezers, bedpans)
were fashioned out of bamboo or wood. Surgeons made use if necessary
of wood saws, clothes needles and pig-killing knives. Due to limited ward
space, many patients were farmed out to families with sheds or animal
stalls and slept on the floor or on plank beds.[14]

In June 1928, the Mao-Zhu forces attacked surrounding counties to
mobilize supplies and gain new adherents. In response Chiang Kaishek
assembled 40,000 soldiers to blockade the Jinggangshan area. Fighting
went back and forth during the autumn, but by December the defend-
ers were beginning to starve.[15] According to Mao's essay on "Struggle
in the Jinggang Mountains," dated Nov. 28, 1928, many members of the
defending army wore only two layers of thin clothing. Because of combat wounds, malnutrition, exposure to cold and other causes, there were
over eight hundred hospital patients, and the need for medications was
acute.[16] In November, Mao told the Sixth Red Army Congress that: "We
must give special consideration to hospital patients, otherwise this could
affect combat morale," adding: "In medical management of wounded and
sick patients the work of nursing aides is very important."[17]

In mid-December 1928 the tenacious new Red Army leader Peng Dehuai
(彭德怀) fought his way through the Nationalist blockade with one
thousand men. Peng had no prior relationship with Mao or Zhu.[18] It was
decided to leave him on the mountain with fifteen hundred men guarding
the sick and wounded while, in January 1929, the main Red Army force
under Mao and Zhu left Jinggangshan, broke through the encirclement,
drew off the enemy, and set up a new base area in southern Jiangxi and
Western Fujian.[19] Once the main Red Army was gone the Nationalist forces

---

[13] Information about drugs is from another on-line article also entitled "Jinggangshan
Hongjun Yiyuan Yiwen." It has much the same text as the previous article cited in note
11 but includes information on drugs not in the previous citation. From http://qkzz.net/
article/7b7e08e4-8be1-43c7-9855-47f79b0e646f.htm.

[14] "Jinggangshan Hongjun Yiyuan Yiwen," (Zhongguo Ji'an web). Information about surgery is from Zhang (1989), 14.

[15] Smedley (1956), 233–235.

[16] Selected Works of Mao Tse-tung, volume 1, 82–83.

[17] Zhang (1989, 15).

[18] Whitson (1973, 32).

[19] i) Smedley (1956), 235–236; ii) Rue (1966), 138; iii) "Jinggangshan Hongjun Yiyuan
Yiwen," (Zhongguo Ji'an web). In a study focusing on healthcare it is not possible to go into

attacked. At least one hundred sick and wounded fighters were captured and questioned as to where the main Red Army had gone and where it had hidden its grain supplies and munitions. When torture yielded no answers, the victims were killed.[20] Mao's comparatively good hospital and the abandoned army barracks were burned.[21]

This disaster proved again that guerrillas needed healthcare adapted to the mobile conditions of guerrilla warfare. In line with Mao's advice, trained teenage nursing aides took care of sick and wounded patients by washing, feeding and hydrating them, dealing with bodily wastes, and bringing problems to the attention of a physician when and if available. In December 1928, after Peng Dehuai's Fifth Army arrived at Jinggangshan, almost all military units set up training courses of varying sizes for nursing aides. Graduates of these courses filled positions in army healthcare units.[22]

Between January 1929 and June 1930 the Mao-Zhu forces set up a small hospital at Donggu and distributed several hundred patients in nearby villages, who were visited by roving health aides. Late in June 1929 Mao came down with a serious case of malaria; he was treated with herbal remedies and looked after by local villagers.[23] As there were no enemy pursuers, the army stayed one month so that its soldiers could bathe, wash clothes, delouse, and deal with frostbite and foot injuries. At this point the army had two biomedical and several Chinese medicine doctors and nurses on its staff. In Fujian the army set up two small hospitals, mobilized local youth as nursing aides, and hired local physicians to treat patients. In November 1929 the hospital moved with the army units but most of the nursing aides were killed in action, leaving only a skeletal staff.[24]

---

the reasons why the Mao-Zhu force should have left so soon after Peng arrived, leaving so many of their soldiers under the care and protection of his limited force. Differences in command priorities between Mao and Peng, as pointed out by Whitson, would suggest that in an emergency Peng would not allow himself to be encumbered with liabilities left behind by Mao. See Whitson (1973), 32–33.

[20] "Jinggangshan Hongjun Yiyuan Yiwen," both sources as in note 13; Smedley (1956), 252–3. The disaster was the consummation of this early encirclement campaign.

[21] Smedley (1956), 252. The numbers of casualties are unclear. Smedley reports that some 6,000 "beleaguered revolutionaries" were slowly dying in their hospital and barracks from starvation, of whom a few crawled away but were hunted down; some seven hundred people survived under the leadership of Peng Dehuai. Zhang reports that the losses were "very great." (Zhang 1989, 21). In an earlier book Smedley reported that the attackers discovered the Red Army arsenal and smashed it. Smedley (1934), 117.

[22] Zhang (1989), 15.

[23] Information on Mao's illness is from Liao Haoping (廖皓平) (2009).

[24] Zhang (1989), 16–17.

At the Gutian conference in January 1930, though political struggles took priority, the conference did affirm that healthcare was an important part of the Red Army's mission. Relations between officers and men, and between medical units and the wounded, must be based on the idea of a revolutionary army and emphasize care for wounded soldiers and commitment to class ties.[25] In short, healthcare required a strategic vision.

One can see the impact of the Gutian conference in the evolution of Peng Dehuai's army health units. After the capture of Da'ye and the formation of the Third Army corps, five medical staff from a Methodist Universal Love hospital (普爱医院) in Da'ye joined the Third Army corps and were welcomed by Peng. Their leader, He Fusheng (何复生 1902–1934) was an underground party member who held long discussions with his colleagues about world politics and China's civil war.[26] The Da'ye Universal Love hospital was run by Dr. Wang Ruiting (王瑞亭), a Chinese Christian and follower of Gandhi, who believed in nonviolence. Under his leadership the hospital treated landlord soldiers openly and Red Army soldiers surreptitiously.

Inspired by Dr. He, his colleagues joined the Red Army. They organized an army hospital, with He as director, to do cleaning of wounds, extraction of bullets, and amputations. The hospital developed an eight-month course for medical aides. Because of constant fighting, severely wounded and sick soldiers were left with volunteers—mainly women—selected from the local Communist Youth League. The women washed soldiers' bodies, took care of medications and food, and disposed bodily wastes. The local government supplied stretcher-bearers and hospital aides.[27]

A more ominous consequence of the Gutian conference was to require Red Armies to engage in more urban insurrection.[28] To prepare for this assignment the First Army Corps set up a small healthcare department, which organized a temporary hospital for reception and transfer of sick and wounded soldiers. Each army had a medical department, and each regimental column had a fairly well staffed healthcare unit with

---

[25] Rue (1966), 178–188; Zhang (1989), 17–18.

[26] A native of Jiangsu and a Communist Party member since 1926, Dr. He joined the Universal Love Hospital in 1927 and the Red Army in 1930. A tireless worker and educator, he was awarded a Red Star medal by the Communist government in 1933, but was killed in 1934 during the fifth Suppression campaign while on front line duty. See He Fusheng biography at http://szb.zhenjiang.gov.cn/htmA/fangzhi/zj/i65.htm.

[27] For information on the Universal Love hospital and He Fusheng and his coworkers, see Feng and Li (1991), biography of Rao Zhengxi, 17–18.

[28] Rue (1966), 211–213; Smedley (1956), 273–276.

biomedical and Chinese medicine officers, as well as health aides and stretcher-bearers.[29] Two base hospitals were available at Donggu in south central Jiangxi and Jiaoyang in southwest Fujian. In 1931 one of the hospitals enlisted seventeen students in a training program in Chinese medicine. Local government helped with the needs of these hospitals.[30]

These healthcare arrangements were upstaged by Central Committee orders from Shanghai to carry out coordinated attacks on Changsha, Nanchang, and Wuhan.[31] Peng Dehuai's Third Army Corps captured Changsha on July 29, 1930, but had to abandon it five days later. The Mao-Zhu First Army Corps failed to capture Nanchang but linked up with Peng's forces for a second attack on Changsha, which also failed, with severe loss of life.[32] At that point Mao and Zhu abandoned the Central Committee plan and led their weakened forces back to Ji'an in central Jiangxi.

After they arrived, Mao wasted no time looking for a medical leader. He heard from an army commander of the work of Dr. Dai Jimin (戴济民; his acquired name means "saves people"). A devout Christian, Dr. Dai spent ten years as a work-study student at a Christian hospital school in Hankou. During and after the 1911 revolution he served with Chinese Red Cross units, but for reasons of health he preferred to live in a country town.[33] Mao brought a delegation of party leaders to visit Dr. Dai. They discussed the medical needs of the Red Army and the medical aspects of "revolutionary humanism" (*geming de rendaozhuyi* 革命的人道主义). Dai agreed to help them. He converted his clinic into a base hospital named the Workers and Peasants Revolutionary Red Hospital (*gong-nong geming hongse yiyuan* 工农革命红色医院), and rounded up seven western trained doctors, several Chinese medicine doctors and teams of

---

[29] According to Rue (212), the First Army Corps consolidated the Third, Fourth, Twelfth, Twentieth, Twenty-first and Thirty-fifth Armies. Zhang (1989) (19) states that according to a central (party) directive of June 1930, the Fourth, Sixth and Twelfth Armies were combined to form the First Army Corps, with a combined force of 15,000 plus men.

[30] Zhang (1989), 19–21.

[31] Whitson's analysis of the warlord, Russian revolutionary, and peasant-bandit military models accessible to the Red Army leadership helps to clarify why Red Army leaders, such as Peng Dehuai and even Zhu De, were willing to keep on attacking cities despite the inevitable losses in human life incurred. Mao's advocacy of peasant guerilla warfare was far from dominant at this time. The models are described in Whitson (1973), 7–23; their implications are discussed in Whitson's accounts of specific campaigns.

[32] The Mao-Zhu First Army Corps was raked by artillery fire while attacking Nanchang, and lost another 3,000 men during the second assault on Changsha. See Smedley (1956), 274–280, 285–286; the Changsha figure comes from Zhang (1989), 34. Losses by other Communist army units were equally severe.

[33] Feng and Li (1991), 341.

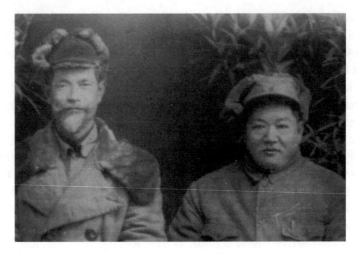

Photograph 3.2: *Dr. Dai Jimin*

Dr. Dai Jimin (left) and General Luo Binghui in Shandong Province in 1946. Dr. Dai Jimin was an ardent Christian and Communist party member, pulled together hospital services to treat Red Army soldiers wounded during 1930 uprisings and became a hospital director. Agreed with Mao Zedong on revolutionary humanism. (*Source*: http://www.luobinghui.com/Article/xwzx/bhzh/200508/4239.html)

nursing aides and stretcher-bearers. They formed into four groups for treating around eight hundred heavily and lightly wounded soldiers, and six hundred patients with leg ulcers and contagious diseases (principally dysentery, malaria and scabies). Although these numbers imposed heavy workloads, the hospital staff was able in little over a month to return 1,000 recuperated patients to their army units. For this achievement Dr. Dai was named one of the "four great golden guardians" (四大金刚 si da jin gang) of the Red Army medical world.[34]

*Healthcare during the First Two Encirclement
and Suppression Campaigns, 1930–1931*

The Mao-Zhu forces now had an army of 40,000[35] to face a Nationalist campaign with 100,000 troops ordered to eliminate Communists from

---

[34] The other three were Fu Lianzhang (傅连暲), Li Zhi (李治), and Chen Yihou (陈义厚). Information is principally from Zhang (1989), 35–36 (based on a personal memoir by Dai Jimin published in 1979); and Feng and Li (1991), 342, 346. There are several documents on line with information about Dr. Dai, Luo Pinghui, and Dr. Li Zhi.

[35] Whitson (1973, 268) estimates that probably "fewer than 25,000" were armed.

Jiangxi province. A short while before occupying Ji'an the Red Armies reorganized the First and Third Army Corps into a First Front Army under the political command of Mao Zedong and military command of Zhu De.[36] Each army corps had a healthcare office. Dr. Duan Zhizhong headed the First Army Corps health office. The regiments had health offices and a rear area hospital, and the medical units nearer the front were strengthened. Hospitals were in Jinggangshan, Donggu (south Jiangxi), Jiaoyang, Caixi, and Longyan (west Fujian). During autumn 1930 Peng Dehuai's Third Army Corps medical office, headed by Dr. He Fusheng, organized training for up to one hundred doctors and several hundred nursing aides and medical orderlies. Dr. He lectured and directed student fieldwork.[37]

The campaign lasted from November 1930 to March 1931. The Mao-Zhu forces carried out a strategic withdrawal, taking with them Dr. Dai's revolutionary base hospital, which regrouped at Futian, near Donggu.[38] Underestimating the danger of the Mao-Zhu forces the Nationalist field commander, Zhang Huizan, led his forces into an ambush. In four hours they were overwhelmed and Zhang was captured, along with large quantities of guns, food, cash and medical supplies. Four days later Peng Dehuai's forces routed a second Nationalist division. The remaining Nationalist forces withdrew, ending the campaign.[39]

To prepare for the campaign Red Army healthcare staff readied two hospitals at Donggu and Chaling as branch rear hospitals and located two field hospitals near Longgang which were responsible for initial treatment and transfer of patients to the rear. These placements depended on the strategy of luring the enemy into the Longgang Mountain defile. Provision of

---

[36] Rue (1966), 217–218. As Rue notes, in the process of opposing the Li Lisan line Mao and Zhu went up against most of the political commissars in the armies over which Mao "was extending his control." But by doing so "he preserved the Red Army's ability to fight again." Mao's interest in Dr. Dai formed part of that larger strategy. Mao was also advancing the strategy of concentration of troops (under his and Zhu's authority), later articulated in his essay on "Strategy in China's Revolutionary War," Selected Works, volume 1, 179–254.

[37] Zhang (1989), 37–38; He Fusheng biography (note 26). The sources have no data on the kind or length of training. The numbers of trainees appear on the large side, but this may indicate that the training was short term. Both sources agree on these numbers. According to his biography, Dr. He was willing to operate day and night and find the medications to treat his patients. In 1933 he received a Red Star medal for his medical work.

[38] Hospital information from Feng and Li (1991), Dai Jimin biography, 342.

[39] Smedley (1956), 285–290, provides a much more detailed account of this campaign. Lessons learned from the campaign are described in Mao's essay on "Strategy in China's Revolutionary War." For general accounts see Whitson (1973), 270; Dreyer (1995), 160–162; and Wei Hongyun (1986), 359–361. The denouement of Mao's conflict with the A–B Corps leadership is discussed in Rue (1966), 231–237.

supplies, nurses, bearers and transportation was assigned to the Southwest Jiangxi workers and farmers people's government.

Such planning demonstrates that Red Army healthcare leaders hoped to avoid the disasters suffered during the retreat from Changsha and were quite successful in their effort.[40] Red Armies captured Zhang's headquarters and destroyed two regiments at a cost of around two hundred casualties, including around thirty-one deaths. The combat units set up first aid and triage stations to rewrap bandages and stabilize fractures before sending casualties across the mountains to the field hospitals, where they were further treated before being sent on to the rear hospital at Chaling. This hospital was spread in homes and temples around a few small villages and hamlets. It had three doctors and eleven nursing aides. The staff had protocols for division of labor and treatment of fractures and care of patients, including changing of dressings and administration of pain relief. The doctors used operations and patient care as a means to train thirty local teenage boys and girls as nursing aides. These actions kept total campaign casualties down to around two hundred and ninety-five and deaths to around sixty-six; they helped compensate for the lack of medical aides[41] and enabled a small fighting force to oppose much larger Nationalist forces.

Undeterred by this defeat the Nationalists assembled 200,000 troops under command of the Minister of War, General He Yingqin (何应钦), and launched a second campaign in April 1931. The armies approached the Central Jiangxi Communist stronghold from four different directions. Although achieving a greater degree of encirclement than the previous campaign, the Nationalist armies were of unequal quality. The Red Army forces moved under cover to the Donggu area, which was the target of the Nationalist Fifth Route Army. After a nerve-wracking wait the Red Army units attacked and disarmed two Fifth Route Army divisions from the rear and then attacked and disarmed most of its remaining two divisions. Some units of the Nationalist 26th Route Army surrendered without firing a shot; the 56th division in Jianning fled precipitately and was cut to pieces by Peng Dehuai's Third Army while crossing the Min River.[42]

---

[40] Zhang (1989), 44–45. This study provides battlefield maps that locate the placement of the medical units.

[41] Zhang (1989), 46–47. The authors note that the statistical data are based on incomplete reports.

[42] Smedley (1956), 295–303; Dreyer (1995), 162–165; Mao Zedong (1936), 227–228; Zhang (1989), 49–50; Wei (1986), 361–362. Both Zhang and Wei identify April 1 as the starting date for the second campaign.

This campaign had a significant impact on civilians. Although large areas of central Jiangxi came under Communist control, the fighting "brought sorrow to thousands of peasant homes" (Zhu De's words as reported by Smedley). Military brutality to civilians increased, allegedly because Nationalist officers forced soldiers to rape, burn, plunder and murder so they would not dare surrender. Red Army forces bore around 2,600 casualties due to wounds, deaths and disappearance. Local Red Guard units also lost heavily.[43]

To prepare for this campaign branch hospitals were located around Donggu, while the central hospital was moved to Futian, nearer the anticipated battlefield. Dr. Dai Jimin, now a Communist Party member, became its director.[44] Army health units replenished their supplies from materials captured during the first campaign and increased their staff with captured medical personnel. Volunteers from local government reported to hospitals as stretcher-bearers and emergency aides, ready to serve on a standby basis.[45]

These preparations improved battlefield medical work. Rescue teams worked with the goal of not losing a single wounded soldier. Army units opened up front line bandage stations to speed up triage of wounded soldiers. Field hospitals were able to staunch bleeding, extract shrapnel and clean wounds. When Red Army forces moved, field hospitals moved with them but left small teams in reserve to handle existing casualties. Volunteer stretcher-bearers moved wounded soldiers across mountainous terrain from the bandage stations to the field hospitals and thence to the Donggu rear hospitals. The general hospital added a third branch hospital at Donggu to increase capacity to absorb wounded patients. This was necessary to handle around nine hundred and thirty casualties created by the first of four major battles. Once the fighting moved further east from Donggu, the field command added more field hospitals and a transport station to facilitate transfer of wounded to rear hospitals.[46]

After the campaign ended the Red Army's General Front Committee entrusted Chief of Staff Zuo Quan (左权) to secure the safety of the Donggu hospitals. Zuo organized local peasant Red Guard units to suppress hostile

---

[43] Zhang (1989), 53; Smedley (1956), 301. Smedley reports 4,000 Red army casualties, and Zhang's numbers are again qualified as based on incomplete reports, thus the actual number of Red army casualties may lie somewhere between these two estimates.

[44] Feng and Li (1991), 343.
(1991), Dai Jimin biography in Feng and Li (1991), 343.

[45] Zhang (1989), 50–51.

[46] Zhang (1989), 51–54.

landlord militias. Because of a conflict within the rear hospitals with elements of an Anti-Bolshevik clique, Zuo moved most of the patients into other facilities. The General Front Committee sent a large amount of medical supplies captured in Jianning to the rear hospitals in Donggu.[47] Medical staff captured when the Red Army entered Ji'an in October 1930 stayed with the Red Army.

In May 1931 the Central Committee in Shanghai sent three biomedical physicians who were Communist Party members to work in the Jiangxi base areas. They were He Cheng, a graduate of Beijing University Medical college and party member since 1925, who worked underground in Shanghai and Wuhan since leaving the Hailufeng base area; Chen Zhifang (陈志方), a graduate of Number One Zhongshan University Medical College in Guangzhou and party member since 1927, who became director of an army medical bureau; and Peng Zhen (彭真, original name Peng Longbo 龙伯), a party member since 1926 who studied at Nanyang Medical University in Shanghai and also in the Soviet Union.

Red Army medical leaders could now draw on party affiliation as well as medical skill. With the establishment of a general hospital in the Fujian-Jiangxi-Guangdong border region Dr. Luo Huacheng (罗化成), a Chinese medicine doctor and party member since 1927, became director, Zhang Lingbin (张令彬) deputy director, and Peng head of medical affairs.[48]

*Advancement of Healthcare during the Third Encirclement
and Suppression Campaign, July to September 1931*

In June 1931 Chiang Kaishek arrived in Nanchang to take charge of a third campaign. Accounts differ as to how it unfolded. According to Mao, Chiang had 300,000 men, while the Red Army had only 30,000 battle weary troops. The Red Army took evasive action but won several victories, slipped out of sight then reengaged Nationalist forces at

---

[47] Zuo was a graduate of the Whampoa Academy and a valued Red Army staff officer. For a brief biography see Boorman (1967), volume 3, 316.

[48] Dr. Lo was born into a Chinese medicine family and apprenticed with his father. Since 1927 he had worked as a political activist; after being wounded in battle he served as hospital superintendent. Zhang was an orphan from a poor peasant family in Hunan with only marginal education. He proved his mettle as a peasant organizer and army section leader and caught the eye of Mao Zedong. See Zhang (1989), 55–57. Information on Dr. Chen is from http://baike.baidu.com/view/1893240.htm. For Dr. Peng see http://wiki .zupulu.com/doc.php?action=view&docid=3966. For Dr. Lo see http://Baike.baidu.com/ view/919857.html?fromTaglist. For Zhang Lingbin see Feng and Li, (1991), 39–46.

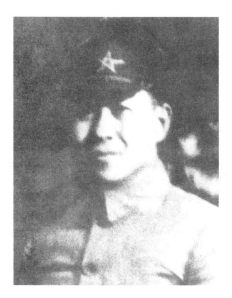

Photograph 3.3: *Dr. He Cheng*
Leading Red Army and civilian health director during Jiangxi period (1930–34), director of a highly successful public health campaign in 1933–1934. Went on the Long March to Yan'an but spent war years (1937–1945) in the Soviet Union and Mongolia. (*Source*: http://tupian.baike.com/a4_11_21_01300000099383121574211906 478_jpg.html)

Gaoxingxi. A two-day battle ended in a stalemate, and the Nationalists got away.[49] On-line Chinese accounts indicate that Nationalist divisions lost over 2,000 wounded and dead while the Red armies lost over 2,200, including two division commanders.[50] Western accounts point out that Nationalist armies continued occupying Communist areas and left only when the Japanese military began seizing northeast China (Manchuria) on September 18, 1931.[51] In the end the Communist forces took over 21 districts with 2.5 million people.

---

[49] Mao Zedong, "Strategy…," 228–230; supplementary details from Zhang (1989), 57–58, and Wei (1986), 362–363.

[50] See, for example, http://www.hsscw.com/newsview.asp?id=144; http://bkso.baidu.com/ view/381103.html?fromTaglist. One account that draws on a Nationalist source notes that the Nationalist commander, Cai Tingkai (蔡廷鍇), reported over 8,000 overall Red Army casualties and the capture of 6,000 guns. Whereas the other accounts of Red Army casualties are admittedly understated by not giving any estimates for the number of losses during the river-crossing battle, the numbers attributed to Cai are almost certainly exaggerated.

[51] Dreyer (1995) 168; Whitson (1973), 272–274.

The extensive battles strained the Red Army's medical relief system. Casualties endured arduous journeys over mountainous terrain while suffering sunstroke, foot injuries, malaria and dysentery. Consequently political teams were organized to boost morale, and local people took in soldiers who were too injured or sick to carry on. Up to ten percent of the force dropped out as a result of casualties, but because of the emphasis on morale a significant number returned to their units. Front line units were instructed to retain lightly wounded casualties for treatment in the field hospitals, while rear hospitals admitted over four thousand patients.[52]

As a result of frequent marching and fighting, and lessons learned from the first two campaigns, Red Army medical units under Mao and Zhu gained valuable experience in rapid removal of casualties to field and rear hospitals. They used trained medical aides for immediate battlefield triage, bearers to carry the wounded back to nursing aides in field stations of a few huts, and finally to rear hospitals, groups of huts with at least a trained doctor. This system was vital to maintaining army morale. The value of reliance on the masses was proved by the willingness of rural people to serve as stretcher-bearers and home care helpers. Treating captives well offered various advantages, including the enlistment of medical personnel with battlefield experience.[53] The Red Army was now assembling healthcare teams combining medical with political skills and biomedicine with Chinese medicine. Typically the biomedical doctors handled the battle casualties and public health work, while the Chinese medicine doctors dealt with disease.

On the downside the Red Army had to deal with around 1,300 deaths and around 1,200 missing, along with ill-equipped hospitals crammed with casualties. There still were not enough trained health workers to keep up with the increasing demands on healthcare imposed by expanded campaigns and larger armed forces, resulting in reliance on hygienically untrained volunteers. The lack of adequate medications, food, and trained personnel, needed to be addressed.

---

[52] Zhang (1989), 60–61. Dai Jimin biography, from Feng and Li (1991) 343. In casualty tabulations, Zhang (1989) gives the numbers of wounded in all five battles as 2,734 on p. 61 and 3,354 on p. 62. In both tables mortalities are listed as 1,319. These reportedly incomplete numbers compare with Dreyer's report of four thousand losses during the two-day battle at Gaoxingxu in September 1931. See Dreyer (1995), 168.

[53] It is unfortunate that Smedley's study of Zhu De lacks any write-up of Zhu's memories of the Third, Fourth and Fifth encirclement and suppression campaigns. Zhu's ability to give eyewitness accounts of what happens on battlefields is missing from more formal studies of this vital era.

Expanding the Scope of Healthcare: Red Army Healthcare School
and Medical Supply Workshops

The Japanese conquest of Manchuria led to a period of respite in Jiangxi, during which the Communist leaders were able to consolidate control over newly acquired districts and develop significant new health services. He Cheng was appointed director of the Red Army's central medical department and Chen Zhifang director of medical affairs. The Japanese-trained doctor Qi Luyu (漆鲁鱼) became director of its health bureau.[54] In December a revolt of the Nationalist 26th Route Army at Ningdu delivered 17,000 soldiers to the Red Army. That army's health services included Chen Yihou (陈义厚), a graduate of the missionary Qilu Medical College in Shandong, who became another of the Red Army's "four great golden guardians"; Ji Pengfei (姬鹏飞), a future foreign minister of China; and eight other much needed physicians. After the 26th Route Army became the Red Army's Fifth Army Corps, Chen Yihou, Ji Pengfei and Liu Ruilin (刘瑞林) took on its top medical positions.[55]

On the civilian front the new base area government set up agencies to make healthcare accessible to 2.5 million people. These agencies worked on control of epidemics and other preventive measures. In due course they established rear hospitals, worker farmer hospitals, hospitals for the masses, poor people clinics, public health clinics, red pharmacies, and health industry cooperatives.[56]

---

[54] Qi Luyu (1902–74) was an orphan who was helped by a kindly uncle. He studied at a private medical college in Chongqing, which soon closed. Qi made his way to Tokyo, studied Japanese and Marxism and spent three years at a special medical college before returning to China in 1928. He joined the Communist Party, did underground work, was arrested but later released, and made his way to the Jiangxi Soviet. At the time of the Long March he stayed behind to take care of the military leader Chen Yi (陈毅), who was badly wounded. In 1935 he was captured by Nationalist forces and again released. Abandoned and friendless, he returned to Sichuan and was reunited with Party units. Information from two online sources: i) http://www.lbx777.com/ywll/r_yzlh/xgzs02.htm; ii) http://www.jjdj.cn/news_show.aspx?id=2465.

[55] Zhang (1989), 84–87. Born to an impoverished landlord family, Ji Pengfei trained at an army medical hospital in Xi'an as a nursing aide and began studying Marxism-Leninism. Through intelligence and industriousness he became an army medical doctor in the service of the Christian warlord Feng Yuxiang and in 1931 was serving in Jiangxi in the 26th Route Army when it transferred its allegiance to the Communist forces. Ji became head of the reportedly well-staffed medical section of the 15th Army. Feng and Li (1991), biography of Ji Pengfei, 12–13.

[56] Information from Gu Xinwei (顾鑫伟) and Liu Shanjiu (刘善玖) (Oct 2006), 807–808.

A long lasting initiative was the creation of an Army Medical School, proposed by He Cheng in November 1931. The Red Army's Central Military Commission accepted the proposal and appointed him Director with responsibility for planning. Chen Zhifang was appointed Dean of Education. The faculty included Peng Zhen and Tang Yizhen (唐义贞), a young woman pharmacologist. The staff advertised for youth who were politically reliable, physically healthy, and with an appropriate standard of literacy. One hundred and fifty applied, of whom nineteen were selected (twenty-five according to several online sources). At the opening ceremony on February 15, 1932, Zhu De noted that the Red Army had expanded but had too few health cadres. "We must train our own army doctors," he declared. "You must study hard to serve our army's officers and men."[57]

The school began with very limited resources. The curriculum was limited to physiology, anatomy and pharmacology. Equipment consisted of one skeleton, a few charts and two microscopes. But practical experience abounded. Before long students were participating in battles, where they learned quickly about management of casualties. They also studied prevention of malaria, dysentery, scabies and leg ulcers. The school moved several times but remained close to the Red Army's general hospital, where Peng Zhen was the Director and the school's Commissar Wang Lizhong (王立中) was hospital Commissar. Several hospital physicians acted as clinical teachers, among them Dr. Li Zhi (李治), another of the Red Army's four great diamond guardians and a graduate of Shanghai's Nanyang Medical College.

After fifteen months of work and study nineteen students graduated. Among them were three who would achieve major positions much later in the PRC. One of them, You Shenghua (游胜华), was singled out by Dr. Norman Bethune as "my most satisfactory surgeon."[58] The school set up classes in medicine, pharmacology and nursing. In October 1932 it changed its name from medical school to Healthcare School (卫生学校), reflecting He Cheng's emphasis on preventive health.[59]

This preventive focus is seen in a Red Army manual for nursing aides completed in June 1933. Sickrooms must be clean and well-aired. The dwelling must be clean, especially the kitchen and latrine and the area outside the sickroom window. Maintaining cleanliness is the duty of

---

[57] Zhang (1989), 94–95; "Changzheng lushang zoulai de hongse yisheng yaolan" (c. 2006).
[58] Reported in Changzheng lushang zoulai (see note 57).
[59] Zhang (1989), 95; Changzheng lushang zoulai.

nursing aides. Food, clothes and patients must be clean. Lightly injured patients can clean themselves, but nursing aides must give seriously injured patients a whole body bath. There are detailed instructions on this, also on how to dispose of bodily wastes and change clothes. Students were taught how to take temperatures, examine breathing and measure the pulse. They learned how to examine excreta, deal with a blocked urethra, administer an enema, and cleanse eyes. They learned that nursing aides are always on duty; if they saw unusual symptoms, they were to inform a doctor. Patients with infectious diseases must be isolated and their clothes washed in boiling water. Students were taught how to guard against digestive disorders and respiratory infections and how to detect and avert suicidal symptoms. Concluding sections dealt with surgical nursing and provision of medications.[60]

In August 1933 the school moved to a location near Ruijin, where it joined with a small medical school begun by Dr. Fu Lianzhang. Chen Yihou took over from Peng Zhen as principal; Wang Bin (王斌), a graduate of Sichuan Special Medical School and just captured from a Nationalist army unit, served as dean. The 13-month curriculum was divided into basic medical sciences, clinical (taught at the Central Hospital in Ruijin) and internship. The school had seven microscopes and an x-ray room. The faculty consisted of five physicians and a foreign language teacher.[61] Training of nursing aides, sanitary aides, pharmacists, and health unit leaders was expanded to five hundred and the number of beds available for bedside teaching to three hundred. Six hundred and seventy students graduated before October 1934. The entire faculty and students went on the Long March; but Dr. Chen stayed behind to lead the remaining health units and was unfortunately killed during a Nationalist army assault.[62]

---

[60] Chen Cheng archive, Stanford University; microfilm in Harvard Yenching Library. There is much more to this text than can be adequately summarized in one paragraph. Chen Cheng's staff collected the archive during the encirclement and suppression campaigns.

[61] They were: Li Zhi (anatomy, physiology and bacteriology); Sun Yizhi (孙仪之, graduate of a missionary hospital school, captured during the fourth encirclement and suppression campaign, and won over by the strong morale of the Red Army medical units; he taught internal medicine, diagnostics and pathology); Li Yannian (李延年, surgery; he and Dr. Peng were killed during the Long March); Zeng Shourong (曾守蓉, pharmacology); Yu Hanxi (俞翰西, ear, nose and throat and skin diseases); and Hu Guangren (胡广仁, foreign languages).

[62] Information from Zhang (1989), 95–97; Chen Yihou biography in Feng and Li (1991), 150–151; and biographies of Sun Yizhi and You Shenghua in Feng and Li (1991), 108–109 and 411–417. Zhu Chao (1988), 135, reports a total of six hundred and eighty-six graduates, consisting of one hundred and eighty-one army physicians, seventy-five pharmacists, three hundred nursing aides, one hundred and twenty-three from health protection classes (who

Development of workshops to produce pharmaceutical and medical supplies was another important initiative. Initially the Red Army health units depended on western drugs such as aspirin, sulfanilamide, and iodine, before coming to rely on herbal medicines. In early 1932 a small medical supplies workshop was opened not far from Ruijin. With simple equipment and few workers the workshop made mixtures from rhubarb, camphor, peppermint and ethyl alcohol. It added workers and started producing ointments, powders and pills. In October the workshop came under the management of Tang Yizhen, the chief of the medical supplies bureau of the Red Army's Central Health Services Department. Although only twenty-three years old, Ms. Tang had spent two years in a medical course in Moscow and made up in energy and vision for what she lacked in experience.[63]

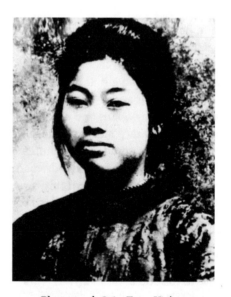

Photograph 3.4: *Tang Yizhen*

Pharmacologist, teacher in Red Army medical school, and very effective direc-tor of Red Army medical workshops. Because of having two young children she stayed in Jiangxi and did not go on the Long March. Martyred in 1935. (*Source*: http://digi.dnkb.com.cn/dnkb/html/2011-06/28/content_172236.htm)

---

subsequently served as regimental health directors or as heads of epidemic prevention sec-tions at the divisional level or above), and seven from a research class (it trained health executives at the divisional level or above).

   [63] She was married to a future minister of propaganda, Lu Dingyi (陆定一), whom she met in Moscow, and gave birth to a daughter at the end of 1931.

Under Tang there were five workshops. A drug workshop produced pills and ointments from locally grown Chinese herbs. Tang came from a family of Chinese pharmacists, so this was an activity in which she had a strong background. Another produced dressings from absorbent gauze and cotton bandages. A third distilled a fiery white colored grain alcohol (烧酒, shaojiu) to produce ethyl alcohol. A fourth produced liquids such as first aid water and tinctures of gentian and iodine. A fifth made forceps, tweezers and scalpels. The factory collected used bandages from rear hospitals and boiled and disinfected them for reuse. Tang encouraged workshops to compete in reaching production goals. By the time the Long March started the workshops had produced sufficient supplies to cover three months. As a result of her work, the Soviet area journal *Red China* (红色中华 *Hongse Zhonghua*) praised her leadership abilities.

But Tang, pregnant with a second child, did not go on the Long March. She persuaded her husband that their friends in Jiangxi could shelter their children. Reluctantly he left, as did the factory, and she stayed and was captured in 1935 by a Nationalist force. She escaped but was recaptured and tortured as to the whereabouts of certain compromising documents. She refused to yield and was taken out and shot. The twenty-six year old heroine has since become an emblem of dedication to a high cause.[64]

The best tribute to Tang and her coworkers lay in the range of their products. Of particular significance was their production of pills and powders derived from locally collected medicinal herbs for treatment of various diseases and battlefield conditions. Their use established the relevance of Chinese medicine to army healthcare. For that reason Red Army forces were always looking to recruit Chinese medicine doctors and pharmacists. So important were Chinese herbal medications to Red Army health that in the army health school physicians trained in biomedicine also studied Chinese herbal knowledge, while those trained in Chinese medicine studied anatomy.[65]

---

[64] i) Zhang (1989), 98–100; ii) Gu and Liu (October 2006); iii) Tang Yizhen biography in Feng and Li (1991), 155–164. The biography of Lu Dingyi in Boorman (1967), was written before information about Tang Yizhen became available outside of China. Apart from her pharmacological expertise and heroism, Ms. Tang was an early fighter for women's rights.

[65] Fan Pu (1988), 134. The Fourth Front Army in the Eyuwan Soviet set up a hospital staffed by forty-nine Chinese medicine doctors.

Campaign against Epidemic Disease

The Red Army health units had three basic problems to address: battle casualties, disease, and daily hygiene and sanitation. During the first three encirclement and suppression campaigns army healthcare leaders developed ways to handle battle casualties and return lightly wounded men to their units in short order. By 1932 disease had replaced wounds as the main cause for depletion of unit strength; and underlying the spread of disease lay the problems of managing hygiene and sanitation. One source reports that over 1,000 people died of infectious diseases in 1932.[66] The dependence of country people on local deities to manage disease did not sit well with the base area health authorities.[67]

The Ruijin government's draft constitution of November 1931 held that laboring people were entitled to free medical help and that the government should implement a health prevention movement. A more urgent statement in March 1932 held that epidemic disease was a serious problem that, if left unchecked, would compromise the revolution. This statement recognized epidemic disease as an enemy to social change. In May 1932 the Communist government's Internal Affairs Ministry decided to carry out a preventive health campaign.[68] The task was entrusted to the Red Army's Central Health Department—no doubt because it already had a track record for getting things done and was under He Cheng's direction.

At a First Front Army healthcare conference in September 1932 the conferees recognized the importance of preventive health and came up with rules for health protection. On the personal side were rules regarding food and drink, bathing, managing hair, cutting nails, changing clothes, sleeping, and early morning exercises. In the public arena several rules called for not spitting freely, discharging human waste only in designated areas, maintaining kitchen, toilet, and living area hygiene, and management of sewage. Hospital rules covered sickroom hygiene, management of dirt, disinfection of clothes, sterilization of laundry of patients with infectious diseases, and burying of corpses. There were also rules for army units on the march. Outbreaks of infectious diseases, whether among the military

---

[66] He Zhaoxiong (何兆雄) (1988).

[67] Three major sources for this section are: 1) Zhang (1989); 2) Gu and Liu (October 2006); 3) Tian Gang (田刚) (2009).

[68] He Cheng's army biography implies that he received a joint appointment as head of the civilian health department of the Ministry of Internal Affairs at (or around) the time the Jiangxi Soviet government was set up, at the end of 1931. Feng and Li (1991), 3.

or residents, should be reported at once. Soldiers should be vaccinated once a year and inoculated against cholera. Water should be protected from contamination. Infected people should not do kitchen work.

To spread these ideas, health personnel held classes each week on basic health knowledge, using blackboards, doing skits and singing songs to get the ideas across.[69] Health knowledge was publicized in popular magazines such as *Red Star* (红星 *Hong Xing*) and *Red China*. The Central Military Health Department's Health Journal (健康报 *Jiankang Bao*) dealt with health management, hospital work, and technical knowledge. *Red Health* (红色卫生 *Hongse Weisheng*), put out by the Red Army Healthcare School, was written for healthcare workers. It carried articles by He Cheng, Chen Yihou, Li Zhi and other faculty members. *Health Talk* (卫生讲话 *Weisheng Jianghua*) was a magazine for soldiers on general health topics. The Red Army Healthcare School published a book for healthcare workers on the four major diseases, emphasizing preventive care. For patients with leg ulcers it recommended washing legs every evening with hot water and getting the patients to do leg movements before sleep. For treatment of malaria it recommended Dichroa root (常山 *chang shan*) and Thorowax root (柴胡 *chai hu*, a fever-reducing drug). To avert dysentery it urged against drinking unboiled water or unsterilized river water.[70] The School prepared handbooks on all major subjects in its curricula, and others on disease prevention for general readers.[71]

In October 1932 the Red Army's Central Health Department launched the health movement instructing all medical units to rename themselves Health Units. The switch from medical nomenclature to preventive health and hygiene (卫生 *weisheng*) is a feature of He Cheng's approach to health management.[72] The goal was to eliminate or control the four destructive diseases, and the plan was to get all troops, political workers and health workers involved. Each catering unit of the First Front Army was instructed to set up a health committee to ensure that troops avoided eating raw, cold or uncleaned food. Individuals were instructed not to go

---

[69] Nationalist public health visiting nurses also used skits to get public health ideas into circulation, e.g. on cutting back incidence of trachoma by having a separate piece of towel for each family member. Information from personal interview with Ms. Zhu Baotian in Taipei.

[70] Information primarily from Zhang (1989), 100–102. Information on anti-malarial drugs from Dictionary of Traditional Chinese Medicine (1984), 152, 154. Two issues of Red Health are preserved in the Chen Cheng archive.

[71] Gu and Liu (October 2006).

[72] He Cheng biography in Feng and Li (1991), 3.

barefoot, not to relieve themselves at will, to bathe regularly, wash their clothes, get their hair cut, help smoke out mosquitoes, and do a thorough cleanup. Inspectors from the Health Department's Health Protection Bureau (保健局 *baojian ju*) were to find out if the masses were paying attention to health. How many sick people were there? Why were they sick? What were the sickroom conditions? To what extent was hygiene an issue? What standards of cleanliness did healthcare orderlies maintain?

To emphasize that civilians were accountable, the political leaders instructed the Internal Affairs Ministry in January 1933 to get directly involved.[73] In March the Ministry put out a directive, which said that: "The purpose of this movement is to get rid of the bitterness of the masses and promote revolutionary struggle." All organizations, urban and rural down to street and village levels, were to develop health agencies and organize teams to push the campaign forward. Government and army units were to mobilize action through night schools, elementary schools, literary classes, clubs, and wall posters. They should teach people how diseases are caused, how to overcome old superstitions, how to get rid of flies and mosquitoes, how to clean up dirt, ventilate rooms, and isolate sick people. Government regulations published in 1933 emphasized prevention of cholera, dysentery, typhoid fever, smallpox, typhus, scarlet fever, diphtheria, plague, and epidemic encephalomyelitis. They listed methods of prevention, reporting systems, and procedures for quarantine, isolation and disinfection. Those who did not follow these procedures were to be punished. Mao Zedong proclaimed that: "It is the responsibility of every base area to launch the movement to eliminate disease."[74]

In October 1933 the Ruijin Communist government acted to prevent spread of contagious disease by blocking travel from any district where an outbreak had occurred and inviting local physicians to participate in control measures. The Red Army sent out healthcare orderlies to vaccinate people against smallpox and help with training programs. In January 1934 civilian and military health leaders convened a second conference. Mao Zedong presented a paper on the wellbeing of the masses, urging political

---

[73] The Ministry's Health Department was also responsible for managing local hospitals, preventing epidemics and infectious disease, investigating carts and boats, public mess halls, review of doctors, pharmacists and drug supplies. Information is from Tian Gang (2009).

[74] Information on diseases listed in government regulations is from Fan Pu (1988), 133, and Fu Weikang (1989), 529.

workers to solve problems facing the masses, such as "food, shelter and clothing, fuel, rice, cooking oil and salt, sickness and hygiene, and marriage." Health leaders put out booklets offering simple guidance on various aspects of public health.[75] In March 1934 a campaign was launched to dredge canals, exterminate mosquitoes and flies, and catch and poison rats. Campaign personnel excavated wells, repaired toilet facilities and buried corpses. All this effort was part of the broader task of mobilizing the masses to advance the healthcare goals of the Communist Party leaders.[76]

This Jiangxi base area health movement was a remarkable effort in social engineering. The ubiquitous local deities serving as arbiters of disease were shunted aside by new world advocates of health and hygiene (*weisheng*), reporting to representatives of a People's government.[77] Mao's distaste for gods and superstitions helped to drive the campaign. However, the campaign focused less on gods and more on the shock troops of pestilence, namely mosquitoes, rats, flies, fleas, and lice, along with the human habits that helped these vectors flourish. As with the Nationalist armies, these enemies were ever present and hostile. One leader, Xiang Ying (项英), contrasted the conditions of "White (Nationalist) areas," in which disease was a feudal enemy holding poor people in thrall, with the liberated Red areas, in which government led the fight against popular oppression. From this perspective liberation from disease was a revolutionary act.[78]

Since the Red Army already operated a public healthcare system its leaders could focus on hygiene. They lacked easy access to biomedical products, thus their strategy was to reduce disease by transforming attitudes towards hygiene, sanitation, and disease causation. It was a grassroots strategy to engage the people on whose lives and energies their future depended. By contrast the Nanjing government's National Health

---

[75] "Be Concerned with the Wellbeing of the Masses, Pay Attention to Methods of Work," part of a concluding speech at the Second National Congress of Workers and Peasants Representatives. Mao (1934), 147–152. The speech is cited by Zhu Chao, Zhong Wai Yixue Jiaoyu Shi, 130. Other information on the congress is from Fu Weikang (1989), 529–530.

[76] Zhang (1989), 110–112, 126–130, and Gu and Liu (October 2006). Zhang focuses on the military health services, while Gu and Liu give more attention to the civilian agencies. Tian Gang indicates how government agencies formulated the policy and points out He Cheng's role in both the military and the civilian agencies carrying out the campaign. Zhang provides a chart (p. 128) which shows how the two branches of government interfaced.

[77] Hsu (1983), provides a classic account of the traditional relationship of local gods to public health.

[78] The article by Tian Gang emphasizes disease vectors.

Administration, although defined as a health and hygiene service, did not have the same authority to intervene in the lives of ordinary people or override local government authority.

What did the Communists accomplish in Jiangxi? According to one source, the rate of disease in two localities in Jiangxi had risen to above eighty percent of the total population. A saying circulating in Jiangxi advised that: "If it's malaria or dysentery, get a piece of land ready" (for a grave). Numbers available to the Red Army in October 1933 indicated that dysentery accounted for sixty-eight percent of the death rate, while the rate of death from malaria was also "very high."[79] But another source reports that the disease rate dropped between 1931 and 1932 by ninety-four percent. Scabies was largely eliminated as a result of the campaign, while incidence of malaria, dysentery and leg ulcers was "greatly lowered." More broadly this source argues that people upgraded their life customs, and young people washed their clothes and quilts and stopped eating unhealthy things. Roaming health units swept places clean, disposed of refuse and dirty water, and cleaned toilets. People figured out that disease was an enemy of the base areas and the people.[80] By seeking to transform people's lives through engaging the leadership and mobilizing the people, the campaign led by He Cheng showed what could be accomplished despite lack of material resources. It even did so while the Fourth and Fifth Nationalist suppression campaigns were occurring.

The Fourth and Fifth Encirclement and Suppression Campaigns, June 1932 to October 1934

Because Chiang Kaishek regarded Communism, not the Japanese invasion, as the chief threat to his regime, he launched a fourth assault on base areas in central China from June to October 1932. During this time Zhou Enlai replaced Mao as chief Army Commissar in Jiangxi, and the Comintern military adviser Otto Braun (李德, Li De) replaced Mao's cautious guerrilla tactics with a strategy of 'active defense,' attacking the enemy beyond the Communist-held borders, even though the Jiangxi Red Army

---

[79] Zhang (1989), 126–127.
[80] Tian Gang (2009), section 4.

only had about 65,000 men to fight an invasion force of around 154,000 plus 200,000 to enforce an embargo.[81]

The Nationalists began their Jiangxi encirclement at the beginning of 1933. Red Army attacks on Fuzhou and Nanfeng were unsuccessful.[82] Nationalist forces moved rapidly south to relieve Nanfeng, forcing the Red Army to withdraw into the Jiangxi base area. By employing the Maoist tactic of using decoys to engage weaker divisions, the Red Army was able during March 1933 to ambush and destroy three Nationalist divisions. News of these successes, and of Japanese incursions in North China, led the Nationalists to abandon the fourth campaign by the end of April 1933.[83]

To prepare for the fourth campaign Red Army healthcare leaders extended the system of healthcare units down to the company level. Army companies were instructed to choose a literate soldier to attend a two-week course on prevention of common diseases, emergency battlefield care, and methods for promoting healthcare. A second short course was for supervisory personnel. The healthcare authorities wanted to ensure that those in charge of recovering casualties sent them back immediately to regimental bandage stations, buried dead bodies after the battle was over, and gathered up captured medical supplies. Company-level health workers were equipped with a bottle of iodine, morphine and opium pills, a bottle of potassium permanganate crystals (water disinfectant), a container of boric acid ointment (antiseptic), various types of sterilized gauze, scissors, tweezers, a probe, and at least ten first aid dressings.[84] Having invested in such preparations, the Central Military Commission forbade

---

[81] Whitson (1973), 275; Dreyer (1995), 186–187. Chinese sources generally estimate the Red Army troops for this campaign at 70,000.

[82] Whitson (1973), 277; Gao Hang (高航) (2005).

[83] 1) Gao Hang (2005). This account blames the 'returned students' for ordering the attack on Nanfeng despite Zhou Enlai's reportedly strenuous efforts to advise against it. After Zhou and Zhu called off the attack they were able to resume control over the battlefield tactics. 2) The decision by the Nationalists to end the Fourth campaign was surely influenced by the Japanese occupation of Rehe in early March 1933. Whitson and Dreyer date the termination at the end of April, after a final campaign along the Gan River. Chinese sources consulted for this study do not mention this campaign and imply that the second successful ambush, occurring around March 21–22 in a mountainous area near Yihuang, was enough to convince the Nationalist armies to pull back. In May 1933 He Yingqin negotiated the Tanggu Truce with Japanese counterparts, buying time for the fifth encirclement and suppression campaign.

[84] From this detailed attention to front line healthcare, it may be inferred that the high level of casualties suffered during the battle of Nanxiong were in part due to limitations in triage of wounded soldiers.

transfer of health workers to other work, or employment of convalescent soldiers as healthcare workers.[85] According to Red Star Newspaper (*Hong Xing Bao*) ten rear hospitals and subordinate infirmaries could handle up to 20,000 patients.[86]

But the strategy of carrying the fight into Nationalist territory made it harder to get sick and wounded soldiers back to rear areas. The assaults took place in the middle of winter, when inadequately clad bearers had to deal with snowstorms and frostbite during hazardous journeys through the mountains to Jianning on the Fujian side of the Jiangxi-Fujian border. To make this journey possible, army health authorities created a system of receiving stations and field hospitals with subunits staffed with a political officer, a medical officer and ten or so nursing aides. A reserve hospital received casualties from field hospitals, keeping the lightly wounded and transferring the rest to the rear hospital in Jianning. Recuperation centers helped get the lightly wounded back to their units, vacating beds for those more seriously wounded. Steps were taken to prepare healthcare units for chemical warfare attacks.[87]

Despite this planning, frostbite took a toll on bearers, leaving Red Army casualties piling up at Jinqi (east of Huwan). Soldiers carried over seven hundred wounded soldiers into the mountains as far as Ziqi Bridge and Laborers carried them on from Ziqi to Jiannin. Once the battles were engaged, triage stations could find themselves covering a distance of up to thirty to forty Chinese li (15 to 20 km) between the front lines and the field hospitals; as a result divisional and regimental healthcare units were unable to deploy sufficient workers to where the battle was engaged, and not enough bandage supplies resulted in loss of blood and infection.[88]

In response to these problems Red Army leaders instructed army group headquarters to maintain close ties with field hospitals, communicate battle plans in advance, and inform field hospitals right away of any changes; the army group health department was to coordinate all healthcare work and have a staff liaison at army group headquarters. The health department set up forward casualty transfer stations to move casualties from front line bandage stations back to field hospitals. Rear healthcare units reached forward to front line units to help move casualties; and regimental health units equipped front line health aides with bandages before

---

85 Zhang (1989), 132–133.
86 Zhu Chao (1988), 131.
87 Zhang (1989), 133–134. A chart of the recovery routes is on p. 135.
88 Zhang (1989), 135–136.

the battle began. They had bearer units organized in advance, and if they needed more bearers they got them from the army.

These measures led to prompt treatment and evacuation of casualties from the two-day ambushes that occurred in late February and mid-March. Serious casualties were carried south to rear hospitals in and around Ningdu. The military success of the ambushes was coupled with better rescuing of wounded soldiers on a rapidly shifting battlefield.[89]

But during the Nationalist army's brutal fifth and last extermination campaign (1933–1934), with a new military strategy under new leadership, the communist's healthcare system broke down. So many lives were lost that finally and abruptly the communist leadership decided to depart on the Long March. They left non-mobile patients as well as hundreds of thousands of country people at the mercy of Nationalist army conquest. The Nationalist government assembled a huge army of between 800,000 to a million men plus two hundred planes.[90] Five hundred thousand men were deployed to invade and destroy the Red Army and the Jiangxi Communist government and the rest directed to intensify the economic blockade. Against this huge force the Red Army could muster only 100,000 trained soldiers and less than 200,000 auxiliary Red Guards.[91]

Yet the Red army leaders again insisted on fighting 'outside the national gates.' They divided their military forces into two parts, sending Lin Biao's First Army Corps to resist invaders from the north and Peng Dehuai's Third Army Corps to campaign on the Jiangxi-Fujian border. Peng had attracted recruits to the Red Army and obtained local material support, as indicated in recently investigated records for Jiangle County in Fujian.[92]

---

[89] Zhang (1989), 136–138. Brief descriptions of these battles, drawn from *Zhongguo Renmin Jiefangjun Quanshi* (中国人民解放军全史 *Complete History of the Chinese People's Liberation Army*) are available on line.

[90] Whitson (1973), 280, favors "more than 800,000 men." Wei (1986), 456, and Zhang (1989), 161, favor 1 million. An official campaign history compiled by the Chinese Ministry of National Defense, dated July 22, 2009, also uses the figure of one million soldiers, with 500,000 assigned to the assault on the Soviet area. See *Zhonghua Renmin Gongheguo Guofangbu* (2009).

[91] These figures are from Wei (1986), 456. Whitson, based on interviews with the former political commissar Kong Chu in 1967, identifies 100,000 soldiers and 50,000 auxiliaries. The Ministry of National Defense official history lists 100,000 regulars but does not offer a numerical figure for the number of auxiliaries.

[92] According to data for this county, two thousand men joined the Red Army during the local revolutionary war period and another eighteen thousand joined mass organizations (including guerrilla and red guard units), amounting to twenty-one percent of the county's population. They contributed personnel, material goods and money, and suffered a good deal of cruelty and devastation, including destruction of twenty villages and loss of

Yet in the heat of the summer, and with inadequate food, his force suffered over 2,000 casualties.[93]

In late September 1933 Nationalist columns advanced south, forcing the Red Armies to withdraw inside the Communist-held perimeter.[94] A revolt in Fujian by the Nationalist 19th Route Army led to a brief abatement of the Nationalist onslaught. Once the Nationalists resumed the Jiangxi campaign in January 1934, they continued moving relentlessly forward. In April a battle at Guanchang inflicted over 5,000 casualties on Red Army forces, representing one-fifth of its defending force.[95] At this point the Red Army leaders began secretly planning the exit strategy that became their Long March.[96, 97]

Strategies pursued by Communist leaders during the fifth campaign made it difficult for army medical units to organize effective relief operations. Lines of communication over mountainous areas were too long to get severely wounded soldiers safely back to rear hospitals. Their armies were often operating well within enemy controlled territory and were unable to plan recovery systems in advance. The weather was bad, the soldiers were camping out in the open, and wound casualties were soon compounded by disease. Wounded soldiers were stranded and many fell into the hands of the enemy.[98] Before the main Red Army force broke through the Nationalist encirclement in October and started on the Long

---

over twelve thousand lives, representing nearly seventeen percent of the population. This and much other information was compiled by the CCP's Central Party Historical Research Institute in or around 2007. Zhongyang Suqu (2007).

[93] Zhang (1989), 163.

[94] Ministry of Defense (2009); Zhang (1989), 160.

[95] Chinese sources consulted for this study give the following casualty figures: for the Nationalist armies, 2,626, for the Red Armies 5,093 (one source gives 5,593, but that is probably a copying error). Cf. Guangchang Zhanyi (广昌战役 Guangchang battle), at baike.baidu.com/view/380979.htm. Given the seventeen-day bombardment that the Nationalist armies mounted against the Red Army garrison, these casualties—while bad enough—seem low. One source notes that the people of Guangchang also made great contributions and suffered martyrdom. It cites an article in *Hongse Zhongguo*, dated May 4, 1934, which reported that the city mobilized three companies of Red Guard units for front line duty. Many citizens helped with transportation, raised large amounts of vegetables, provided two fat pigs, 300 kg of tofu, and 5,000 pairs of straw sandals. See ks.cn.yahoo .com/question/1306110123119.html.广昌战役.

[96] The details are discussed in Benton (1992), 13ff.

[97] Brief summaries of these engagements (and many others) can be found in "Guo Gong Neizhan Zhandou Liebiao" (国共内战战斗列表) Chart of Nationalist and Communist Civil War Battles). Information on losses of senior officials is from Whitson (1973), 280.

[98] Zhang (1989), 163–165.

March, plans were made to distribute a minimum of ten thousand hospital casualties in "safe" locations—and possibly double that number.[99]

For the healthcare leaders who had invested so heavily in spreading healthcare in the Red Army and the civilian base area, this debacle must have been wrenching. The mishandling of resistance to the Fifth campaign resulted in undermining almost everything these health leaders had striven to achieve. It is easier to see how mistakes in strategic planning led to the battlefield disasters, less easy to see why military leaders did not react sooner to policies which led to so many defeats and resultant losses in life, military effectiveness and morale. The party leadership left a modest force in Jiangxi with leaders adept in guerrilla warfare. Such a force could not prevent the Nationalist armies from occupying Ruijin on November 9. Zhu De claimed that: "They never succeeded in conquering the countryside... they did succeed in slaughtering hundreds of thousands of people."[100] Benton's account of the conquest indicates that the victors came down like a firestorm, scattering households, killing wounded soldiers, killing or capturing disoriented guerrillas, and leaving one-third of the arable land in the old Central Communist base area idle.[101]

For the Communist forces it was a dreadful denouement. During the crisis of departure there was no time for reflection, and as Benton points out, there was little incentive among official Chinese or in Western accounts to review what happened, or credit the survival and rebuilding of guerrilla forces in Jiangxi and Fujian provinces. The surviving healthcare units organized a detachment to protect central party leaders and marchers (including Mao again sick with malaria) on the dangerous, ill-defined journey ahead;[102] they left a core group of healthcare workers in Jiangxi to keep the immobile wounded alive and preserve an ongoing guerrilla operation.[103]

---

[99] Zhang (1989), 165–168. Zhu De, as reported years later by Smedley, said that 20,000 casualties were left behind. Benton (1992, 68) concludes that it was up to 30,000 or more.

[100] Smedley (1956), 309.

[101] Benton (1992), 32, 55, 68. This view is adopted also by Sun Shuyun.

[102] At the time of the exodus Mao was ill at Yudu. Local doctors could not diagnose the problem. Alerted by Zhang Wentian, Dr. Fu Lianzhang hurried over by mule to Mao's side, diagnosed malaria and in three or four days got his fever under control so that he could travel. See i) Feng and Li (1991), 75; ii) Dong Ping (东平) and Wang Fan (王凡) (2007). Mao praised his rescuer effusively.

[103] The population of Jiangxi, which was estimated at 17.16 million in 1930, dropped to 12.68 million for the benchmark year of 1949. This is by far the largest gross population decline of any province during that period, during which China's overall estimated

Health Care during the Long March from Jiangxi to Northwest China

The Long March from Jiangxi began in October 1934 and continued for some marchers until late in 1936. Fighting began early and escalated at times into brutal conflicts. In between, marchers spent time traveling at night to avoid plane attacks and circumventing enemy armies by doubling back on their tracks, thus extending the march by thousands of miles.

To prepare to break through the enemy encirclement, health leaders organized hospital services in the mountains south of Ganxian. Guerrilla forces covered the withdrawal of wounded soldiers along two assigned routes. That system worked for four tense days, during which farmers transported the heavily wounded. Thereafter no more wounded were sent back. The lightly wounded accompanied the main force, while heavily wounded were carried in a mobile hospital and treated on the march. If not soon cured, they were escorted to the Guangdong-Jiangxi border area, left with a rural family, and supplied with eight yuan to defray expenses of recovery. The army marched on into the Guangdong-Hunan border area, severing the last connection with Jiangxi.[104]

A crisis occurred at the end of November 1934 when the marchers crossed the Xiang River in the face of a large army of Nationalist and pro-Nationalist forces organized by Chiang Kaishek. The battle was a bloodbath and the Red Army suffered severe losses. Having begun the march with around 80,000 people, by the end of this battle the Red Army had around 30,000. What happened to the lost 50,000? The position in official texts is that the majority fell during the Xiang River battle, while an unknown number became sick or wounded while crossing through Guangdong and southern Hunan. A position more common in English language texts is that desertion was a significant factor. In Whitson's view homesickness, dysentery, and fatigue so undermined raw recruits in the 8th and 9th Corps and the Central Column that the army lost 25,000 men even before it arrived at the Xiang River.[105]

---

population increased from 453 million to 541.6 million. See Tian Xiang Yue (2005). How to allocate this critical decline to several potential causes is unclear, but the fifth encirclement campaign was certainly one major cause.

[104] Zhang (1989), 177–178. Benton (1992, 25) notes that some of these casualties were subject to an ongoing political purge after being sent back.

[105] Whitson, 1973, 282. A recent Chinese source that analyzes the ill-fated Xiang River battle in detail argues that the Red Army had already lost over 20,000 casualties while passing through the first three enemy blockades in Jiangxi and Southern Hunan. It attributes

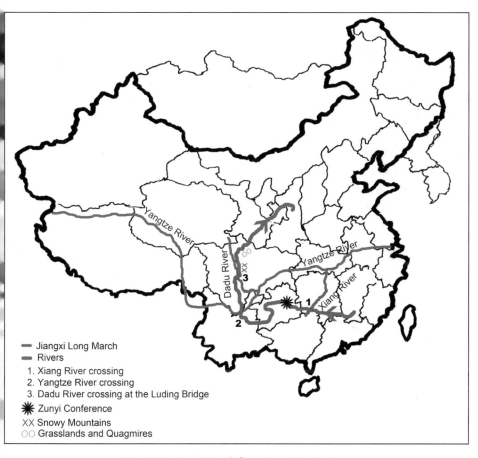

Map 3.2: *Long March from Jiangxi to Bao'an*
The Jiangxi Red Army Long March of over 12,000 kilometers from Yudu in Jiangxi Province to Bao'an and Yan'an in Shaanxi Province is the most famous of three Communist Long Marches on foot from locations in southeast and central China to locations in the northwest. The journeys were tortuous and very dangerous. 80,000 started while barely 7,000 arrived at Yan'an with Mao. Physicians, nurses, and medical aides managed to obtain supplies and treat marchers despite losing many of their own workers during the journey. If the healthcare service had crumbled, the prospects of the marchers would have been much more dubious. (*Source*: J.R. and A.S. Watt.)

To aid seriously wounded marchers the Health Department had one hundred and twenty stretchers and four hundred and eighty bearers. Whenever the marchers passed through populated areas healthcare workers looked for quinine and other drugs.[106] The Central Column contained a convalescent company headed by the party official and educator He Changgong (何长工), with Dr. Li Zhi as medical director. It served elderly and women soldiers, an assemblage of leading cadres including twenty-four women leaders, and army commanders from the company level on up.[107]

A memoir by a former Red Army health school student describes health work on the march.[108] During nighttime travel health workers accompanied the walking wounded to keep an eye on them; the seriously sick and wounded had doctors available. During day travel they might send nursing aides ahead to prepare hot water or gruel for a meal during rest periods. According to this source, western medicines were used during the march. Before reaching the Xiang River, three convalescent companies served rank and file soldiers. Small operations, such as extracting bullets or setting fractures, could be performed in transit.

After crossing the Xiang River the depleted army climbed over several steep mountains. Seriously wounded soldiers had to get off their stretchers and either "crawl or be pushed, dragged, or carried up" a steep cliff, while the lightly wounded made their way with the aid of a stick. Although lacking adequate food, clothing or shelter, the marchers kept going. Women workers "helped the men in their care without once showing any sign of weariness" and even took over from stretcher-bearers. Political workers sang revolutionary songs and set up tea stations. Senior cadres gave up their horses for use by sick and wounded people. Revived by this energy the army arrived on December 15 at Liping in southeast Guizhou province.[109] At a conference the following day a revived Mao Zedong persuaded Central Military Commission members to march into Guizhou, which was weakly defended and offered a chance to set up a base area. After adjusting military and healthcare units to improve

---

these losses to the panic-stricken flightism and incoherence of Bo Gu (博古) and Li De. See "Xiangjiang Zhanyi" (湘江战役 Xiang River Battle) (no date).

[106] Smedley (1956), 311–314. The Xiang River battle is not mentioned in Smedley's account, which may mean that Zhu De could not bring himself to talk about it.

[107] Information mainly from biography of Dr. Yu Hanxi (俞翰西). See http://baike.baidu.com/view/580437.html?fromTaglist.

[108] Li Haiwen (2006): "Changzheng zhong Weisheng Jiaoyu he Yiliao Gongzuo."

[109] Zhang (1989), 180; Smedley (1956), 314.

fighting mobility at the front, the marchers defeated a Guizhou force and on January 7 occupied Zunyi.[110]

Zunyi, known for the conference that restored Mao to a position of authority, was a place where the Red Army could rest, eat proper meals, treat its sick and wounded, and reorganize. Health workers took time to review work during the battles and cure the sick and wounded. According to statistics of that era, the cure rate was reportedly eighty percent.[111] To aid mobility healthcare units were moved out of the rear echelon and attached to regimental units. Divisional rear field hospitals were shut down and their workers joined regimental health units. In addition the healthcare school resumed classes taught by Wang Bin, Sun Yizhi, Li Zhi, Hu Guangren, and Yu Hanxi.[112] Two hundred individuals attend classes on battlefield triage, disease prevention, and health essentials on the march. During the Zunyi conference two military leaders from Sichuan proposed that southwest or northwest Sichuan would be a better setting for a base area. The conferees approved this proposal and the 37,000 strong Red Army set off towards the Chishui River.[113]

The journey from Zunyi to the Luding Bridge in West Central Sichuan, was marred by serious military losses. The army had barely arrived at

---

[110] Zhang (1989), 181–182; Whitson (1973), 283; Chinese Academy of Social Sciences, Communist Youth League News Bureau and Institute of Modern History, Liping Huyi (黎平会议) http://changzheng.china1840-1949.net.cn/jghy2.htm. The Li De-Bo Gu group attempted a last ditch effort to aim for the other Red Army groups in Sichuan by planning to maneuver the Central Red Army back into western Hunan, where Chiang Kaishek was assembling yet another force to demolish it. This plan was rejected at a one-day leadership conference in Houchang on January 1, which brought Mao back into a triumvirate managing Red Army affairs. See http://changzheng.china1840-1949.net.cn/jghy3.htm. (Unfortunately the jghy urls are now largely inaccessible).

[111] Zhang (1989), 182.

[112] Dr. Yu was a graduate of the Zhejiang provincial special medical school, who joined the Red Army in 1933. He became an instructor in the Red Army health school, and served as an attending physician in the Central Column's convalescent company. A close associate of Dr. Li Zhi, he was killed by a Nationalist bomb in April 1935. Decades later Dr. Li Zhi arranged for the erection of a memorial to him in his home county. See http://baike.baidu.com/view/580437.html?fromTaglist.

[113] Sun (2006), 123; Zunyi huiyi de ziliao (遵义会议的资料 Zunyi Conference Materials), accessible through changzheng.china1840–1949.net.cn/jghy4.htm; this url is no longer available but many others provide details on Zunyi conference materials. See also http://luanyunfeidu.blog.hexun.com/6820259_d.html. This url is still online (April 2013). Whitson, writing in 1973, argued that the decision to move on to Sichuan was "probably not made at the Tsunyi conference," but this position is evidently incorrect. The Conference materials source listed here presents an orthodox account and includes the conference's adoption of Sichuan as a site for a base area. The blog offers reasons. Sun's account summarizes and adds to these perspectives.

Tucheng, in north central Guizhou, when it ran into dangerous opposition from a Sichuan warlord army. Its rear echelons were ambushed, resulting in significant loss of life among health personnel. Badly wounded soldiers were left with local villagers. After Red Army leaders discovered that Nationalist forces were blocking the route to the Yangtze River, the army returned to Zunyi, where it successfully beat off a Nationalist attack. A convalescent unit treated several heavily wounded casualties.[114]

During March and April, Red Army units searched for a safe way to cross the Yangtze River, settling on a route through Yunnan to the Golden Sands River—the Yangtze's main upstream course. While passing through Guizhou, night marching became necessary. In Yunnan the journey was easier but health workers had to guard their charges against heatstroke and intestinal disease and pay special attention to camp hygiene. From May 3–9, the main force found ferryboats at Jiaopingdu and crossed to the Sichuan side.[115] At the end of May they successfully crossed the Luding Bridge across the raging Dadu River and continued north.[116]

The marchers now climbed the formidable Jiajinshan Mountains. Their diet of corn was indigestible, and in the higher reaches their hands and lips turned blue and men froze to death. They were harassed by enemy planes, and while traveling to a meeting with medical colleagues Dr. Peng Zhen was struck by a bomb and killed.[117] By the time the column descended from the high mountains it had "so many sick and exhausted men" that the leaders decided to take a rest.[118] Over the next three weeks Zhang Guotao and Xu Xiangqian (徐向前), leaders of the Fourth Front

---

[114] Zhang (1989), 185; Li Haiwen (李海文) (2006): Changzheng zhong Weisheng Jiaoyu, http://vip.book.sina.com.cn/book/chapter_40933_25324.html. Both sources include details of surgical operations.

[115] i) "Qiaodu Jinshajiang" (巧渡金沙江 Skillful Crossing of Jinsha River) http://changzheng.china1840-1949.net.cn/jg4.htm; ii) Zhang (1989), 185–187. The name where this force crossed the river is also given as Shujiedu.

[116] Account summarized from the following sources: i) Zhang (1989), 187–188; ii) Qiangdu Daduhe (强渡大渡河 Forced Crossing of Dadu River), http://changzheng,china1840–1949 .net.cn/jg5.htm; iii) summary of account by the vanguard political commissar Yang Chengwu (杨成武, 飞夺泸定桥 Swift Capture of Luding Bridge), http://dangshi.people. com.cn/GB/170835/175705/175709/10505102.html; iv) Changzheng Zhuanzhe Jieduan, Jan 15–June 14, 1935, (长征转折阶段 Transitional Stage of Long March), http://cyc69.cycnet .com:8090/xuezhu/changzheng/dsj.jsp?ar_id=8572&subchannel_id=52&page=1.

[117] Peng and Li (1991), 149, biography of Peng Zhen. He was on his way to a meeting with He Cheng, Chen Zhifang, Wang Bin, and Ji Pengfei to discuss how to manage the next phase of their work. His colleagues rushed to his aid, but there was nothing they could do to save him.

[118] Smedley (1956), 325–326.

Army, and Mao Zedong and Zhu De argued about how to proceed, and the First Front Army's healthcare school resumed classes.[119]

During the next month differences between Zhang Guotao and Mao came to a head, leading to the formation of two distinct columns combining elements of both armies.[120] This arrangement allowed Mao to retain hold over the political leadership of the Red Armies. Dr. He Cheng was assigned to the group led by Zhu De that marched in the left column with Zhang Guotao. Zhu and He did not reach Yan'an until late in 1936, a year later than Mao's force. Dr. He's biography insists that he struggled against Zhang Guotao's "splittism," indicating that the doctor might have been vulnerable to such a charge.[121] Although the leading Communist physician in Jiangxi, He surprisingly played no role in the Yan'an era and instead was ordered to accompany the injured party leader Wang Jiaxiang to the Soviet Union.[122]

To prepare for crossing the high grasslands, healthcare staff collected supplies of barley and wheat for the wounded and sick during what promised to be a daunting passage. They packed dried meat and cheese, lamb fleeces, containers of drinkable water and supplies of gauze, cotton swabs, tweezers, probes and a sterilized operating knife.[123] Before departure Zhou Enlai, who had been unwell during much of the march, came down with a high fever and fell into a coma. A team of physicians diagnosed amoebic dysentery with liver abscess. Treatment with emetine, and the care of several leading physicians, brought him back to health.[124]

On August 21 Mao's column set off across the high swamp-ridden grasslands with most of his First Front Army and elements of the Fourth Front Army under Xu Xiangqian. The Mao-Xu column proceeded rapidly and arrived at Banyou in the extreme north of Sichuan five days later, having

---

[119] Feng and Li (1991), 112, biography of Sun Yizhi.

[120] Chen Yi's comment on the Zunyi Conference resolutions indicates that he thought along some of the same lines as Zhang Guotao. He remarked: "How can there be military mistakes divorced from political mistakes? The military mistakes happened under the influence of the political mistakes." Benton (1992), 11.

[121] Feng and Li (1991), 5.

[122] Ibid. Wang returned to Yan'an in 1937 but He Cheng remained in the Soviet Union till 1941 studying at Soviet Party Far Eastern Research Centers. Then on the way home he stopped in Ulan Bator and spent the rest of the war as a physician at its Central Hospital. For Wang see Borman (1967), volume 3, 365–66.

[123] Zhang (1989), 191–192.

[124] Feng and Li (1991), biographies of Wang Bin, 174–175, Dai Jimin, 344, Li Zhi, 353. The attending physicians were those three doctors plus Dr. Sun Yizhi. Dr. Dai's services were requested by Mao Zedong. Emetine (also known as ermentine) was a treatment for amoebic dysentery and amoebic liver abscess. See Akinboye and Bakare (2011).

lost a good many men to quagmires or freezing weather. According to Sun Shuyun, four hundred men were lost from the First Army group, and its medical staff dropped from 1,200 at the beginning of the Long March to 200 by the time they emerged from the high grasslands.[125] During August 29–31 the right column fought a critical battle at nearby Baozuo with a Nationalist division from the army commanded by Hu Zongnan, capturing much needed supplies and driving the enemy away with substantial casualties. A week of fruitless telegramming followed, after which Mao quietly separated his forces from those of Xu and went on north with his First Front Army, now reduced to 8,000 men or less.[126] Xu led his group back to Songpan, where eight hundred men were recovering from the Baozuo battle.[127] Mao's decision to abandon Xu meant that those who went with Mao, including twenty-one top political and military leaders and most of the remaining healthcare workers from Jiangxi, had thrown in their lot with him.[128]

Arrival of Red Army Forces in Northern Shaanxi and Revival of the United Front

Mao's forces now pressed on northeast and arrived at Wuqi (Baoan County) in Shaanxi province on October 19.[129] To their dismay, it was a desolate, primitive settlement where "the people were poor and the wolves hungry."[130] There was not enough food, clothing or housing, and winter was setting in. But for Mao Baoan was a place from which to resist Japan. His forces joined with the 15th army corps from the Eyuwan base area to form an army of around 11,000 soldiers. An attempt by Chiang Kaishek to launch a suppression campaign, fought by divisions from the Northeast army of Marshal Zhang Xueliang (张学良), was neutralized at Zhiluozhen in November 1935. The Red Army captured 5,300 men and

---

[125] Sun (2006), 189, 194.

[126] Whitson (1973), 147–148, 287; Sun (2006), 174–179. The occurrence and timing of Mao's early morning departure is provided by Sun. See also http://cyc69.cycnet.com:8090/xuezhu/changzheng/dsj.jsp?ar_id=8572&subchannel_id=52&page=1 for a detailed chronology of the Long March.

[127] Whitson (1973), 149.

[128] See Whitson (1973), 62–65, 145–148; Sun (2006), 172–177.

[129] Account reconstructed from Long March chronology, 8/5–6 to 10/19 (for access see note 126); Zhang (1989), 192–194; Sun (2006), chapter 8; Whitson (1973), 148–149, 287.

[130] Sun (2006), 206, citing memoir by Wang Bing.

3,500 guns. They indoctrinated the prisoners by strongly supporting the war against Japan and sent them home to spread the word.[131]

Needing more supplies, Mao obtained Central Committee agreement to launch an expedition into Shanxi province. The army set off in February 1936. The weather was frightful but Mao was undaunted. He wrote one of his most famous poems to celebrate the event. Amidst the snow the mountains "danced like silvery snakes." "Wait until a sunny day," he promised; "all (the great emperors) have passed away... brilliant characters are still to be seen."[132] The expedition carried out significant "resist-Japan" propaganda among the population in Shanxi and added a sizable number of recruits to the Red Army.[133] Seeing the Communist forces as potential allies against Japan, Marshal Zhang began discreetly supplying cash and guns.

Meanwhile the Left Column led by Zhang Guotao and Zhu De spent the winter in Ganzi in northwest Sichuan and in June 1936 met up with the Second Route Army led by He Long. The party center in Shaanxi developed a plan to open up a connection with the Soviet Union through Ningxia province and sent Peng Dehuai and the First Front Army to cross the Yellow River at Jingyuan in Gansu province. The three Front Armies met just south of Jingyuan on October 8. For the next two weeks they made plans to cross the river. But Chiang Kaishek called on the Gansu Moslem cavalry to defend the left bank of the Yellow River and assembled a large army and a bomber group to attack the main Red army force. At first the Communist leaders stuck to the Ningxia plan. Their ground forces were able, with great difficulty, to move 21,800 Fourth Route Army soldiers under Xu Xiangqian across the huge river during October 26–29. At that point, with a Nationalist attack imminent, it became necessary to change plans. The west bank force, now renamed West Route Army (Xilujun 西路军, also known as Western Legion) was ordered to proceed into Gansu to attack the Moslem cavalry base.[134]

---

[131] Zhiluozhen Zhanyi (直罗镇战役), at http://baike.baidu.com/view/133254.htm.

[132] Zhang Chunhou, (2007), 192–198.

[133] Whitson estimated "perhaps 5,000 recruits;" a Chinese source puts the number of recruits added at "over 8,000." See Whitson (1973), 65; Li Ji (李吉) (2002): "Hongjun Dongzheng" (红军东征) at www.tydao.com/suwu/2002/1223-3.htm.

[134] This account follows a detailed analysis of the river crossing in "Hongse Fangmianjun zai Jingyuan Qiangdu Huanghe," (红色方面军在靖远强渡黄河 The Red Front Army Crossing of the Yellow River at Jingyuan) at http://61.178.146.167/jfq/shownews.asp?nid=639 dated March 18, 2010.

From then on the West Route Army fell victim to a tragic underassessment of the size, capability, and resentments of the Moslem cavalry.[135] The army suffered its first major defeat in mid-November 1936. As a result of countervailing orders it moved slowly west into the barren Hexi corridor, where the Gobi desert provided no refuge or local support. Outmaneuvered and outgunned, the army was relentlessly cut to pieces. Only a few hundred soldiers escaped. A woman's regiment of over 1,000 soldiers was decimated, and those still alive were hunted down and distributed as sex slaves.[136]

For decades hardly a word of this disaster made it into Long March mythology. The campaign was condemned as an example of Zhang Guotao's right wing opportunism and flightism. Early in 1937 Mao Zedong and the Party leadership denounced Zhang and the verdict was incorporated into Mao's writings.[137] But in the early 1980s Li Xiannian (李先念), PRC President from 1983–88 and a West Route Army survivor, was encouraged by party elders Deng Xiaoping (邓小平) and Chen Yun (陈云) to look into the matter. The archives revealed that Mao and the Party Central Committee had ordered the doomed army to set up a base area in Gansu and take on the Muslim cavalry. Zhang's hands were not clean, but he was not solely responsible for the loss of his army.[138]

But for the Center, lack of supplies and Nationalist attack were of more immediate concern. The Red Army forces that did not cross the Yellow River returned to Shaanxi and defeated the pursuing Nationalist forces at Shanchengbao on November 21. During this battle three Red Army rear hospitals were able to treat 330 casualties. Ten days later the army headquarters group, led by Zhu De and Zhang Guotao, arrived in Baoan.[139] By that time Chiang Kaishek's decision to fly to Xi'an to supervise what he hoped would be the final suppression of the Communist forces changed everything. On December 12 Chiang Kaishek was captured by troops of

---

[135] Sixty years previously a major Hui rebellion had been decisively suppressed by the Qing Governor General Zuo Zongtang. While peace was restored, memories rankled.

[136] Account reconstructed from Whitson (1973), 148–154, and Sun (2006), chapters 11 and 12. Whitson's account was constructed before access to survivor memoirs became available. Sun's account of the destruction of the West Route Army is detailed and chilling.

[137] See for example Selected Works of Mao Tse-tung (1936), 193, and "On Tactics against Japanese Imperialism," note 22, Vol. 1, 175–176.

[138] Information from Li Qingying (李庆英) (2005). The author notes that Xu's memoirs, published in 1987, shed light on the army's fate, but commentators were reluctant to study the issues for fear of being charged with attempting to reverse the verdict on Zhang. It was not until the 1990s that this restraint eased.

[139] Zhang (1989), 234–236; Whitson (1973), 152.

Marshal Zhang and his ally General Yang Hucheng (杨虎城), who could no longer tolerate further civil war. Ironically it was the Communist team, led by Zhou Enlai, which came to Chiang's rescue. The deal was a new united front against Japan and incorporation of the Red armies into that alliance.[140]

Having secured this huge concession, the Communist leaders set up their headquarters in Yan'an. Mao's strategy of resisting Japan prevailed over his party and Nationalist opponents. It would bring thousands of young people, including hundreds of medical workers, to Yan'an to help fight the foreign enemy.

Summary

Chinese Communist leadership in the Jiangxi area began with a health delivery system geared to survival and protection of military forces. It peaked with a thoroughly planned and executed civilian health drive. The fifth Nationalist suppression campaign neutralized the results of that health drive and forced the Communist armed forces to leave Jiangxi and revert to survival mode during the Long March. Nevertheless Mao's forces arrived in northwest China with functioning military health services and a functioning health school, agencies that played a vital part supporting the Communist Eighth Route Army in the war against Japan.

We have seen that from 1928–1937 the Jiangxi Communist leaders were focused on establishing important health priorities despite being constantly under fire from far larger numbers of their Nationalist counterparts. Red Army focus on infectious disease, training of local young people as bearers and aides to help provide triage for saving the wounded, and incorporation of Chinese medicine into their health system made the Red Army an ally in the onslaught on social oppression. Chinese medicine doctors, pharmacists and teenage nursing aides, became part of the social system that would bring rural China into a post-warlord, post-landlord, post-demonic, and post-witch doctor era.

Before that era arrived the Chinese people had to face a far more formidable and ruthless military opponent than any they had experienced since the Manchu conquest in 1644. There were also huge floods and famines.

---

[140] Account largely reconstructed from Sun (2006), chapter 11, and Zhang Chunhou (2007) Li Ji (李吉) (2002): "Hongjun Dongzheng," (红军东征) at www.tydao.com/suwu/2002/1223-3.htm.

The loss of life during the War of Resistance against Japan (1937–1945) was staggering. Yet the Chinese people found ways to rise to this daunting challenge. We will explore this part of the story through two chapters dealing with military lifesaving, one with initiatives undertaken by civilian health administrators, and one on military and civilian initiatives by agencies of the Yan'an government headed by Mao Zedong.

CHAPTER FOUR

JAPANESE INVASION, ARMY MEDICINE, AND THE CHINESE RED
CROSS MEDICAL RELIEF CORPS (CRCMRC), 1937–1942

*It was not until the War of 1914–1918 that military hygiene really came
into its own; and it was only then, and since then, that worthwhile results
have been achieved.*
                                   —Field Service Hygiene Notes, India, 1945

The Japanese invasion in 1937 precipitated the most serious military crisis
in China since the outbreak of the Taiping Rebellion in 1851. The invaders
were determined to punish the Nanjing government and its people and
had a huge array of 20th century weapons with which to do so. Despite
Chiang Kaishek's determination to defend Shanghai and Nanjing, the
Japanese military, with their superior firepower, were able to overwhelm
stubborn Chinese resistance. When Chinese armies retreated to Nanjing,
only to abandon it in mid-December, the Japanese pounded their way
into the capital, reduced much of it to rubble and subjected its Chinese
inhabitants to a bloodbath.

These shocking developments exposed China's unreadiness for all-out
war. China's armies had only marginal health services incapable of dealing
with the Japanese onslaught. Its fragile civilian public health services were
in no position to support so many wounded soldiers and terrified civilian
refugees. Unknown tens of thousands were abandoned on battlefields or
left to die by the roadside. The government, struggling to reorganize in
Wuhan, would within a year move much further west to Chongqing, surrendering east China to the enemy. Millions of east China's people were
left to shift for themselves.

It is not often that large populations are subjected to such massive
destruction and chaos. What resources did China have within its great civilization to respond to such a battering? Here is where the modern health
reformers met their greatest test. They did respond, and with considerable
effect, using the CRCMRC to come to the rescue of China's soldiers. But
in doing so they ran into damaging opposition from both domestic and
foreign sources. Chapters four and five explore these struggles to assess
what was accomplished and at what cost.

PART I: CONSTRUCTING A MODERN MILITARY HEALTHCARE SYSTEM

Army Medical Services up to 1937

Modern army medical service in China began with the founding of the Beiyang (later Naval) Medical College in Tianjin in 1893 and the Beiyang Military Medical Academy (*Beiyang junyi xuetang* 北洋军医学堂) in the same city in 1902. By 1912 the upgraded Army Medical School (陆军军医学校) had graduated 136 physicians from a four-year program and 18 pharmacists from a three-year program.[1] During the early years of the Republic (1911–1949) the Army Medical School moved to Beijing, where it added graduate departments and a clinical training program. But with the onset of warlord power struggles, the School suffered constant turnover in leadership, and in 1932 the Naval Medical College closed.

In 1929 the new Nationalist Government set up an army medical office at Nanjing in the Ministry of Military Affairs (军政部军医司), under the direction of Dr. Hao Zihua (郝子华 Hou Tzu-hua).[2] The former PUMC director Dr. Liu Ruiheng (刘瑞恒) was appointed to supervise the medical office attached to Chiang Kaishek's headquarters.[3] Later that year Dr. Liu appointed the PUMC-trained physiologist Dr. Lu Zhide (卢致德 C. T. Loo) head of the medical department of the Central Military Academy in Nanjing, to upgrade military medical training.[4]

As a result of Japanese military incursions into north China, the Army Medical School moved to Nanjing. It organized an ambulance corps and began preparing for a war of resistance. In 1934 Dr. Liu Ruiheng became its director as well as head of a Military Medical Planning and Supervisory Commission (军事委员会军医设计监理委员会). A strong opponent of German medical practice, he discharged the existing faculty, overhauled the curriculum, and appointed the American-trained surgeon and hospital administrator Dr. Shen Kefei (沈克非) dean of studies. In 1935 the government merged the Military Commission's medical affairs unit with the Ministry of Defense's medical office to form the Army Medical Administration (*junyishu* 军医署 AMA), placing it under Dr. Liu's direction.[5]

---

[1] Wong and Wu (1936), 479, 519–20, 543; Zhang Jian (张建) (1984).

[2] Dr. Hao was a graduate of the Army Medical School; he served in various warlord armies in the 1920s but joined the Northern Expedition as surgeon general and chief of a field hospital. China Weekly Review (1936), 78–79.

[3] Wong and Wu (1936), 763. This office would have gone to Dr. Jin Songpan, had he not disapproved of the White Terror and made himself unavailable.

[4] Bowers (1972), 160.

[5] Yang Wen-tah (1989b), 123.

Dr. Lu Zhide was sent to Britain's Imperial Medical College and to the U.S. to study modern military medical services.[6] The Army Medical School initiated an emergency training class for army medical personnel; the Central Military School started a similar class.[7]

By 1936 the Army Medical School had graduated 1,045 physicians and 300 pharmacists, most of whom were serving in the three armed services (army, navy, air force) or in various army hospitals, and it had a current enrollment of 108 students.[8] Then in February 1937—a few weeks after returning from the dramatic Xi'an negotiations—Chiang Kaishek took personal control of the school as part of a consolidation of military agencies under his direct control. He discharged the pro-American Drs. Liu Ruiheng and Shen Kefei and appointed as dean of studies Dr. Zhang Jian (张建), a graduate of the Army Medical College (AMC) with advanced study at Berlin University, whom he had met during a brief visit to south China. A small military medical school in Guangdong where Zhang was working became a branch agency of the Central Army Medical College in Nanjing.[9]

By the time the War of Resistance erupted in July 1937 a small cadre of military medical officers and pharmacists existed to serve centralized military medical agencies and a few urban-based hospitals. These agencies were not positioned to provide modern medical field services for Nationalist China's three million or more soldiers. In addition, no integrated "service of supply" system existed to support the field armies. Thus the task of saving lives in the face of Japanese military invasion fell on medical units controlled by each individual group army and its subordinate divisions.

Army Healthcare Units in Wartime: The Early Phase

Nationalist China's War of Resistance began with epic military confrontations in east central and north China, during which divisional medical personnel handled battlefield triage. To appreciate the magnitude of this task, we have to understand the kind of war unleashed by the Japanese

---

[6] Liu Siqin (1989), articles by Chen Tao (63–65), Yang Wen-tah (65–69 and 121–127), P'an Shu-jen (167–169), and Liu Jui-heng (309–313). New York Times obituary (p. 361) has Dr. Liu's date of appointment as army surgeon general as 1931.

[7] Zhang Jian (1984), 10.

[8] *CMJ*, 51, 4 (April 1937): 554.

[9] Zhang Jian (1984), 11. Chiang had mistakenly understood that Dr. Zhang was a graduate of Tongji Medical College with advanced study in Japan. His status as an Army Medical College alumnus with advanced study in Berlin made him an ideal candidate to be dean of studies under Chiang's authority. See Zhang Li'an (张丽安) (2000), 86–92. The author is Dr. Zhang's daughter.

military. Although it never declared war, The Japanese government treated the Lugouqiao incident (卢沟桥事变 Marco Polo Bridge incident) in July 1937 as a war provocation.[10] In the 1930s the Japanese emperor's status and leadership increasingly defined the role of the military as guardian of Japanese sovereignty, culture, and divine authority, and as instrument for achieving regional supremacy. Consequently the punishment inflicted by the Japanese military in China acquired the status of a holy war against mutinous forces. This attitude also drove Japanese military attempts to suppress Chinese Communist forces.[11]

To this one should add arguments about the use of military force on civilian populations that are a central feature of John Tirman's study on "The Deaths of Others."[12] Tirman's analysis focuses on American military killing of civilians in Korea, Vietnam, Iraq and Afghanistan. This provides a context for recognizing that Japanese and Chinese military killing of civilians in the 1930s and 1940s is a characteristic of military conduct during the last century. Tirman's argument focuses on the distinction between "us" and "others." Civilians as "others" are expendable. Arguments blaming Japanese killing on an over militarized *bushido* (武士道 way of the warrior) culture do not account for widespread killing of civilians by soldiers of other countries, nor for regrets later experienced by soldiers involved in killing civilians.[13] In effect a stance of justified ruthlessness drove the Japanese invasion, against which the Chinese armies and their front line medical units had little to offer. To save lives the health reformers would have to inject a similar tenacity into China's army medical units.[14]

During the early campaigns Nationalist armies relied on a traditional system for supplying medical personnel. Under this system each divisional commanding officer appointed the chief medical officer. The

---

[10] The bridge (*qiao*) is near Beijing.

[11] Studies of divine mission accorded to the Japanese military by Japanese policy makers and public opinion in the 1930s include Herbert Bix (2000). This outstanding work provides a detailed analysis of the themes summarized here. Ishikawa (2003) offers a literary treatment of this subject. Honda (1999) is an unforgettable account of Japanese military slaughter from the East Coast to Nanjing. Tanaka (1998) deals with Japanese military war crimes.

[12] Tirman (2011).

[13] For example, Gen. Li Hanhun (立汉魂) preserved the diary of a Captain Nakajima. The Captain wrote: "for whom am I perpetrating all this cruelty?.... In my conscience, I dare not face my parents." See Virginia C. Li (2003), 104. On the other hand another Japanese soldier's diary reported without comment the execution of thirty young men arrested in a "dangerous" village. See Smedley (1938), 122–123.

[14] The distinction between "civilian" and "soldier," so important to U.S. nongovernmental agencies, became blurred as the war progressed and was replaced by the distinction between "patriotic" and "unpatriotic."

divisional medical officers were responsible to the divisional commanders but held no military rank. Due to low military pay and the low status of the military in traditional Chinese culture, the position seldom attracted graduates of modern medical colleges.

The divisional medical officer received a budget for supplies and the authority to enlist personnel. The latter were usually recruits with poor physique considered unsuitable for combat. Nurses, dressers and stretcher-bearers were commonly untrained coolies or peasants. Each division was entitled to have two 'sanitary' companies consisting of nine medical officers and 87 subordinates. In practice many such companies were much smaller and were unfit to administer first aid or carry off the severely wounded.[15] Stretcher-bearers were to evacuate non-ambulatory casualties to field dressing stations and field and base hospitals. But during the critical early campaigns of 1937 the force of the Japanese invasion overwhelmed the military medical relief system. According to a report by the missionary physician Dr. Harold Balme:

> Many divisions were absolutely destitute of skilled surgical aid or of proper medical appliances. Ambulances, stretchers, splints, surgical dressings, anti-tetanus serum, drugs—all were at a minimum or, more often, simply non-existent, and after most battles great numbers of the wounded were left untended in the field, or crawled away to die in some place of hiding.

Aerial bombardment of cities added to this misery, rendering thousands of people homeless and spreading infection, especially cholera. In many hospitals available stocks of dressings, anesthetics and drugs were quickly used up.[16]

This picture is supported by Agnes Smedley:

> Very few of the severely wounded reach any dressing station or any hospital... Owing to bad organization, indifference and incapacity, the Army medical service itself does not, and cannot, evacuate most of the wounded. This work is done by soldier comrades... In places where mobilization of the people is allowed by the authorities, the people help evacuate the wounded.[17]

---

[15] i) Freda Utley (1939), chapter 4; ii) Evans Fordyce Carlson (1940a); iii) Agnes Smedley (November 1938), 475–476; iv) "ABMAC, box 2, Army Medical Administration, The Army Medical Service," undated report (by Dr. Lin Kesheng 林可胜) c. August 1938; v) ABMAC, box 5, Cheng Pao-nan folder, "The Army Medical Service and Some of its Problems," by General Loo Chih-teh (Lu Zhide 卢致德), dating towards the end of 1939 or early 1940.

[16] Balme (April 8, 1939): 836–839.

[17] Utley (1939), Smedley (1938).

Sick and wounded soldiers who reached receiving stations and field hospitals were not necessarily better off. Such hospitals were generally situated in primitive collections of abandoned huts and temples and staffed with individuals untrained to treat severe injuries and diseases. This account of a receiving station is by Utley:

> ... A cluster of ancient, dirty, low-ceilinged houses. In the dim light of our electric torches we crept through these hovels over the bodies on the floor. The wounded lay in their filthy, blood-soaked clothing, their wounds roughly bandaged, but with no one there to attend to their wants—no one even to give them a drink in the hot August night ... It was as grim a sight as I saw during my stay in China ...[18]

Auden and Isherwood recorded similarly harrowing descriptions.[19] Utley found one of the best army hospitals where the wounded lay on bamboo beds and even had sheets and pillows. They still wore dirty, bloodstained clothes.[20] Smedley reported that operating tables were often boards covered with pieces of unbleached cloth. Medical and surgical supplies were at times almost nonexistent. Most of the wounded were emaciated. Yet this was an improvement over conditions a year earlier, due to the tireless labor of a few capable Army and Chinese Red Cross doctors.[21]

Accounts such as these indicate that the Chinese military leaders had learned nothing from the lessons on military hygiene gained at huge cost during World War One, although the information was readily available in translatable handbooks. For example, Dr. Frank Keeper wrote a handbook on elementary military hygiene and sanitation, published in 1918, that provided detailed information on diseases, nutrition, management of food, camp and march sanitation, categories and rates of battlefield casualties, care, training, and fitness of troops, and disposal of wastes.[22] Another book by Dr. W. W. Keen on treatment of war wounds, published in 1917, provided meticulous information on evacuation of war wounded and management of infection.[23] The surgical skills described by Dr. Keen were not available in China's combat divisions, but other procedures, such as collection and evacuation of wounded and those dealing with hygiene

---

[18] Utley (1938), chapter 3.
[19] Auden and Isherwood (1939).
[20] Utley (1938), chapter 5.
[21] Smedley (1938). Williamsen (1992, 147–153) provides a similarly bleak account of military medicine.
[22] Keeper (1918).
[23] William Williams Keen (1917).

and sanitation, could have been part of any competent army medical field-training program in the 1930s.

A few Nationalist army commanders did take an interest in army medical work, recognizing that it could help preserve the combat efficiency of their troops. Utley reported that Generals Li Hanhun (李汉魂 also known as Li Hanyuan) and Tang Enbo (汤恩伯) were interested in the problems of the wounded and were aware that men would fight better if assured of proper care of casualties.[24] Tang was able to get his sick and wounded men off the Xuzhou battlefield by transporting them on litters on the backs of donkeys.[25] Tang was again cited by the American army surgeon L. S. Powell for his interest in medical training and provision of rations.[26]

But in matters of health management Nationalist China's armies were unready for total war. The central army medical administration had no influence on the staffing, training or supplying of army divisional medical units, and those units were unable to train or supply themselves effectively. Any strengthening of army medical services could only come from outside the military system.

The Chinese Red Cross and War Relief

The Chinese Red Cross, through its Medical Relief Corps (MRC), played a unique role in the early years of the War of Resistance. It provided a way to overcome the resistance of educated youth to war work and bring their patriotism and skills to the aid of front-line soldiers. The MRC was led by a group of elite medical school graduates with aid from patriotic overseas Chinese principally from the Dutch East Indies. It obtained substantial funds and equipment from overseas Chinese groups in Southeast Asia and North America, and from relief agencies in the US, Canada, Britain, Australia and New Zealand. Until 1942 it was the driving force in bringing modern healthcare to Chinese battlefronts.

The Chinese Red Cross (CRC) was formed in Shanghai in 1904 to aid the people of southern Manchuria during the Russo-Japanese War.[27]

---

[24] Utley (1939), chapter 4. Virginia C. Li (2003) provides a vivid account of her father, General Li Hanhun's military and civilian careers. There are also accounts of his life on line. http//:hudong.com/wiki/李汉魂 has a helpful assessment of his achievements.

[25] Belden (1944).

[26] Lyle Stephenson Powell (1946), chapter 8.

[27] For a major study of the origins and development of the Chinese Red Cross, see Reeves (1998).

It achieved a significant record of war relief that carried on into the 1930s.[28] When the Japanese attacked Shanghai in January 1932 it organized a relief corps providing twenty first-aid teams, forty temporary hospitals and five refugee centers.[29] In 1933 it came to the relief of Chinese armed forces resisting Japanese encroachment in the Shanhaiguan region north of Beijing. It appointed a North China Medical Relief Commission under the direction of Dr. Liu Ruiheng and sent thirteen teams to the front to relieve the wounded or to perform operations in field and base hospitals. Because army units had few officers capable of carrying out surgical operations, the teams collectively performed over 1,300 operations and treated around 7,500 casualties. Front line teams provided emergency relief and sorted out casualties needing immediate evacuation. Several individuals who would subsequently play important roles during the War of Resistance with Japan got their first experience of battlefield, healthcare during this conflict, among them Drs. Lu Zhide, Zhang Xianlin (张先林), Fan Rixin (范日新 J. H. Fan), Rong Qirong (容启荣 Winston W. Yung), and Wang Kaixi (旺凯熙 Mark Wang). At the end of June 1933, when a truce was declared, all but one of the Red Cross units was disbanded.[30] However, the PUMC, which supplied a good many students to the Red Cross units, set up a medical officers field training program to have medical officers available for future military needs.[31]

After hostilities broke out in Shanghai in August 1937, the Chinese Red Cross organized a provisional Medical Relief Commission. It put together twenty-two rescue and first-aid teams, twenty-four emergency hospitals and ninety-eight ambulances, and engaged sixteen public and private hospitals to support the front line troops. In October it set up a 3,000-bed hospital on the campus of National Central University in Nanjing under the direction of its General Secretary Dr. Pang Jingzhou (庞京周

---

[28] The Canadian missionary physician, Dr. Omar L. Kilburn, who was a cofounder of the West China Union University Faculty of Medicine, was also an organizer of the Chinese Red Cross organization in Sichuan and provided months of battlefield relief under its auspices. Hensman, (August 1967), 471–483.

[29] Wong and Wu (1936), 710, 764–765, 857; *Zhongguo Hongshizi Hui* (1947), 3. The latter text mistakenly sets the outbreak of the Shanghai war on January 28, 1931.

[30] *Zhongguo Hongshizihui Huabei Jiuhu Weiyuanhui Baogao* (c. 1934). In 1936 the CRC organized a relief commission in Suiyuan, which set up refugee centers and temporary hospitals and supplied over 200,000 first aid dressings. *Zhongguo Hongshizi Hui* (1947), 4.

[31] Owing to copying restrictions at the time this material was collected, the author only obtained information on college affiliations of members of four out of thirteen Red Cross teams. In those four teams PUMC students constituted a little under half of the medical personnel.

C. C. Kohlhaus Pang). This hospital had a staff of over three hundred physicians and nurses and over four hundred orderlies; it could perform up to seven operations concurrently.

Tragically, the Nanjing hospital had to be abandoned when the Japanese armies closed in on Nanjing and precipitated the Nanjing Massacre. Enemy soldiers killed wounded patients unable to get out in time, along with a number of doctors and nurses. Around seven hundred Red Cross personnel escaped, of whom a number were killed while in transit.[32] The catastrophe indicated how little the Shanghai Red Cross leaders knew about modern warfare. The survivors retreated to Hankou, far from their base of support and without the guidance of the Medical Relief Commission. New leadership was required to reorganize these Red Cross workers. The Combined Health Services Minister, Dr. Liu Ruiheng, called on his former PUMC colleague Dr. Lin Kesheng to respond to this need.[33]

Lin Kesheng and the Chinese Red Cross Medical Relief Corps

We now approach the fascinating irony of an overseas Chinese physician being called to lead a critical response to a Chinese national emergency. Dr. Lin Kesheng (林可胜 Robert K. S. or Bobbie Lim, 1897–1969) was a leading figure in the Chinese biomedical world. He was born in Singapore in 1897 of Fujian parentage. His father Dr. Lin Wenqing (林文庆 Lim Boon Keng) was a noted physician, Confucian scholar, business leader, and first president of Xiamen University. His mother's sister married Dr. Wu Liande.[34] When he was only eight years old Lin was sent to attend schools in Edinburgh, Scotland, and followed his father in taking a medical degree at Edinburgh University. After a period of postgraduate study in

---

[32] i) Information on CRC response in Shanghai and Nanjing is from *Zhongguo Hongshizi Hui* (1947), 4–5, and He Tao (何涛) (1987), 134–5; ii) Information on deaths of patients and personnel was provided by Dr. Berislav Borcic to Agnes Smedley and reported in Smedley (1943), 213.

[33] ABMAC Box 23, National Red Cross Society of China, "Confidential Memorandum on the History of the Medical Relief Corps, May 15, 1941," *Zhongguo Hongshizi Hui* (1947), 5, without mentioning Dr. Liu's role, states that Lin was invited to serve as general manager of the Medical Relief Commission and general director of the Medical Relief Corps, adding that the latter was formed in the spring of 1938. Many texts refer to Dr. Lin as Dr. Robert K. S. Lim; mainland Chinese texts refer to him as Lin Kesheng (林可胜).

[34] http://libportal.nus.edu.sg/media/media/databank-linkesheng.pdf: Online source of the library of the National University of Singapore (text in Chinese).

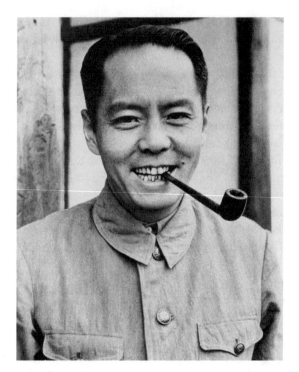

Photograph 4.1: *Dr. Lin Kesheng*
In British army medical service during earlier years of World War I, Professor of
Physiology at Peking Union Medical College, Director of Chinese Red Cross Medical Relief Corps 1938 to August 1942, out of service from August 1943 until end of
1944, In 1945 became Army Surgeon General. (*Source*: ABMAC Archive)

Scotland and the U.S., he was invited to join the PUMC faculty and soon
appointed chair of its Department of Physiology.[35]

Dr. Lin was one of only two Chinese professors to become department chairs during the early years of PUMC. He was an ardent Chinese
patriot who took to the streets in 1925 during anti-British demonstrations. Lin founded the Chinese Physiology Society and edited its journal;
he also became President of the Chinese Medical Association. His studies of gastrointestinal physiology and the central nervous system gained

---

[35] The information that Lin went to Scotland at the age of 8 is from an appraisal of
his scientific work by the noted gastroenterologist Horace W. Davenport. See Davenport
(1980).

him international recognition and awards from scientific communities in China, Europe and the U.S.[36]

But it was his experience as a wartime medical officer that made Lin the obvious choice for the CRC assignment. Before enrolling at Edinburgh University medical school in 1916 he underwent British officer cadet training. During the early years of World War One he served with the Indian army in France and England as a private, NCO and later as warrant officer, ending as a lieutenant in the Royal Army Medical Corps. As a professor at PUMC in Beijing he organized the student medical officer training corps. He led a Red Cross unit in the fighting around Shanghai in 1932 and then served as head of the personnel division of Chinese Red Cross's North China Relief Commission. In that capacity, and with help from his former student and colleague Dr. Lu Zhide, he organized twelve mobile medical teams and a small transport and supply service and led senior students during the hostilities with Japanese forces at Gubeikou on the Great Wall. These units worked up standardized first aid kits, treated around 20,000 casualties, and developed an orthopedic service.[37] Under his inspiration PUMC students produced in 1937 a field service manual sponsored by the CRC Beiping branch. This manual provided detailed training information for Red Cross army field medical workers. It has considerable information on gas warfare, which the Japanese military used in China, and detailed information on management of hygiene, sanitation and disease in military contexts.[38]

In 1937 Lin was due for academic leave. He was on his way to Europe to do research when an urgent telegram from Dr. Liu Ruiheng reached him in Singapore. He cancelled his plans and returned to Hankou via Hong Kong and Nanjing.[39] Arriving in Hankou around the end of 1937,

---

[36] According to an ABMAC eulogy he was elected Honorary Member of the Deutschen Akademie der Naturforscher, Halle, in 1932; Honorary Member of the American Gastro-enterological Association in 1946; and Honorary Fellow of the American College of Surgeons in 1947. See Davenport (1980).

[37] i) *Zhongguo Hongshizihui Huabei Jiuhu Weiyuanhui Baogao* (c. 1934); ii) *Huashuo Lao Xiehe* (1987), articles by Fan Rixin (446–450) and Wang Kaixi (451–455); iii) Xue Qingyu (薛庆煜) (1987), 39. T. V. Soong (宋子文 Song Ziwen) was reportedly amazed that students performed better than army regulars. (biography by Sze-ming Sze in ABMAC box 15, Lim, Robert K. S., miscellaneous).

[38] i) Confidential Memorandum, May 15, 1941, ABMAC box 23; ii) *Jiuhu Shouce* (1937); iii) personal interview with Dr. Yang Wen-tah. Gas warfare is treated in chapter 7.

[39] Liu Yung-mao (刘永懋) (1970): 95–98. Liu travelled with Lin from Singapore to Hong Kong, along with other Chinese medical students returning from overseas study. Dr. Grant states in his 1937 diary (August 18) that he advised Lin to take his furlough as planned. In his oral history memoir he recalled that after the Nationalists lost Shanghai

Lin summoned to his aid former students and junior colleagues from the earlier CRC military assistance teams.[40] Together they took charge of the surviving Red Cross personnel from Nanjing and made plans to continue their military relief work. Lin began this task without endorsement from the CRC Board of directors or general secretary, who were immobilized in Shanghai.[41] By now the military front extended for hundreds of miles and the Army Medical Administration had already placed over two hundred hospitals in the war areas. As further evacuation was inevitable, it was decided to organize small mobile units consisting of three physicians, six nurses, and nine dressers. The MRC sent out twenty such units, armed with equipment from Nanjing, to supply army hospitals.

Meanwhile Lin created a headquarters office with departments of supply, transport, and general administration. Initial funding came from the Ministry of Health (NC 200,000) and the Russian Red Cross (R 100,000) through the Soviet Consul in Hankou. Supply depots were organized, and through the initiative of Drs. Lin and Lu Zhide, emergency supplies for treating wounded soldiers in the field were packaged into a large number of standardized kits.[42] MRC transport convoys sent up supplies and helped bring casualties back to base hospitals. MRC medical units attached to base hospitals took charge of operations and of two hundred of every thousand beds containing the most serious cases. In addition, a number of preventive and x-ray units were organized. The latter worked with medical field units while the former carried out anti-epidemic work.[43]

---

he received a cable from Dr. Liu asking him to persuade Lin to join the Red Cross and set up a relief corps to take care of wounded soldiers. When Lin's ship docked at Kowloon Grant met him and showed him Dr. Liu's cable. Lin disembarked and went up to join the retreating Red Cross forces. Grant, *Oral History*, 485–487.

[40] Dr. Yang Wenda was one of those who responded to the call. He traveled from Nanchang to Hankou, met with Lin and slept on his tabletop for one night. The next day Lin sent him back to Nanchang to head up the 71st Medical Relief Unit. See Hsiung (熊秉真) (1991), 33.

[41] ABMAC box 23, National Red Cross Society of China, Unit Reports, "Confidential Report on the Medical Relief Corps, Transport, Training etc., June 28, 1941;" "Confidential memorandum."

[42] This initiative is noted in Smedley (1943), 219, and with growing respect on p. 430.

[43] "Confidential Memorandum"; see also ABMAC box 2, Army-General Medical folder, "China Information Committee, Daily Bulletin 66," June 21, 1941. Yu Shifa (余世法) (1987), 111–113, describes the work of field x-ray units and the x-ray service at Tuyun'guan.

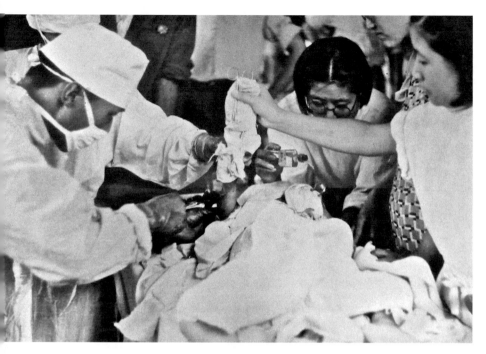

Photograph 4.2: *Medical Relief Corps (MRC) Surgical Team*
Dr. Lin attracted hundreds of young medical school graduates from China and the Chinese diaspora to bring medical relief to China's soldiers. Many later had distinguished medical careers in Mainland China and Taiwan. (*Source*: ABMAC Archive)

Organization of Emergency Medical Service Training School (EMSTS) (Zhanshi weisheng renyuan xunliansuo 战时卫生人员训练所)

In May 1938 the National Health Administration directed Lin to organize a medical training school to serve the medical and anti-epidemic corps of the NHA, the MRC and the Army Medical Services.[44] The first such school, organized by Medical Relief Corps staff with assistance from the Army Medical Administration and the National Council for Rural Reconstruction, opened in Changsha. Funds were provided from the British Boxer Indemnity Fund and the National Council for Rural Reconstruction. The school had seven departments: military, medical, surgical, nursing,

---

[44] ABMAC box 2, EMSTS folder, "ABMAC, report on EMSTS of Ministry of War" by Pao-san Chi, ABMAC Chinese Secretary, January 1942.

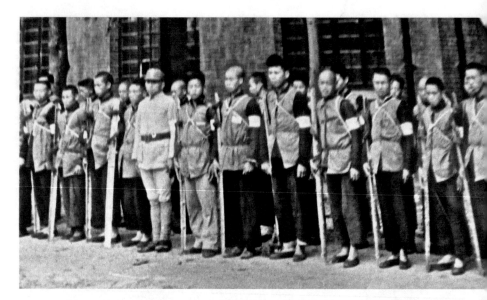

Photograph 4.3: *Early Graduates of Emergency Medical Service Training School (EMSTS).* The School provided basic health care training for thousands of young men as front line bearers and medical aides, giving them a vital role in the defense of China. (*Source*: ABMAC Archive)

preventive medicine, sanitation, and general administration. Initially it set up four-week courses to train four types of field units: first aid, nursing, curative, and preventive. The courses were practical but stressed military discipline and "socio-political understanding." Between May–December 1938, 1,432 students graduated from these courses, including army physicians ordered by Chiang Kaishek to attend the school.[45] These numbers indicate the importance attached by higher officials to this school. Colonel (later General) Stilwell, who knew Lin, attended the first graduation ceremony.[46]

After Hankou fell to the Japanese in October 1938, the school and the MRC headquarters withdrew to Qiyang, Guilin and finally to Guiyang in February 1939, where it remained for the rest of the war. A location was found at Tuyun'guan just outside Guiyang. Buildings were constructed from bamboo fence, mud and rice straw. Before long what had been a

---

[45] ABMAC box 2, EMSTS folder, "EMSTS of the Ministry of War: First Report," May 1938-June 1942; ABMAC box 22, National Red Cross Society of China, Robert K. S. Lim, "Memo on EMSTS and the Orthopedic Centers," dated March 3, 1941.

[46] Smedley (1943), 221–222. Lin's English language secretary Wang Chunjing also reports this visit and says that Stilwell had known Lin in Beijing and appeared to be dropping in without any specific purpose. See Wang Chunjing (王春菁) (1987), 117.

tiny hamlet grew into a market town harboring one of Nationalist China's major wartime medical centers.[47]

After setting up at Tuyun'guan, the EMSTS developed four basic courses of two to three months duration for medical officers, assistant medical officers, medical subordinates, and medical orderlies. Until August 1939 the school remained under the aegis of the National Health Administration, at which point the government's Military Affairs Commission ordered it transferred to the joint control of the Ministry of Internal Affairs (in which the NHA was then located) and the Ministry of War. In 1940 it was reestablished under the Ministry of War with Lin as director and staffed by MRC personnel. The school was told to plan courses for a long war that would have some value for postwar reconstruction, and to develop branch schools, so that its influence could reach throughout China's war areas.[48]

Growth of Medical Relief Corps Work, 1938–1940

During 1938–1940, the Red Cross MRC grew into a substantial agency supplying field armies with on-the-spot training, surgical, medical and sanitary services. The MRC obtained its senior-level work force from medical college graduates and young Chinese volunteers from Southeast Asia, especially Java and its capital Batavia (now Jakarta).[49] Until the Japanese military took over Southeast Asia, significant financial aid came from Chinese communities in the Dutch East Indies.[50] There were two other major sources of financial and material support in these early years. One was the American Bureau for Medical Aid to China (美国医药援华会 ABMAC). Organized in New York in the fall of 1937 by three patriotic overseas

---

[47] *Honghui Jiuhu Zongdui* (1937), 77, 107–108, 118–119, 167.

[48] ABMAC box 2, EMSTS folder, "Emergency Medical Service Training Schools of the Ministry of War, First Report, May 1938-June 1942."

[49] Lin's father, Dr. Lin Wenqing, was a close associate of the overseas Chinese business leader and philanthropist Tan Kah Kee (陈嘉庚 Chen Jiageng). A native of Fujian province who went to Singapore at the age of 16, Tan was one of the chief overseas Chinese leaders mobilizing support for the War of Resistance against Japan. Various European (mainly Jewish) physicians, including a number who had served on the Republican side during the Spanish Civil War, also joined the MRC.

[50] ABMAC, "Confidential memorandum." Since Dr. Lin had not lived in Southeast Asia since the age of eight, his father's connections must have been helpful. Dr. Lin senior was a cofounder in 1914 of the Ho Hong Bank. Headquartered in Singapore, the bank soon opened branches in Batavia and Palembang in the Dutch East Indies. In the 1920s it opened branches in Hong Kong and Shanghai. In 1932 it merged with two other banks to become the now well-known OCBC Bank. (Information on Ho Hong bank from Wikipedia). As well as providing funds, the Ho Suk Hua-chiao Chiu-hu Tuei (of Batavia) provided medical supplies and vehicles. ("Confidential Memorandum.")

Chinese (two of them physicians), it rapidly enlisted support from Chinese communities in the U.S. as well as from leaders in the American medical profession with Chinese ties. Several of its directors had been professors at PUMC. Aid also came from British organizations, principally the British Fund for the Relief of Distress in China (formerly the Lord Mayor's Fund), and the Chinese Medical Aid Committee.[51]

Articles by Lie Chen-Ie and Koh Keng-We provide a vignette of contributions by overseas Chinese Java medical teams to the work of the CRCMRC. After the Lugouqiao Incident in July 1937, a number of Chinese organizations and individuals in Batavia, led by Dr. Kwa Tjwan Sioe (柯全寿 Ke Quanshou),[52] raised funds and put together an ambulance unit of four physicians, fifteen nursing aides and nine ambulances, equipped with medical supplies and instruments and led by Dr. Go In Tjhan (吴英璨, Wu Yingcan). Lin met with this team in Hong Kong. They traveled north to Changsha, and then on to Xuzhou, Xuchang (Henan) and Xinyang (south Henan) before retreating to Wuhan. The team was unsuccessful in getting Nationalist army divisions to take advantage of its services and eventually headed back to Batavia, leaving its equipment with Communist military medical organizations.[53]

Dr. Kwa was part of a network of overseas Chinese leaders who took an interest in the welfare of Chinese people in China and abroad. In 1931, during the Yangtze flooding in Hubei, he sent a team of people and medical supplies to Wuhan to help with flood relief and two physicians from his convalescent hospital to participate in flood relief and preventive health work. After war erupted in 1937 he joined other overseas leaders

---

[51] For the British organizations, see Balme (1939), "The Medical Emergency in China." The League of Nations sent three teams in 1938 to engage in anti-epidemic work. These teams were assisted by CRC medical units but were required to limit their services to the civilian population and to maintain strict neutrality. See i) Lasnet (1939), 300–317; ii) "Medical Help for China," (1939), 616.

[52] I am grateful to Cheong Wai Yin of the Chinese Heritage Centre in Singapore for supplying me with the characters for Dr. Kwa's name and other information.

[53] Dr. Go was subsequently imprisoned by Japanese invaders in the Dutch East Indies for organizing medical assistance for resistance forces. Lie Chen Ie (2003), 28–31; Yinni Huayi Mingyi Ke Quanshou (2010). Lin mentioned in his Confidential Memorandum that he had received a gratifying response to his appeal for trucks, largely due to the efforts of Dr. Kwa in Batavia and Dr. Co Tui of ABMAC in New York. After the Dutch East Indies stopped sending funds to China through the Chinese Red Cross, Dr. Kwa arranged with Bishop Ronald O. Hall of Hong Kong for funds from the Batavia Overseas Chinese Committee and the Dutch East Indies government's Minister of Finance to be sent to the 'International' Red Cross Committee in Guiyang for relief purposes. See ABMAC box 23, National Red Cross Society of China Reports, "Confidential Report on the Medical Relief Corps, Transport, Training, etc.," June 28, 1941.

to organize emergency relief units to provide front line relief and plan long-term relief and fundraising. Advertisements elicited four hundred volunteers, from which came the team led by Dr. Wu Yingcan. Fundraising by Dr. Kwa, Hong Yuanyuan (洪渊源) and Situ Zan (司徒赞) between July 1937 and December 1941 yielded 50 million Hong Kong dollars (roughly equivalent to US \$6.2 million in currency values of 1940).[54] Some funds were used to buy badly needed medicines and ambulances, and the proceeds were divided between the Chinese Red Cross (Lin's Medical Relief Corps) and the China Defense League organized by Madam Sun Yat-sen (宋庆龄 Song Qingling). This illustrates the level of overseas Chinese support that Lin could count on in developing the CRCMRC.[55]

Lin's reports identify three phases in the MRC's development. In the first the units were chiefly attached to army base hospitals. With the second, beginning in summer 1938, the units pushed nearer the front, and some were sent to large field hospitals. The third began after the fall of Hankou in October 1938 and the Nationalist government's adoption of defense in depth (up to 150 km). This involved destruction of highways and railways to obstruct Japanese mechanical transport. Creation of roadless areas forced hospitals further to the rear, creating a gulf between casualties and treatment centers. Only bearer transport could bridge it, so local peasants were rounded up to fill out the Army's bearer units. As bearer transport was slow, serious and moderate casualties deteriorated en route, and many wounded soldiers died before reaching a rear hospital.

To address this problem the MRC reorganized its teams into smaller units of 1 physician, 1 nurse and 4 subordinates, with up to 10 bearers and sanitary assistants. A unit was assigned to an army corps to help each division organize a field hospital and clinic, sanitary routines, regimental medical posts and training routines for divisional medical personnel. The EMSTS developed simple manuals of standing orders covering the basic areas of medical and sanitary work, to assist field training.[56]

A problem for the MRC and other relief agencies had to do with the waves of refugees created by rapidly advancing mechanized armies. The Canadian missionary physician Dr. Robert B. McClure argued that the object

---

[54] See Latter (2004).

[55] Yinni Huayi Mingyi Ke Quanshou (2010).

[56] ABMAC box 23, National Red Cross Society of China Unit Reports, "Confidential Memorandum," May 15, 1941. Lin's strategies were reported to American health specialists by Robert Baird McClure (1941), 640–645 and Thomas Malone (1942): 256–260. Malone's article describes MRC work and the plight of refugees fleeing Canton at the time of the Japanese invasion in 1939. Smedley (1943, 507) reports that Lin was staying up late writing these manuals while she was staying in his cottage in 1940.

of this warfare was to destroy civilian morale and spread disease by creating waves of terrorized civilians. Cholera, typhus and scabies were diseases that could be generated and rapidly spread in this way. Antidotes, such as cholera vaccines and isotonic saline solution for cholera victims, were available, but delivery required a mobile transport system to get help to victims fast. Malnutrition, especially lack of salt, was another problem requiring a planned solution. Although Drs. McClure and Lin had an uneasy relationship, McClure saw that Lin and his aides were able to provide the needed relief. In McClure's judgment, "The fact that Dr. Lin did as well as he did in quickly putting a medical relief corps into service can be attributed only to the outstanding fortitude and courage of his handful of doctors and nurses." That was partially correct, as was Lin's ability to create a system through which they could do their work.[57]

Under Lin's leadership the MRC grew rapidly in size and scope:

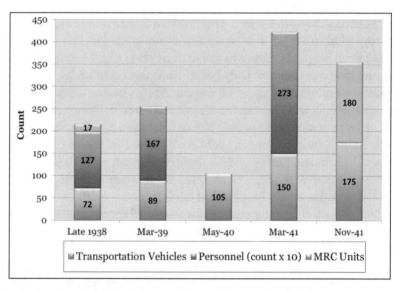

Graph 4.1: *Growth of Medical Relief Corps (MRC), 1938–1941. (Sources:* 1) ABMAC box 21, NHA 1940–41, "Health Program of NHA: Wartime Medical Relief," broadcast by Dr. F. C. Yen (Yan Fuqing), March 1939; 2) 1940 data are from materials found in the Jiangsu provincial archives in Nanjing and collected by Priscilla Armstrong; 3) ABMAC, box 22, National Red Cross Society of China, general folder, "Memorandum on the CRC-MRC, March 3, 1941." The latter report gives the growth in medical personnel; the greatest increase was in bearers and orderlies.)

---

[57] McClure (1941). As Graph 4.1 indicates, "handful of doctors and nurses" did not give an accurate sense of the number of people working for the MRC in November 1941.

During this period statistics compiled for ABMAC fundraising purposes reported that between January 1938 and December 1940 MRC units carried out 67,000 operations, applied 3.9 million dressings, treated almost 500,000 people for infectious diseases (mostly louse and mosquito-borne) and another 334,000 for special diets, and deloused some 450,000 soldiers and 2.5 million articles of clothing.[58]

MRC units also dealt with epidemics. In spring 1938 a cholera epidemic broke out in Guangdong, Hunan and Henan. Around twenty percent of those sick at the Yangtze River front suffered from dysentery and another ten percent from other enteric diseases. In August whole regiments were infected with malaria and an entire division stopped in its tracks. During that year the MRC distributed over fifteen million anti-malarial quinine tablets. Seventy percent of patients appearing at health stations had scabies; a number had the louse-borne relapsing fever.[59]

Medical Relief Corps accounts of patients in military hospitals recorded the sanitary conditions.

> Most hospital wards are untidy and the floors messy. Patients' clothes appear pathetic and uncared for. Their bodies are unwashed, their hair long and nails uncut, and their quilts covered with lice. The dysentery or diarrhea cases lie in beddings soaked with excreta...Many are infected with scabies...Numbers are also suffering from nutritional disturbances.[60]

Because of such conditions, prevention of disease through sanitation became an urgent aspect of MRC work. In September 1938 the MRC started a delousing, bathing and scabies (DBS) program serving military hospitals, and put seven DBS stations into operation. This grew by June 1940 into two hundred and two DBS units spread throughout the war areas along with others established by Army medical services.[61] At first, resistance

---

[58] ABMAC box 23, National Red Cross Society of China, Reports, "Memorandum on the CRCMRC, March 3, 1941." The data in the memorandum are given down to the last unit. However another series drawn from a 1943 source and covering the same period offers generally larger, but in the case of operations smaller, totals. Thus the figures should be taken as orders of magnitude.

[59] Ibid., "National Red Cross Society of China, Medical Relief Commission, Third Report, August-December 1938."

[60] Ibid.

[61] ABMAC box 2, "EMSTS...First Report, May 1938-June 1942,"; ii) ABMAC box 23, "Third Report," (see note 59); iii) Liu Yung-mao (1970). Lin's letter of April 25, 1939 to CRC President Wang Zhengting mentions that several MRC units served as instructional centers for training hospital staff to learn DBS and special diet procedures. See ABMAC box 22, Robert K. S. Lim, 1939. Around December 1939 the Central Military Commission gave Lin $105,000 to establish 222 DBS stations. $20,000 was sent to Guo Zuyuan (过祖源 T. S. Kuo)

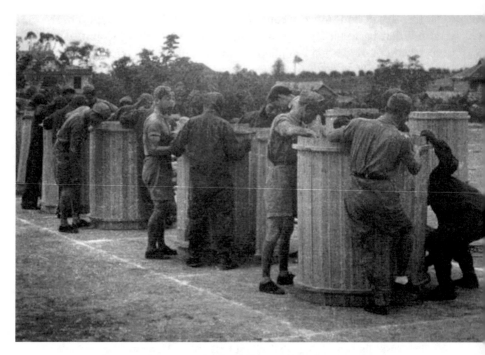

Photograph 4.4: *Medical Relief Corps (MRC) Delousing Station*
Pioneered in China by Dr. Lin and his sanitary engineering colleagues, the stations provided
low-cost means of keeping typhus, relapsing fever and scabies under control. (*Source*: ABMAC
Archive)

to DBS stations was quite widespread among rank and file soldiers. In
1939–40 the former warlord Feng Yuxiang (冯玉祥), now a nominal government minister, visited Tuyun'guan and received an account of Medical
Relief Corps training in preventive and sanitary care, along with a lecture
on the history of typhus and its catastrophic effect on modern European
wars. Feng exhorted trainees to make good use of such "new knowledge"
and thus contribute to military health and victory against Japan.[62]

In spring 1940, Lin and several of his staff traveled by foot through the
front line areas. Their aim was to protect soldiers from epidemic disease
by improving camp hygiene. By this time the war with Japan had entered
into a protracted stalemate, and wound casualties were giving way to

in Baozheng to set up DBS stations in the Northwest. Lin to Wang etc, December 14, 1939,
in ABMAC box 22.
    [62] Guo Zuyuan (1987) 9–10.

losses principally from malaria and gastrointestinal diseases.[63] To counteract the latter Lin and his engineering staff developed a Waste Water Control program to improve drinking water and management of human waste. This program was introduced in the Changsha military region and extended to other front line areas. In southwest China and along the Burma Road, where malaria was endemic, they started a malaria and mosquito control program using prophylactic drugs and instructions on how to cover the body at nighttime. To retard mosquito breeding some ponds were drained and water covered with kerosene. Many of these techniques were adapted from British army hygiene manuals.[64] So important did Lin view this work that he required all his medical and nursing staff to go through basic sanitary training.[65]

In the early war years MRC units traveled widely through the war areas. The first curative unit, set up in Hankou in December 1937, went to Zhengzhou with two other small units. Unit One was assigned to two base hospitals in Luoyang, where patient problems were mostly chronic. In February 1938, it moved to a base hospital in Xi'an with one thousand wounded soldiers, two hundred of them severely. The patients were lying on the ground with very little bedding, and the wards were dark and swarming with flies. In April it was ordered to Xuzhou in northwest Jiangsu province, where bitter fighting had been going on, and assigned to an evacuation hospital where the team was busy day and night. On May 13, Unit One and three other Medical Relief Corps units retreated by hospital train to Zhengzhou. The journey took three days with Japanese

---

[63] Liu Yung-mao, 1970; ABMAC box 22, Lin to Wang Zhengting, etc, April 20, 1940. A memorandum dated March 3, 1941, states that wound casualties were reduced to about a third of those during the first year of the war, but losses due to sickness had increased fourfold and were growing.

[64] According to Liu Yung-mao, these included such sources as the British army manual *Field Service Hygiene Notes*, second edition (New Delhi: Government of India Press, 1940), and Robert Svensson, *A Handbook of Malaria Control* (London: Raven Press, 1943). Examination of the 543- page 1945 edition of the *Field Service Hygiene Notes* indicates that this is a very thorough manual covering hygiene organization, climate and health, food and nutrition, water supplies, disposal of waste, hygiene of the camp and on the march, control of diseases, specimens, sick rates and statistical data. It has 32 pages of information on malaria control. The book also devotes many pages to the connections between nutrition and military fitness. Of dysentery it says, "bacillary dysentery, and its poor relation diarrhoea, have always been *the* diseases of armies in the field...The least carelessness in camp sanitation will be punished by an epidemic of dysentery." (338–339). Evidently Lin made good use of the *Hygiene Notes*.

[65] Liu Yung-mao (1970).

machine-gunning planes in pursuit. After crisscrossing central China, Unit One arrived in December 1938 in Luqi in Northwestern Hunan.[66]

The 46th "Java" Curative Unit, organized in Guangzhou in May 1938, had five doctors, seven nurses, one quartermaster, and four assistants. Its job was to assist the Guangdong provincial department of health with anti-epidemic and health propaganda work. In one place, where flies were abundant, it stressed sanitation and put on a play entitled "Guard my Health" at the local stadium. In Heyuan the people were better informed about hygiene and accepted inoculations. Japanese capture of Guangzhou in October 1938 forced the unit back to Qiyang, where it provided sanitary training. It was then assigned to the 172nd base hospital in Guilin. Other units were sent to Yan'an and to various places in Jiangxi province.[67]

The emphasis on hygienic training was by design. Several interviewees mentioned that Lin saw it as a chance to instill basic preventive health techniques in a large cadre of military health workers, who after the end of the war could carry this knowledge back to their home counties and contribute it to postwar reconstruction.[68] In fact he expected MRC units to help look after "civilian farmers" as well as the military units. "No one looks after their health," he noted, "so the work of our units in this regard is very important."[69]

Lin believed that the purpose of engaging in preventive and sanitary work was to preserve and build up the fighting strength of China's armed forces.[70] In view of the United Front patched up between Nationalist, Communist, and Northeastern military forces, he concluded that Red Cross medical relief units should remain politically neutral. He justified sending MRC teams to Communist military units by saying that: "The really important roles in the defense of the country which the 8th Route and New 4th Armies play justifies the measure of support they are (both)

---

[66] National Red Cross Society of China, Unit reports, in ABMAC, box 23.

[67] ABMAC, box 23, ibid.

[68] Interviews with Wang K'ai-hsi, Liu Yung-mao and Yang Wen-tah. See also Liu Yung-mao (1970).

[69] ABMAC box 22, Robert K. S. Lim, 1939, Lin to Co Tui August 27, 1940. In a letter of December 13, 1940, to the distinguished American medical missionary Edward Hume, Lin said that he had taken steps to coordinate his training programs with those of the NHA's Public Health Training Institute, so that similar methods would be taught and both organizations work towards the *common goal of placing modern medicine firmly in rural areas.* (also in ABMAC box 22; emphasis added).

[70] Liu Yung-mao (1970); Chen Tao (陈韬) (1987), 191–198.

getting."[71] It was this attitude that got him into trouble with the Nationalist high command, for whom destruction of Communist forces remained a major concern throughout the war with Japan.

PART II: POLITICS PREVAIL OVER HEALTHCARE

Reorganization of Chinese Red Cross Headquarters and Downgrading of Lin Kesheng

The Chinese Red Cross had become an agency of the Nationalist government as early as 1932.[72] At the first Board meeting held in 1934 Wang Zhengting (王正廷 former minister of foreign affairs) was appointed president, and Liu Hongsheng (刘鸿生 O. S. Lieu, at that time general manager of China Merchants' Steam Navigation Company) and Shi Liangcai (史量才, a newspaper publisher later assassinated in November 1934) were appointed vice presidents.[73] Chiang Kaishek took the position of honorary president, and several party and government leaders became honorary vice presidents.[74] In 1936 the CRC was repositioned under the National Health Administration.[75] From May 1937 to September 1938 Wang Zhengting was ambassador in Washington, D.C., and for six months after that in Hong Kong working for the Bank of Communications before moving to Chongqing in 1939.[76] By that time the CRC had its general representative office in Hong Kong. In early 1940 the office moved to Chongqing and started operating there on April 1.[77]

Under this arrangement Dr. Liu Ruiheng was within his authority to designate Lin to head up the MRC; but with Liu's exit from government in

---

[71] ABMAC box 22, Robert K.S. Lim 1939, Lin to Co Tui, April 28,1939. According to Guo Shaoxing, two MRC units were sent to aid the New Fourth Army on the advice of Agnes Smedley. See Guo Shaoxing (郭绍兴) (1987), 7.

[72] At that time it was under the War Ministry for war operations and the Interior and Foreign Ministries for famine relief and foreign activities. Lamson (1935), 488.

[73] Because he was highly critical of Chiang Kaishek's Japan policy, Shi was eliminated by agents of Dai Li's secret police organization. See Eastman (1991), 29, and biography of Shi in Boorman (1967), III, 126–128.

[74] They included Huang Shaoxiong 黄绍雄, an anti-Communist general serving as Interior Minister, and Wu Tiecheng 吴铁城, Mayor of Shanghai and from 1941–1948 Secretary General of Guomindang party headquarters.

[75] Information is from Zhongguo Hongshizihui Bainian (2004), volume one, 52–55, 61, 464. I am indebted to Christina and Peter Gilmartin for making this work available to me.

[76] Boorman (1967), III, 364.

[77] Zhongguo Hongshizihui Bainian (2004), 61.

early 1938 Lin was left without effective party or government patronage. Wang's return to the helm of the Chinese Red Cross in early 1939 was a move by Chiang Kaishek to restore party and government control over CRC headquarters and operations.[78] The most influential directors by then were Mr. Wang and the two vice presidents, Du Yuesheng (杜月笙 Y. S. Doo, the powerful Shanghai gangland leader) and Liu Hongsheng, who had business ties. Under their leadership the Red Cross office in Hong Kong became the primary funnel for overseas funds and supplies. The secretary general, Dr. Pang Jingzhou, was authorized to control all correspondence, finance and supplies and to liaise between the MRC and the Board. Everything now had to "pass through his hands."[79]

These changes soon cramped Dr. Lin's management of the MRC. The MRC was repositioned, wrote Lin, as a subunit of the Board of Directors "in which none of us is represented."[80] In May Lin informed Dr. Frank Co Tui (ABMAC cofounder, executive vice president, and Lin's chief American confidant), that the CRC Directors had suddenly issued many new regulations and told him not to bother about funds or corresponding abroad.[81]

Around the beginning of 1940 Dr. Pan Ji (潘骥 C. Pan, also known as Pan Xiao'e 潘小萼), was appointed CRC secretary general.[82] A graduate of the Harvard School of Public Health and cousin of the influential New Life leader Huang Renlin (黄仁霖 J. L. Huang), Pan had previously served as acting Chief of Bacteriology and Epidemic Disease Control at the Central Field Health Station and then as Commissioner of Health of Jiangxi Province, giving up a "comfortable position" to work with "country people." According to Huang, Pan had organized a group of student volunteers and with their help got rid of malaria and cholera in that province.[83]

---

[78] I am indebted to Caroline Reeves for pointing out that Guomindang control over CRC began as early as the early 1930s; in the 1940s it extended from policy to membership.

[79] ABMAC box 22, C. Y. Wu to Co Tui, April 8, 1939, in. In 1937, when Dr. Liu Ruiheng was Minister of the Combined Health Services Ministry and in charge of all CRC relief organizations, he detached Dr. Wu from the National Health Administration and sent him to Hong Kong with CRC Board approval to take charge of forwarding supplies.

[80] ABMAC box 22, Lin to Co Tui, personal and confidential, April 21, 1939.

[81] Ibid., Lin to Co Tui, May 8, 1939.

[82] Dr. Pang Jingzhou found a position as chief of the Yunnan-Burma railway medical service. See Lin to Co Tui, August 26, 1941, in ABMAC, box 22. Note: Dr. Pan Ji has the same name as a man who served in the Red Army in Jiangxi and Fujian provinces and died a martyr's death in 1931.

[83] i) For Dr. Pan's CFHS position, see Central Field Health Station (1934); ii) for Harvard degree, relationship with Huang, and work with Huang as health consultant to the War

This change was highly damaging to Dr. Lin and his work. As a well-connected Guomindang official with public health credentials, Pan's job was to assist Wang Zhengting in restoring CRC control over Lin's operation. In his confidential report to ABMAC, Lin claimed that since 1940, when Pan was appointed secretary general, the MRC was restricted in every way. Budget revisions were delayed and work programs had to be submitted for Board approval, despite the Board's lack of technical expertise. Medical and transport units could not recover costs in reasonable time because of red tape in the MRC accounting department (appointed and controlled by Chinese Red Cross Headquarters (CRCHQ)). Lin himself was authorized to make local purchases only up to NC 1,000 (US $53). Larger amounts required approval from the Hong Kong purchasing committee.[84]

Other restrictions, felt as personal slights, came down on Lin. In June Wang Zhengting advised him to "delay no further your supplying this office MONTHLY and REGULARLY with GOOD photographs of accomplished things and a SUMMARY of WORK in both Chinese and English (two copies for each)."[85] To ABMAC Vice President Dr. Co Tui he wrote: "Dr. Lim (Lin) has exceeded his powers by making direct appeals to you... All appeals... have to be made to your Bureau ONLY from the general office of this society and not from any of its subordinate officers. I am writing to Dr. Lim and other officers of this organization to this effect."[86] In August 1940, when Japanese encroachment in Southeast Asia was making the supply situation increasingly precarious, Lin telegrammed Chinese ambassadors in the U.S. and U.K. to urge Haiphong and Rangoon to permit MRC medical supplies to pass through. This elicited a rebuke from Wang:

> You know of course that I have a very high opinion of your work as head of our Relief Commission from the technical and medical point of view. Your administrative side has many weak points, the most serious of which is your inability to play the game as a TEAM. Your recent action in wiring direct to our embassies in London and Washington is a very clear evidence. I must

Area Service Corps, see Huang (1984), 28, 63–64, 118. The claim of ridding Jiangxi of both cholera and malaria with a group of student volunteers is not credible.

[84] When the Ministry of Education was setting up the National Zhongzheng College of Medicine late in 1936, it appointed Lin chair of a planning commission for the college and Pan Ji as a commission member in his capacity as Jiangxi Commissioner of Health. When Pan left that position he also left the Commission. No mention of this liaison was found in the Lin correspondence, but it points to a prior history between the two men before trouble over management of the CRCMRC surfaced. See Xu Shusheng (徐书生) (2008).

[85] ABMAC box 22, Wang Zhengting to Lin, June 20, 1940.

[86] ABMAC box 23, Wang Cheng-ting folder, Wang to Co Tui, April 4, 1940.

say I was very much surprised as well as grieved over such an action which amounts to insubordination.

Seething from this criticism, Lin fired off a long confidential letter to Dr. Co Tui. Of his relationship with Wang he said: "I am not to 'appeal' for funds, supplies or help of any kind, only the Directors can do so. So my 'appeal' for the Vaccine Plant and my telegrams to various people...fell foul of the Presidential fist." Lin added that he might be fired, but that whatever happened he would still continue working for the army and the people at the front through the Emergency Medical Services Training Schools. He concluded: "This is China and it is part of her troubles."[87]

Lin's Ambitions for the EMSTS and the MRC

Despite problems with Red Cross Headquarters, Lin Kesheng continued to work on developing an integrated healthcare training and service network (essentially a public healthcare system) throughout the various war areas. Only a few months after the initial training school settled down outside Guiyang, the Central Military Commission ordered him to begin establishing branch training schools. In due course he set up five branch schools at Baozheng, Shaanxi (August 1939), Yiyang, Jiangxi (October 1940), Junxian, Hubei (October 1941), Qianjiang, Sichuan (May 1941), and Dongan, Hunan (Autumn 1942).[88]

The branch schools carried out much the same programs as the central school. For example, the third branch school set up six training departments and provided clinical services to the 17th army corps hospital. The school concentrated on nursing and provided three-month basic and advanced courses. It provided a sanitation course covering chlorination, food sanitation, construction of latrines, night soil disposal, mosquito and rat control, and delousing. The trainees spent a little over one month working in the two hundred-bed hospital. They led a frugal life, having two meals a day and sleeping on wooden mattresses. The director, Dr. Ma Jiaji (马家骥, PUMC 1935), reported that they were "excellent material"

---

[87] ABMAC box 22, Lin to Co Tui, August 27, 1940.
[88] ABMAC box 2, EMSTS...First Report, May 1938–June 1942. According to Lin to Wang Zhengting (June 3, 1939) the instruction to set up the first branch school came in the Central Military Commission's order number 6720.

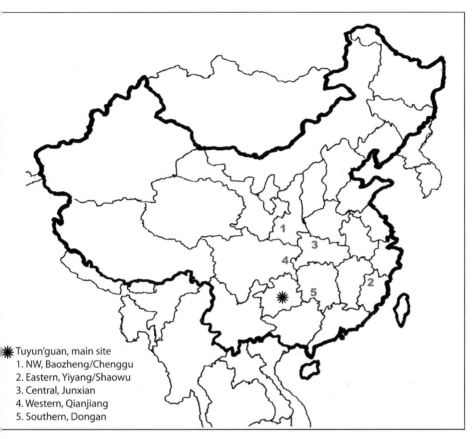

* Tuyun'guan, main site
1. NW, Baozheng/Chenggu
2. Eastern, Yiyang/Shaowu
3. Central, Junxian
4. Western, Qianjiang
5. Southern, Dongan

Map 4.1: *Locations of Emergency Medical Service Training Schools (EMSTS) 1938–1942*
The EMSTS schools were the means by which Dr. Lin Kesheng built up a corps of well-trained army medical aides. Lin used army medical training manuals developed in British India from experience during World War One, to provide trainees with state of the art training. By 1942 there were six schools. Two more were added later to help China's soldiers prepare for the recapture of Burma. Altogether 16,000 or more people (predominantly soldiers) received healthcare training through Dr. Lin's training schools. (*Source*: J. R. and A. S. Watt)

and if given a course in public health after the war would make competent rural health officers.[89]

The central school in Guiyang set up a six hundred bed training hospital. In September 1939 it added an orthopedic center with two hundred

---

[89] ABMAC box 2, EMSTS, Third Branch EMSTS First Annual Report, June 1941–June 1942.

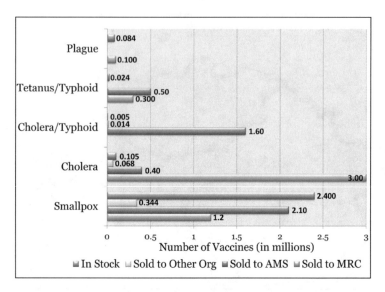

Graph 4.2: *Medical Relief Corps (MRC) Vaccine Plant Production and Sales, March 1941–1942*
The vaccine plant director was Dr. Chen Wengui; the MRC administered around 500,000 cholera doses purchased during January 1941 to March 1942. *Note* AMS is Army Medical Service, referring to the agency headed by Dr. Lu Zhide. (*Sources*: ABMAC Archive, box 2, EMSTS First Report, May 1938–June 1942; details in ABMAC box 8, items #10 and #11.)

beds, a physiotherapy service, a machine shop for making artificial limbs, and an occupational training program. The school linked up with the Chinese Industrial Cooperatives (Indusco), for vocational training.[90] By November 1940 there were two orthopedic centers and a third being organized.[91] From ABMAC Lin obtained a vaccine plant, which between March 1941 and June 1942 produced six million doses of smallpox vaccine and 6.2 million of other vaccine (see Graph 4.2).[92]

---

[90] i) Note on orthopedic hospital and physiotherapy service from ABMAC box 2, EMSTS, First Report, May 1938–June 1942; ii) note on collaboration with Indusco from ABMAC box 22, Lim correspondence, Memorandum on the EMSTS and the Orthopedic Centers, March 3, 1941. That link did not last, but the main center did provide vocational training, in which shoemaking and carpentry courses attracted interest. See ABMAC box 8, EMSTS 1940–42; iii) One of the patients treated at the orthopedic center was Dr. Xie Xide (谢希德), later to become President of Fudan University. She was ten years old at the time. (Personal communication).

[91] ABMAC box 22, Lim to Co Tui, November 18, 1940.

[92] ABMAC box 2, EMSTS First Report, May 1938–June 1942; details in ABMAC box 8, items #10 and #11.

In 1941 a department of medical equipment was organized and a library established with a printing press for putting out future publications. Between February 1939 and June 1942 the central training school trained 2,750 students and the branch schools another 2,000.[93]

To raise army medical standards Lin planned a staged six-year program to convert assistant medical personnel into physicians. Even by 1942–43 only eighteen percent of the Army's evacuation and base hospital staff and only eleven percent of its divisional staff were graduates of qualified medical schools, while only one hundred medical school graduates a year were willing to join the army medical services. Lin and his staff felt that they were more motivated and competent to train army physicians than existing medical schools.[94]

During this period the MRC transport system began to bring in supplies along the Burma Road as well as distribute them to military units. From the railhead at Lashio (in Burma) to Kunming, trucks traveled 715 miles crossing the Mekong and Salween rivers. Drivers negotiated severe grades rising to elevations of 8,500 feet and many dangerous turns along a dusty roadbed averaging only nine feet wide. The road to Guiyang was another 415 miles and from Kunming to Chongqing another 700 miles, and another 480 miles to Luzhou on the upper Yangzi. It took two tons of gasoline to bring one ton of goods to Chongqing. Impressed by the MRC system of fuel and repair stations along its transport network, the American Red Cross representative Walter Wesselius recommended in 1941 provision of a year's gas and oil credit along with a supply of spare parts.[95] With trucks and ambulances supplied by overseas Chinese and through ABMAC and the American Red Cross, the Medical Relief Corps developed a transport system almost equal in size to the Army Medical Administration's, which helped to move the Army's as well as the MRC's medical supplies.[96]

---

[93] ABMAC box 2, EMSTS . . . First Report, May 1938–June 1942.

[94] ABMAC box 2, EMSTS, Report by Dr. Isidore Snapper (undated but sometime during 1943). According to Snapper, the plan was "wholeheartedly" supported by AMA director Lu Zhide but opposed by General He Yingqin. See Lin to the Rockefeller Foundation representative Dr. R. C. Balfour, June 18, 1941, in ABMAC box 22, National Red Cross Society of China.

[95] ARC archive, file 985, box 1394, *China War Relief*, volume 1, appendix 51–55, Walter Wesselius letter 110; A. N. Young, "Overland Transportation and Distribution . . ." August 15, 1941, appendix 56; Walter Wesselius, document dated December 12, 1940, appendix 60–61. Wesselius noted in letter 110 that Lim "made a very masterful presentation of his program . . . and a very favorable impression on the (Chongqing) ARC committee."

[96] i) ABMAC, box 22, Robert K. S. Lim, 1939, Rong Dushan (荣独山, T. S. Jung) to Co Tui, May 4, 1940; ii) report of November 20, 1940, to China War Relief Association of

In the field Lin promoted a broad range of diagnostic, preventive and curative services, backed by coordinated supply and transport systems and reinforced at the front by a continuing emphasis on field training by MRC units. Because of the prevalence of malnutrition, MRC field units developed a special army dietary service. In the 18 months up to the end of 1940 its kitchens in army hospitals served 236,000 patients.[97]

Problems in Army Medical Management

The divisions of labor and turf in the Nationalist government's Army Medical operations present a sharp contrast to Lin's unified system for managing and transporting personnel, supplies and services. After the government settled on defense in depth, the duties of army medical care were allocated as follows: In the combat zone, divisional and regimental medical units remained in charge of medical relief. In the intermediate communication zone, responsibility for receiving stations, ambulance convoys and field hospitals lay with the Quartermaster General's office in the Board of Supply and Transport. The Army Medical Administration had charge over medical units in the rear zone. It provided base hospitals (up to one thousand beds), orthopedic centers, hospitals for severely wounded, and medical supply depots. It also had charge over fieldwork in the communication zone.[98] Since August 1938 the direction of the AMA had passed to Dr. Lu Zhide, Lin's close associate at PUMC.[99]

Such a division of duties seriously endangered the lives of wounded soldiers moved from front lines to rear hospitals. When Dr. Lu returned to China, he was tasked to set up the receiving stations and field hospitals, and put in charge of medical evacuation but lacking power to enforce orders on army group commanders. Lu spent much time in the field devising ways to speed up evacuation of the wounded and criticizing field medical staff for not moving the wounded faster or keeping their units

---

America, San Francisco, in same folder; iii) memo of October 31, 1941, on medical transportation, in Lim (correspondence) folder.

[97] ABMAC box 22, Lin to Professor T[homas] Addis, December 4, 1940. A graduate, like Lin, of Watson's College and Edinburgh University Medical School, Addis (1881–1949) became an internationally respected specialist in renal disease and the application of dietary therapy to its treatment. A member of the Stanford University faculty, he became sympathetic in the 1930s to left wing causes. See Kevin V. Lemley and Linus S. Pauling (1994).

[98] Carlson (1940a), chapter 10; Utley (1939), chapter 4.

[99] Carlson (1940b).

clean.[100] He worked with Lin to standardize supplies, prepare sterilized first-aid dressings and helped set up the emergency training school. Writing in 1939, Carlson concluded that the Army medical administration was still far from satisfactory in its handling of wounded and diseased soldiers, "But tremendous progress had been made ... since the beginning of hostilities at Shanghai" in 1937.[101]

To staff 292 military hospitals, 127 receiving stations, and the medical units of 250 divisions required 12,000 or more physicians. But only twenty-two percent of army medical personnel had such a qualification; the rest were nurses and dressers doing physicians' work. Few had prior wartime experience. Lack of stretcher-bearers in the field, where the average minimum casualty rate per engagement was ten percent of fighting strength, was overwhelming. The AMA had to find civilian 'volunteers' to transport wounded and sick soldiers.[102]

Lu wanted to reorganize the AMA, establish a standing medical corps (which he observed on his visit to Britain), and have the EMSTS recognized as the principal army medical field training centers. Research was needed to study malnutrition and defense against chemical and bacterial warfare. Lu had many other proposals, but he knew it would take "not months but years" to solve such problems. His enthusiastic support of the MRC and the Medical Training Schools reflected his frustration over problems with the established Army medical units.

Yet the problems did not lie solely with army personnel or management. Chinese armies were fighting a twentieth century war with the attitudes and methodology of a bygone era. One of the serious problems was the lack of educated, middle class leaders in the armed forces. The Army, wrote Utley, was thought of by Chinese middle and upper classes as an army not of their sons, husbands and brothers, but of coolies and peasants (in other words illiterate 'others'). Armies were generally all-male organizations, in which officers often disciplined the rank and file with beatings.[103] With a few bright exceptions one rarely found women in nursing or even visiting army hospitals. Until the educated and wealthy mobilized for war service, the old conception of the Army as apart from the nation would not disappear.

---

[100] For an example, see Smedley (1943), 430.
[101] Carlson (1940a), chapter 10.
[102] ABMAC, box 5, Cheng Pao-nan folder, "The Army Medical Service ..."
[103] Lary (1985), especially chapter 4.

Lin's Move to Convert EMSTS and MRC into Centers
of Modern Medicine

In 1939 the United Front against Japan was still functioning. The MRC
continued to attract educated youth and increase its technical services
to Army medical units. Lin and his senior associates, especially his original deputy Dr. Peng Damou (彭达谋), worked with field commanders
on plans to develop closer cooperation between the MRC and the field
armies.[104] Following his two-month tour of front line areas during spring
1940, Lin reported that despite evidence of widespread sickness, treatment
of wounds had improved and better preventive and curative services were
found among the frontline divisions.[105] In November 1940 he reported
that the EMSTS was recognized as an official government agency.[106]

The new regional EMSTS training schools had the capacity to train army
hospital and medical field personnel and act as a base for MRC front line
units. By this time Nationalist China's armies had some 20,000 medical
officers and 280,000 medical aides, most of them still largely untrained.[107]
By March 1941, the EMSTS were redefined as War Area Medical Centers
(WAMC), responsible not only for training but also for technical services,
anti-epidemic work, and treatment of medical and orthopedic cases. Lin
felt that prevention of disease had become so urgent that it was helping to "diminish economic loss and prevent social and political unrest."[108]
Throughout 1941 Lin continued to promote the war area medical center
concept, saying "I feel this is a great opportunity to set up in each of the
War Areas a center for modern medicine, which will serve not only during
the war but in the days following to help in reconstruction and to continue the spirit of service for the people and the State, which is now ... the
essential duty of military service."[109]

---

[104] ABMAC, box 22, Lin to Wang Zhengting, December 5, 1939; Lin to Roger Greene,
November 11, 1941.

[105] ABMAC box 22, National Red Cross Society of China, Lin letter dated June 14, 1940,
(filed in correspondence for the year 1941).

[106] ABMAC box 22, Lin to Co Tui, November 5, 1940, and November 18, 1940.

[107] Ibid., Lin to Co Tui, November 18, 1940.

[108] ABMAC box 22, Lim folder, Memo of March 3, 1941, on the EMSTS and the Orthopedic Centers.

[109] Ibid., Lin to Co Tui, August 8, 1941, and August 9, 1941. In a letter of June 8, 1941,
to the Rockefeller Foundation China representative Dr. M. C. Balfour, Dr. Lin equated the
military medical structure, from the WAMC down to army and divisional units, with the
civil structure of provincial to county (*xian*) civilian health centers, arguing that the former
would serve the latter in a postwar reconstruction period.

Lin's next idea was to integrate the CRCMRC into the overall WAMC strategy. In a memorandum to Dr. Co Tui, he noted that the MRC had strengthened the Army medical units technically, provided transportation and supplies, and lent staff to the training schools and divisional medical units. It was now essential, he argued, to regularize the MRC as auxiliary to the Army medical services and to place it under the direction of the Army Medical Administration.[110]

Political Troubles Assail Dr. Lin

Lin's desire to integrate the MRC into the Army medical services illustrates the conflict between his military-oriented field command and the civilian and party-managed leadership at CRC Headquarters. I will now summarize the process by which Lin's relationship with CRCHQ and certain political and military leaders became increasingly strained and in due course ruptured.

According to Lin's confidential report of June 28, 1941, reports surfaced in 1940 charging him and his staff with pro-Communist activities. In August 1940 Lin was summoned to the Generalissimo's office to explain the charges. As a result of this meeting Chiang decided to set up a political department at Tuyun'guan. A party official by name Wang Qiamin (王洽民) led a group of political workers to Tuyun'guan to carry out this order.[111]

From December 1940 to March 1941 accusations mounted. This was during and subsequent to the bitterly contested Southern Anhui Wannan Incident (皖南事变) on January 7, 1941, between 9,000 troops of the Communist New Fourth Army, including a large medical contingent, and a Nationalist army of over 80,000 men. Lin again defended his conduct before Chiang, who continued to express support but said he feared Communist infiltration of the MRC.

Articles by Guo Shaoxing (郭绍兴) and others, published by the Chinese Red Cross in 1987, clarify the extent to which Chinese Communist Party underground members penetrated the MRC.[112] Following the Nationalist government's retreat to Hankou in early 1938, contact was made between Lin and Ye Jianying (叶剑英), the Eighth Route Army agent in Wuhan.

---

[110] ABMAC box 22, Lin correspondence folder, letter dated October 31, 1941.
[111] Wang Youchun (汪犹春) (1987a), 106, 113.
[112] See especially Guo Shaoxing (1987), 3–8.

In summer 1938 local CCP leaders set up a secret MRC party branch with Guo Shaoxing as branch secretary. Before long the branch had over ten party members and over twenty members of a people's vanguard corps.[113] In April–May 1939 the branch convened a secret meeting led by its new regional supervisor Yuan Chaojun(袁超俊). The meeting set up a general CCP branch with Guo as secretary and three sub-branches, one attached to the MRC transport unit. The acting transport director was the Qinghua engineering graduate and CCP underground member Zhang Wenjin (章文晋). Zhang arranged for distribution of Marxist-Leninist literature and other 'progressive' books and magazines to some seventy MRC units in northwest, southwest and central China.

As a result of these initiatives the CCP team persuaded many MRC workers to sympathize with their war aims. They got over twenty MRC teams sent to Yan'an and other CCP base areas. They garnered support from progressive youth, foreign doctors (many from the Spanish Civil War) and international antifascist fighters, notably Agnes Smedley. As well as doing publicity for the MRC, she collected supplies and funds for medical units of the Eighth Route and New Fourth Armies and was able to get two MRC units sent to help the New Fourth Army. According to Guo, she visited Tuyun'guan during the summer of 1939 and met with Mao Huaqiang (毛华强, an underground party member) in Lin's office to discuss his political work in the EMSTS.[114]

In 1940, the Guomindang initiated counter measures by sending a special agent to the EMSTS to set up a political department and undo the work of the CCP underground organization. This was Wang Qiamin. It appointed political leaders for the EMSTS branch schools, set up MRC-EMSTS party branches, enlisted party members and carried out anti-CCP propaganda.[115]

Lin had for some time been the object of venal gossip in missionary and bureaucratic circles, fed by his success in accumulating drugs, equip-

---

[113] Guo Shaoxing (1987), 4.

[114] Guo Shaoqing (1987), 5–7. Zhang Wenjin acted as interpreter. Smedley does not mention this visit in *Battle Hymn*. A year later, when Smedley was in Chongqing with deteriorating health, Dr. Lin took her to Tuyun'guan and personally took care of her before sending her on to Guilin and Hong Kong. See Smedley (1943), 506–509. It is possible that Guo's memory is off by a year; but given the Guomindang high command's close scrutiny of the MRC in 1940, it would be surprising if Smedley had used Lin's office to engage in conversations that could have hugely embarrassed him and endangered a young CCP party member. See also Wang Youchun (1987a), 101–103, where Smedley is reported as visiting Tuyun'guan in the spring of 1940, while Lin was away visiting the front lines.

[115] Guo Shaoqing (1987), 8.

ment and funds for the MRC.[116] Around the middle of 1940 Dr. Pan Ji initiated an underground attack against Lin, designed to undermine his control over the MRC and his credibility as a leader. While attending a dinner party in Chongqing in summer 1940 Smedley heard a foreigner and a Chinese discussing a secret memo reportedly delivered by Pan to Dai Li (戴笠), the dreaded head of the Guomindang's secret police. This allegedly accused Lin of being corrupt and of using Red Cross trucks to transport Communist literature into China. Smedley angrily accused two or three members of the Red Cross Board of "trying to drive Lin from his position and make room for one of their own henchmen."[117]

It is not clear to what extent Lin was aware of the CCP initiatives within his organizations. But 1940 was a watershed year in which these competing party initiatives within the MRC came to a head. Because of the charges raised by Guomindang and CRC leaders, Lin decided to resign at the CRC annual meeting in February 1941. An effort by Madame Chiang to forestall this rift failed and Lin announced his resignation. But the directors were ordered by the Generalissimo not to release him and to resolve the difficulties. Lin requested the return to the MRC of much of the autonomy it once enjoyed. However, his request was tabled at a Board meeting one-month later in Chongqing.[118]

In May 1941, Lin met with Chiang Kaishek to counter the charge that he was a Communist who had organized one hundred and fifty units to work with the armed forces on the instructions of the CCP and was using the EMSTS to propagate Communist doctrines to students. The Generalissimo told Lin he didn't know about this charge, although according to Lin the Central Military Commission, of which Chiang was the head, had relayed it to all armies and army organizations.[119] Chiang again expressed

---

[116] For a sampling see Smedley (1943), 216.

[117] Smedley (1943), 501, 515.

[118] An interesting commentary on Lin's attempted resignation is worth noting. Dr. Lin had a close relationship with Mrs. C. M. Chen (wife of the Guomindang martyr Chen Qimei), as did the Guomindang security chief Dai Li. Mrs. Chen's nephew was Zhang Wenjin (whose underground name was Chang Hongdao). Zhang enjoyed Dr. Lin's support, and at one time all the faculty wrote a note denying Zhang's CCP affiliations. Because of their mutual friendship with Mrs. Chen, Dai Li "was very good" to Dr. Lin but suggested that he should resign his MRC position. Zhang later became Zhou Enlai's English language secretary in Chongqing. Information from interview with Dr. Wang Kaixi, August 27, 1987.

[119] It could have been relayed in routine reports not brought to Chiang's attention. In a letter to Drs. Van Slyke (ABMAC President) and Co Tui dated November 10, 1942, Dr. Lin charged that personal relations between Dr. Pan and certain members of Chiang's HQ (this would include the New Life leader Huang Renlin) facilitated the submitting of such

confidence in Lin, but General He Yingqin told Lin he suspected that Communists were trying to influence the troops through the medical officers. In his correspondence with Americans Lin attributed these attacks to the mentality of Chinese officialdom.[120]

However the charges of Communist infiltration of the MRC are confirmed by Guo's 1987 account. During the second United Front period (basically 1937–1940) Lin sent Medical Relief Corps units to work with the Chinese Communist Party's Eighth Route Army and New Fourth Army. He signed up the team of left wing European doctors from the Spanish Civil War, several of whom were Communist party members. He accepted support from the pro-CCP China Defense League led by Song Qingling. He was friendly with Agnes Smedley, and he had prewar professional ties with Dr. Shen Qizhen (沈其震), the leader of the Communist New Fourth Army medical service. In autumn 1939 Shen stopped in Guiyang to ask Lin to send two medical teams and a large supply of anti-malarial medicine to the New Fourth Army.[121] Lastly, several Qinghua University engineering graduates in the MRC transport services were suspected rightly of being CCP members or sympathizers.

Lin added to these suspicions by insisting on the neutrality of the MRC and downplaying the Guomindang's fear of Communism. The Red Cross icon became for him the symbol that medical work should serve all, and he transmitted this idea to the younger people who came to serve the MRC out of respect for his leadership.[122] In sum, Lin Kesheng stood fast on combining idealism and medical science to save lives of wounded people regardless of their political affiliation. But this stance ran up against the struggle in top Guomindang circles over whether the Nationalists should focus more on resisting the Japanese or on overcoming Chinese Communism. The main Chinese opposition to Lin came from those in the Guomindang who embraced the latter cause. Even the Generalissimo, who is sometimes depicted as trying to straddle this division, was vexed by Lin's neutralism. At one of their three meetings the following dialogue is reported to have occurred:

---

charges and their dissemination as routine reports from General HQ. See ABMAC, box 38, correspondence folder.

[120] ABMAC box 23, Confidential report, June 28, 1941.

[121] See biography of Dr. Shen in Feng and Li (1991), 128–132. Dr. Shen undertook research at PUMC on neurotransmission under Dr. Lin's direction.

[122] A characteristic statement of this idea can be found in Shi Zhengxin (1987), 81.

Chiang: Why do you send medical units and drugs to the Eighth Route Army
and the New Fourth Army?
Lin: The Red Cross is an international organization...
Chiang (sternly): This is China![123]

Chiang concluded that although Lin was medically essential he was politically naive. He ordered Wang Qiamin to take over management of Lin's
office, set up political study activities and get rid of left wing propaganda.
In 1942 the political departments were reorganized as Guomindang party
branches. Overtly the political workers taught the Three People's Principles and the Five Power Constitution, provided exhortations on Sun-
day mornings and supervised weddings. Their real job was to monitor
suspect political activities and build up party membership. According to
Israel Epstein, they were "soon thriving on the sale of foreign donations
of drugs."[124] Because the political conditions were becoming unfavorable,
the CCP underground leadership dispersed its MRC members to safer
locations.[125]

Fights over Control of Assets, Lin in Burma and India, and Lin's Resignation from the MRC

Another dispute between Lin and CRCHQ was over deployment of CRC
and MRC assets. At the beginning of the war these amounted mainly to
east coast hospitals and urban clinics, which soon fell under Japanese control. Lin's success in organizing the MRC and his ability to raise support
from overseas Chinese, North American and British sympathizers, had
created a flow of funds, equipment and supplies to the MRC. In 1939 Lin
was forced to ask Dr. Co Tui of ABMAC to address contributions intended
for him directly to the MRC.[126] Wang Zhengting is said to have been an
ineffective fundraiser,[127] but he was able to get MRC resources back
under Board control, and in November 1940, when the effects of wartime

[123] Lin Jingcheng (林竞成) (1987), 70.
[124] Israel Epstein (1947), 135.
[125] Guo Shaoqing (1987). See also Wang Youchun (1987), 106, 113; and Lü Yunming
(吕运明) (1987), 190. While he was ambassador in Washington, Zhang Wenjin credited his escape from Guiyang to Dr. Zhou Shoukai, a PUMC graduate and one of Lin's
trusted lieutenants, who died in 1970 during the Cultural Revolution. This revelation
occurred during a conversation with Dr. Zhou's widow. See http://www.xmnn.cn/dzbk/
xmrb/20070710/200707/t20070710_252123.htm.
[126] ABMAC box 22, Lin to Co Tui, April 21, 1939.
[127] Ibid., Co Tui to Lin, April 11, 1939, in Lim correspondence folder.

inflation were keenly felt, Lin again had to ask Co Tui to indicate clearly the destination of ABMAC supplies, otherwise they would be distributed by CRCHQ "at its discretion."[128]

Early in 1941 the American Red Cross (ARC) became a major potential source of aid, replacing the Dutch East Indies Chinese communities, whose financial help was dwindling and would soon be cut off. On March 5 Wang Zhengting signed an appeal to the ARC, prepared by the MRC, to provide one year's medical supplies and transport facilities. The response of China's ARC director was lukewarm, proposing only a three-month transportation budget. Lin met with Roosevelt's personal envoy Lauchlin Currie in Hong Kong and was dismayed to be told, "I know all about you—you do not take orders."[129] Fortunately the ARC field director, Walter Wesselius, agreed to support the appeal.[130]

Meanwhile the National Health Administration, which had been paying Lin a salary since 1937, removed him from its payroll. The CRC Headquarters insisted that he go on their payroll, and he was obliged to agree.[131] With Lin now in a state of financial subordination his relations with Wang Zhengting improved, and the CRCHQ promised support for the MRC field program for the next year.[132] In October 1941 Lin reported to ABMAC that Wang was doing his best to make things go smoothly, but that Pan Ji was "apparently still responsible for noncooperation." In November he complained to Roger Greene (the former PUMC executive) of the ill effects of price increases, defection of personnel, and efforts by Pan to "shipwreck the MRC."[133]

After the outbreak of the Pacific War in December 1941, Medical Relief Corps problems were intensified by the rapid Japanese occupation of Southeast Asia and the loss of support from overseas Chinese. Early in

---

[128] Ibid., Lin to Co Tui, November 18, 1940.

[129] ABMAC box 22, National Red Cross Society of China, Memo of June 28, 1941. Currie became the Lend Lease administrator for China. See Tuchman (1970), 221.

[130] ABMAC box 22, Memos of March 3, 1941, and June 28, 1941. See also Lin to Co Tui May 2, 1941.

[131] Lin to Co Tui, June 3, 1941, July 12, 1941, (handwritten), and August 8, 1941. Since 1938 Lin had been nominally director of the NHA's Central Field Health Station, but in his words the only direct work he did for it was to organize the anti-epidemic corps. The correspondence does not indicate why the AMA, from which Lin also held an appointment, did not apparently offer a stipend. According to the ABMAC field director Cheng Baonan, who was a strong supporter of Lin, the NHA took this action as a result of the charges of pro-Communism against Lin. Cheng Baonan to Co Tui, June 20, 1941, in ABMAC box 5.

[132] Lin to Co Tui, August 9, 1941, in ABMAC box 22, National Red Cross Society of China, Robert K. S. Lim 1939.

[133] ABMAC box 22, Lin to Co Tui, October 6, 1941, and to Roger Greene, November 11, 1941.

the War the MRC had agreed with the government to be responsible for wounded soldiers and restrict fundraising to overseas communities, allowing refugee agencies to fundraise within China.[134] With the MRC now in a financial crunch Lin counted on the American Red Cross to make a cash grant of $250,000, 90 percent of which would go to the MRC. In March 1942 he wrote to Dr. Co Tui that: "so far I have not received any of these funds. Dr. C. Pan (Pan Ji) is largely responsible for this state of affairs."[135] By then fuel was getting scarce and supplies could not be distributed. The MRC was trying to convert twenty trucks to operate by burning charcoal. Fearful that volunteer support would no longer sustain the MRC, Lin tried to get the MRC placed under the Ministry of War. This would relieve his problems with CRCHQ and at the same time, qualify the MRC for the assistance of a "semi-governmental body" such as the American Red Cross. But this was contrary to CRCHQ's own agendas as well as ARC policy, which had restricted its aid to nonmilitary groups.[136]

A new crisis blew up with the Japanese threat to cut the Burma Road. The collapse of British resistance and the Japanese occupation of Rangoon in early March 1942 threw the onus of further resistance on Chinese forces. A Chinese expeditionary force (CEF) was sent to resist the Japanese invasion of Burma. Fighting began in mid-March and continued till the end of May. Several of the Chinese divisions put up strong resistance, but lack of equipment, air cover, and vigorous leadership proved decisive. The expeditionary force struggled out to India or Yunnan, where it went into training for future operations.[137]

The Expeditionary Force required medical assistance. In the middle of March 1942 the director general of the Indian Medical Service, Sir Gordon Jolly, recommended that Drs. Lu and Lin visit Burma to investigate the CEF medical facilities. The Ministry of Defense, at Stilwell's request,

---

[134] ARC Archive, file 985.08, box 1394, Phillips F. Greene to Richard Allen, May 26, 1942, in *China War Relief*, volume I, appendix, 62–65. Greene wrote that the agreement for CRC to solicit outside of China and the Government not to do so held more or less until December 7, 1941. With the fall of the East Indies and Singapore, a large part of the financial support for the CRCMRC was cut off.

[135] ABMAC box 9, EMSTS, Robert Lim folder, Lin to Co Tui, March 10, 1942.

[136] Cf. ARC archive, file 985.08, box 1394, *China War Relief*, volume I, 36, L.M. Mitchell to David Price, May 22, 1941: "The ARC cannot expend Government funds for medical supplies for the general use of the armed forces of China. Medical and other supplies purchased with Government funds and shipped to China are restricted to the use of refugees made destitute by hostilities. This point is apparently not clear to the Chinese representatives who are seeking to secure contributions through the ARC."

[137] Hsu Long-hsuen and Chang Ming-kai (1971); Tuchman (1970). See chapter 5 for further discussion.

authorized the visit.[138] As the MRC had agreed to send three units and one convoy to assist the CEF, Lin must have welcomed an opportunity to escape the pressures on his leadership of the MRC and reengage in front line medical care.

Drs. Lin and Lu set off for Burma on March 22. When they arrived they found only two medical units serving the Chinese Expeditionary Force—a base hospital at Mandalay (曼德莱) and a receiving station at Myitkyina (密支那). The MRC units arrived at Lashio (腊戍)—the railhead for the Burma Road—just three days before the hospital was bombed and destroyed. Five hundred wounded were trucked up to Lashio, where the civilian hospital was already crowded. Lin got hold of a residence, supplies and cash and in 24 hours improvised a hospital to accommodate the casualties.[139]

During the ensuing military retreat MRC units were able to bring the casualties back to Yunnan, but a rapidly advancing Japanese column cut off Lin and his immediate associates. They retreated north, joining another Chinese unit with many casualties on stretchers. Eventually they got through to Ledo (利多 in northwest Assam 阿萨姆, India), arriving in Dibrugarh (迪布鲁加) at the end of May. From there Lin went on to New Delhi to arrange for the establishment of a medical training service for the CEF forces at Ramgarh (莱姆加). In mid-July he returned to Kunming and continued on to Chongqing to report to CRCHQ. He returned to Guiyang in August after an absence of over four months.[140]

While Lin was in India, the CRCHQ seized control of the MRC supply depot in Guiyang. The pretext for this coup was provided by charges the previous year that MRC supplies had been turning up in the Guiyang commercial drug market. Preoccupied with medical education plans, Lin noted that some leakage was inevitable and at least the supplies were being put to some use,[141] but he called in a British administrator to make an inventory and set up guards for the depot.[142] He also sent a "petition" to CRCHQ reporting the losses and "voluntarily requesting punishment."

---

[138] ABMAC box 5, Cheng Baonan to Co Tui, March 26, 1942; ABMAC box 38, "Originals," Interview with Robert Lim, September 4, 1943.

[139] ABMAC box 9, EMSTS, Robert Lim, "Welcome to Dr. Robert K. S. Lim...on his Return to Kweiyang," August 1, 1942.

[140] i) Xue Qingyu (1987), 46; ii) Wang Youchun (汪犹春) (1987) 177–186; iii) ABMAC box 9, EMSTS, Robert Lim. Lin Report to General Stilwell, and "Welcome..." August 1, 1942.

[141] Wang Congyan (1987), 133; also the writer's interview with Dr. Wang Kai-hsi.

[142] ABMAC box 3, Dr. George Bachman to Helen Kennedy Stevens (ABMAC executive director), May 12, 1942.

The CRC leadership drew up a document reprimanding him, dismissed the acting chief of the supply depot and authorized CRC's representative, Dr. Tang Lizhou, to take charge of the depot. Document in hand, Tang arrived at Tuyun'guan on May 6 and delivered it in person to Lin's deputy Dr. Rong Dushan.[143]

Demoralized by Lin's absence the MRC staff found no way to avert this takeover. CRCHQ now controlled a large depository of supplies made all the more valuable by the closing of the Burma Road. Wang Zhengting followed up this move by ordering that all supplies sent to the MRC via India or Kunming must receive a permit from him before they could be released. To further demoralize his staff, Lin's enemies circulated rumors that he had been dismissed by Chiang Kaishek, requested a post in the British army, and was buying bonds under his own name and permitting the sale of drugs and gasoline on the black market. These tactics, designed also to undermine Lin's reputation among his American supporters, found a ready ear from the new ABMAC field director Dr. George Bachman. He reported them all to New York adding, "Such is the story. Until I know Lim (Lin) and see for myself, I am content to listen well and believe nothing."[144]

In another move to undermine Lin's leadership the CRCHQ used its control over funds to squeeze the Medical Relief Corps into submission. Lin reported in early March 1942 having not yet received any of the promised ARC funds, which at the official exchange rate of around US $1 to NC¥ 18.71 would have amounted to around NC¥ 4,677,500. According to information made available by Pan Ji to the ARC representative Dr. Phillips Greene and the ABMAC representative Dr. Bachman, CRCHQ was supposed to forward from its ARC grant five monthly installments of NC 935,672.55. These, according to Pan, were distributed as follows:

---

[143] Ibid., Bachman to Stevens, July 21, 1942, enclosure 3. The document said, "The Society shall directly assume control of the depot and shall immediately send Director Tang Li-chow to take over charge and to devise new measures of careful management in order to safeguard official property." Bachman had written to ABMAC on May 12 that Wang Zhengting had promised not to take over the stores until Lin returned, but this promise was a dead letter even before Bachman reported it. On June 11 Bachman reported that Tang was acting head of the MRC supply department and head of the MRC's Central Depot for "safekeeping of supplies against theft, fire, air raids." The ARC representative Dr. Greene reported that Tang was in charge of the MRC supplies when he visited there on August 14 (after Lin's return). See ABMAC box 1, ARC folder, Greene to Allen, letter 74, August 26, 1942.

[144] ABMAC box 3, Bachman, George W, Bachman to Stevens, May 15, 1942, and Bachman to Van Slyke, June 24, 1942.

Table 4.1: Chinese Red Cross Planned Distributions to
Medical Relief Corps, February to July 1942

Month/usage	Amount in NC¥
February	750,000
March	850,000
April	850,000
May	850,000
June	850,000
July	128,362.74
Gasoline	400,000
Total	4,678,362.74

Source: ABMAC Archive, box 3, Bachman, George W., data from Enclosure #1 (National Red Cross Society of China, C. Pan to Dr. Phillips F. Greene, dated June 14, 1942), in Bachman to Stevens #13, July 21, 1941.

The July budgeted amount was supplemented by NC¥ 761,637.26 from a British Red Cross grant of £81,000. However, when Greene examined the accounts at Tuyun'guan in August 1942 he found the following picture (see Graph 4.3).

Greene reported that: "If these (figures) are correct it lends support to Dr. Lim's earlier claim that Headquarters was delaying transmission of our funds at a time when he urgently needed them." He assured the American Red Cross leadership in Washington that the whole amount had been spent "legitimately."[145] During this period, wrote the ARC assistant director, costs were escalating: candles costing 90c at the end of 1941 were up to 6.50 only three months later, and salaries paid to white collar workers had become fictitious and misleading.[146]

The medical community in Chongqing knew that a showdown between Lin and CRCHQ was only a matter of time. At the end of August Lin tendered his resignation as director of the MRC. The Chinese Red Cross Board reportedly declined it and suggested that Lin take a six month leave, allowing Dr. Pan Ji to take over as acting head in Chongqing while Dr. Tang and another staff member took over management at Tuyun'guan.[147] Determined

---

[145] ABMAC box 1, American Red Cross, Phillips F. Greene to Richard F. Allen, letter number 74, August 26, 1942.

[146] ARC archive, file 895.08, box 1394, Reports, Statistic, Surveys and Studies, 1942–1943.Albert Evans report, March 31, 1942.

[147] This is Dr. Tang Lizhou (Tang Li-chow). In Xu Zhi (1987), 150, his name is given as Tang Yizhou (汤彝舟); but the archival materials give his name as Tang Li-chow without noting the characters.

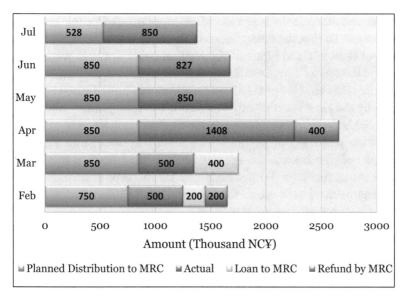

Graph 4.3: *Comparison between Chinese Red Cross (CRC) Planned and Actual Financial Distribution to Medical Relief Corps, February to July 1942.* (*Sources*: 1) ABMAC Archive box 3, Bachman, George W, Enclosure #1 (National Red Cross Society of China, C. Pan to Dr. Phillips F. Greene, dated June 4, 1942), in Bachman to Stevens #13, July 21, 1941. 2) ABMAC Archive, box 1, American Red Cross, tabular data in Phillips F. Greene to Richard F. Allen, letter number 74, August 26, 1942.)

to retain his position as head of the Emergency Medical Service Training Schools, Lin turned down this proposal and insisted on acceptance of his resignation. He handed over his duties on September 1, 1942.[148]

Conclusion: Outcomes in the Balance

The breakdown between Dr. Lin and the Chinese Red Cross Headquarters was more than a rupture between a few individuals. As an organization led by patriotic and medically trained volunteers, the Medical Relief Corps injected vision and competence into provision of front line military healthcare. Lin's equation of patriotism with service to the military, his refusal to be confined by party allegiances, his interest in the health of China's common people, and his plans for China's future healthcare services, set a style of leadership that both attracted the support of his

---

[148] ABMAC box 3, Bachman to Stevens, September 4, 1942, September 28, 1942.

juniors and aroused the suspicion of his superiors and people envious of his success. During the emergencies of the early war years, Lin's improvisational skills enabled him and the Medical Relief Corps to work around the weaknesses of China's military medical units and challenge them to do better. The rupture of the Guomindang-Communist United Front, signaled by the New Fourth Army Wannan Incident of January 1941, underlined the breach between Lin's science-focused humanitarian values and the power politics gripping the top leadership in Chongqing. The repercussions of this breach, though less obvious than those resulting from the Wannan Incident, did not bode well for the lives of men depending on army medical services, or for the balance in China's future between humanitarian and ideological visions.

The departure of Lin from the Red Cross also affected overseas Chinese priorities. Although the Nationalist leaders were successful in clearing the underground Communist party cell out of the Medical Relief Corps, they paid a price. Lin was a champion not only for PUMC's scientific worldview but also for the ardent patriotism and anti-colonialism of overseas Chinese elites. Japanese occupation of Southeast Asia temporarily removed the overseas Chinese leaders from engagement with the struggle in China, but it intensified their resistance to colonialism. For such anti-colonial modernizers, Yan'an's fierce hostility to Japan would become a bigger draw than Chongqing's prevarication.

The divisions that emerged between leaders of a humanitarian, science-based and internationalist approach to modernization and political leaders vying for ideological supremacy over a traditional society were deeply rooted. Lin's efforts to democratize healthcare would not carry much weight with individuals trained in Japanese military schools. But the differences were not simply personal. At the end of 1937 a curtailed and compromised Dr. Liu Ruiheng was about to be squeezed out of the leadership of the NHA; after the Long March Dr. He Cheng was finessed out of the leadership of the Red Army health services; and in 1942 Lin was pressured into resigning from the CRCMRC. Other Chinese medical and public health leaders of this era would find themselves passed over or squeezed out. These fissures were not just due to personality conflicts, or to the naiveté of scientific and humanitarian reformers. Rather they reflected basic issues dividing scientific and humanitarian vision from the driving forces of political ideology. But in 1942 the outcomes still hung in the balance. As the next chapter will indicate, the political leaders still faced many handicaps, and the health reformers still had resources to come to their support.

CHAPTER FIVE

HOW RIGIDITY, DISEASE AND HUNGER UNDERMINED NATIONALIST CHINA'S MILITARY MEDICAL REFORMERS

An army marches on its stomach.
                          —Attributed to Napoleon

There are no bad regiments; there are only bad officers.
                          —Field Marshal William Slim

His achievements should go down in history (said of Lin Kesheng)
                          —Wu Hongzi[1]

The crisis caused by Lin Kesheng's resignation from the MRC demonstrated that civilian auxiliaries such as the Red Cross Medical Relief Corps could not compensate for deficiencies in Nationalist China's military medical systems. This is the basic problem that the military medical reformers could not overcome and that left Nationalist China's soldiers in the lurch. But there were larger problems in Nationalist China's military command system that caused its leaders to criticize and downplay Lin's pioneering military medical work. Care of wounded and sick soldiers was not high enough in their scale of values to warrant the degree of resource mobilization and organizational empowerment that Lin had accomplished. We have already explored this problem in relation to Communist penetration of the MRC, but the problem is larger than that. It is reflected in the unwillingness of the military leaders to feed Nationalist China's soldiers properly, or to operate a legitimate conscription system, or to concentrate resources on defeating the Japanese military.[2] Although the military medical reformers found ways to work around these obstacles, they could not overcome them.

This chapter explores that basic problem, beginning with its impact on Dr. Lin's work and its impact on the MRC. We will look at ways in which the medical reformers, aided by American logistics, worked around

---

[1] Wu Hongzi (吴宏字) (1987), 141.
[2] Thus the observation of a military historian, that "no general ever won a war whose conscience troubled him or who 'did not want to beat his enemy too much.'" Dixon (1994), 15.

the military leaders in Chongqing and then examine the problems of nutrition and conscription that beset Nationalist Chinese armies in the last year of the war. The replacement of He Yingqin by Chen Cheng as Minister of Defense in December 1944 provided a last ditch opportunity for the military medical reformers to work with a leader sympathetic to their work.

Eclipse of Lin Kesheng and the MRC

The eclipse of Dr. Lin, beginning with his resignation from the CRCMRC in September 1942, continued with his removal from the Emergency Medical Service Training Schools in August 1943 and with the resignation of his friend and colleague Dr. Lu Zhide as director of the Army Medical Administration at the end of 1943. A major decline in the front line outreach of the Medical Relief Corps went along with the ouster of Dr. Lin from leadership in the field of army healthcare until after Chen Cheng became Defense Minister. The differences that helped to bring him down were over values, goals and resources, as well as a need expressed by his staff for more rewarding work.

For General He Yingqin the problem boiled down to insubordination. Traditionally army medical personnel were untrained and had no professional status. Their main job was to get wounded bodies off the battlefield. What happened to the bodies after that was of little concern to army authorities. Dr. Lin, however, not only trained healthcare rank and file but brought in professionally certified physicians, surgeons and nurses, in other words educated people, to take charge of the rescue and care of wounded and sick soldiers. In a meeting on November 5, 1942 with Dr. Phillips Greene (American Red Cross), Dwight Edwards (United China Relief) and Dr. George Bachman (ABMAC), General He Yingqin reportedly told these American civilian health representatives why, during the previous year, the Emergency Medical Service Training Schools (founded by Lin) had been an increasing thorn in his flesh, "as it was giving rise to a new group of men within the army medical program but having a political color of their own and proving rather unwilling to cooperate and quite outside army discipline."[3]

---

[3] Phillips F. Greene to Richard F. Allen, Vice Chair, American Red Cross Insular and Foreign Operations, letter 245 dated February 3, 1943, in ABMAC box 8, EMSTS 1942–1946.

Let us parse this remark. Dr. Lin supported the United Front between the Chinese Nationalists and Communists while General He didn't. Lin equated patriotism with healing of front line soldiers; the General's vision was strategic. Lin raised far larger amounts of money from patriotic overseas Chinese than the top Nationalist leaders had anticipated and also enjoyed significant support from medical leaders in the U.S. and the U.K. Especially galling for General He and the top Nationalist military brass was the fact that Stilwell recommended Lin for an American Order of Merit along with the Generalissimo and General He. Lin needed to be cut down to size.

In August 1943 General He told Edwards, Bachman and John Nichols (new ARC representative), much to their satisfaction, that Lin had been removed from all offices under the Army Medical Administration. No doubt Lin saw this move coming. General He also told them that Lin's friend and colleague Surgeon General Lu Zhide had been instructed to go to Anshun and turn authority over the EMSTS over to the AMC. That remark was a fabrication; but it sufficed temporarily—and inexcusably—to demean both medical leaders.[4]

Around the Board of Supply and Transport—the agency responsible for furnishing military supplies and transporting wounded soldiers to rear hospitals—an attitude of blatant indifference prevailed. In October 1944 Shi Hualong, the Board's Quartermaster General, visited the Third EMSTS Center and told its staff that there was a general tendency in army circles to look on medical service as a benevolent enterprise rather than integral to army work. By that time the Japanese military were advancing into southwest China and soldiers, army recruits and refugees were sick and starving by the tens of thousands. The Board had a reputation for corruption; it may not have attacked Lin, but it offered no support for his work, and showed no interest in wounded soldiers and civilians at a critical time.[5]

---

[4] Confidential Notes on an Interview with General Ho Ying-chin on the part of Messrs D. W. Edwards, George W. Bachman and J. D. Nicols, August 16, 1943, in ARC Archive, 985.5, China Health Activities. Since Dr. Lu was a person of impeccable integrity plus a devoted student of Dr. Lin's, the idea that he would have turned over the EMSTS to a school that practiced German-style medicine is not possible. PUMC professors had a poor view of the quality of training going on at the Army Medical College.

[5] ABMAC, box 9, Financial Reports, EMSTS, Semi-annual Report of Third Branch EMSTS, July to December 1944. The Central Military Commission's Board of Supplies and Transport (后勤部 Houqinbu Rear Area Services Ministry, it handled transportation, supply depots and evacuation and treatment of wounded) was one of the more problematic agencies in the Nationalist military system. General Yu Feipeng (俞飞鹏), a relative of

A major problem for Lin was his willingness to send MRC units to assist Communist as well as Nationalist armed forces. We have seen in chapter 4 that Red Cross Secretary General Pan Ji alerted Dai Li, head of the Nationalist Party's Secret Police, to MRC activities and noted that Dai advised Lin in 1941 to resign from the MRC, which he offered to do. In his book *The Unfinished Revolution in China*, published in 1947, Israel Epstein states that he found Lin in 1940 "confused, discouraged, and weakly surrendering the position on which he had built up his service," namely, the allocation of supplies and personnel to fronts where war operations against the Japanese were most active. As Epstein saw it, Lin was so often forced to go to Chongqing to explain that the MRC was not a conspiracy to overthrow the government, that he had little time to do his job. Moreover he was forced to take on politically reliable but medically and morally unqualified employees, who were soon thriving on the sale of foreign donations of drugs. The campaigns to cut off Lin from his foreign supporters and delay his budget appropriations were followed by direct campaigns to oust him and investigate his accounts. By 1944, according to Epstein, Lin had been thoroughly broken. He had spent months "at the penitent's bench" as medical adviser to Dai Li's secret police and now shook with trepidation in the presence of high officials. His enemies not only broke Lin; they also succeeded in wrecking the MRC.[6]

American representatives of civilian relief agencies accused Lin of syphoning funds away from their priorities. According to Dwight Edwards, funds were sent directly to Lin "and upon his request the Red Cross was ignored and its authority denied." EMSTS, in Edwards' view, had an expensive plant and large staff making unnecessary demands on American funds and cramping medical activities of other very deserving work. He claimed that the funds controlled by ABMAC had been used to advance projects desired by a very small group of Chinese and not approved by the responsible Chinese groups concerned (e.g. the Ministries of War and Education).[7]

Chiang Kaishek, was the director; he was one of the officers most distrusted by Stilwell as not having the interests of China's soldiers at heart. For Yu's appointment see Chinese Ministry of Information (1943), 323; for functions of *Houqinbu* see Hsu and Chang (1971), 274–279; for Stilwell's views, see Tuchman (1970), 237, 275, 389. General Yu was a graduate of the Military Commissariat School (军需学校) founded by Dr. Sun Zhongshan. He served in various capacities as commissariat aide to Chiang Kaishek. For Wedemeyer's comments on the Military Commission's Services of Supply see below. Quite likely Mr. Shi was expressing the sentiments of his boss.

[6] Epstein (1947), 132–135. Epstein's claims concerning Dr. Lin and Dai Li are undocumented.

[7] ABMAC, box 8, folder 2, Dwight Edwards, Confidential Report on the Emergency Medical Service Training Schools and the Medical Relief Corps, May 1943.

The Chinese Red Cross agents in Chongqing and ABMAC's medical representative Dr. Bachman largely supported these views. Bachman, no friend of Lin's, regarded EMSTS as an "extravaganzia." The President of ABMAC, Dr. Donald Van Slyke, sent a blistering response to Edwards, and Bachman was recalled to the US and resigned his post. Unfortunately these actions did not stop this line of criticism.

Troubles at Tuyun'guan also attracted negative attention. Critics of Dr. Lin could not help comparing the makeshift appearance of the Tuyun'guan campus with the well-constructed and orderly appearance of the AMC wartime campus at Anshun in Western Guizhou. In the middle of September 1942 a huge fire swept through Tuyun'guan's hospital buildings causing further disruption, though fortunately the patients and much of the equipment were saved. Another problem resulted from the loss of the Burma Road to the Japanese in May 1942. This closed down China's backdoor pipeline, left the Chinese military short of transportation fuel and made it difficult to get army medical personnel into central EMSTS training programs. Several years of doing little else than teach elementary courses to junior middle school graduates in Tuyun'guan were taking a toll on Lin's highly trained EMSTS staff. They longed for the laboratories enjoyed by their competitors at Anshun. To meet this need Lin initiated a six-year staged plan to train army medical aides as physicians. While the small number of medical college graduates volunteering for military service justified the plan, this move raised a host of additional complaints from Lin's critics, some financial, some organizational.

All this unease added fuel to complaints about the MRC's aid to Communist armies and suspicion that Dr. Lin harbored Communist party members in the MRC. After the Wannnan Incident of January 1941 blew up the fragile Nationalist/Communist United Front, support of Communist Chinese forces was no longer a viable stance for a leader reporting to the Nationalist government. Some of his "slanderers" even believed that Lin's thinking was left wing and pro-Communist.[8]

Lin's friends—and he had many—had an entirely different view of his contributions. Among his numerous junior colleagues it was his war service, his often acclaimed patriotism, and his abilities as a teacher, scholar and organizer that attracted their loyalty. Peers admired his administrative skills and his commitment to the health of China's unprivileged people. He was known for working long hours and making do with four or five hours of sleep. What was undeniable to all of them was that he

---

[8] Wu Hongzi (1987), 148.

gave up a flourishing scientific career to serve China in its time of need. But even they could see that during 1942 his energies and administrative skills flagged.

If Lin was flagging during 1942 so too was the CRCMRC. While it had 2,726 personnel in March 1941 and nearer 3,000 by November 1941 (see Graph 4.1), by July 1943 its numbers were down to 678.[9] About one third left after their leader resigned, and many more left for other reasons.[10] Partly this could be due to the funding crisis, which hit the MRC before Lin's resignation but continued on after it. The pressure the Red Cross leaders put on Lin after his resignation undoubtedly caused more slippage of personnel, as Epstein pointed out. But in a few months that would change.

In February 1943 Chiang Kaishek removed Wang Zhengting and Pan Ji from leadership of the Red Cross and replaced them with Jiang Menglin, a former Minister of Education, and Hu Lansheng, a former AMA Surgeon General.[11] In October 1943 Dr. Hu made an astonishing report to John Nichols that sheds light on this change of personnel. Dr. Hu stated that when he became Secretary General the Red Cross was in terrible shape and utterly discredited. He had put it on an honest, respectable and effective basis. The Chongqing hospital, which he inherited as an extravagant monument, had been made an efficient running organization. The transport section, which was in shocking condition, had been rehabilitated and put in running condition.[12] If this and more is what Dr. Hu did and said, then he was indicating that Wang Zhengting and Pan Ji had much to answer for.

The most important thing they had to answer for was the damage done to the Medical Relief Corps. The MRC had grown as a result of Dr. Lin's commitment to the medical relief of China's soldiers and his ability to raise funds and medical supplies. In his view physicians could practice civilian medicine in times of peace, but in times of war their country

---

[9] ABMAC Box 22, National Red Cross Society of China, General, Military and Technical personnel July 1, 1943.

[10] For one third figure see ABMAC box 22, National Red Cross society of China, General Arthur Kohlberg, Report to ABMAC Directors November 22, 1943.

[11] Jiang Menglin (蔣夢麟 Chiang Monlin) was at the time Chancellor of Peking University and co-director of the wartime Union University in Kunming. Hu Lansheng (胡蘭生, Woo Lan-sung,) was a graduate of St. John's University Medical School in Shanghai.

[12] ARC Archive 985.08, China War Relief Volume II, Summary Report of ARC Operations, January 1943 to January 1946, Memorandum from John D. Nichols to Philip E. Ryan, ARC Director of Civilian Relief, dated October 25, 1943.

needed them, and front line wounded soldiers especially needed them. It is likely that Lin's views were influenced by the many British physicians who volunteered to serve in the military during World War One, 740 of whom died in that war. In any case he made this perspective the center-piece of his personal philosophy and the focus of his six years of work for the MRC. Lin's exit and the shrinking of the MRC was thus a devastating blow not only to Lin but to China's frontline service and "national life-line" (国家命脉).[13] After noting Lin's six years of war service up to 1943, a contributor to the Red Cross volume of War of Resistance reminiscences wrote that Lin's successors diverted MRC resources into the luxurious Red Cross general hospital in Chongqing and into civilian air defense rescue work, thereby diminishing MRC's commitment to "our brave offi-cers and men."

Although he could do nothing about the MRC, Lin's former student, Surgeon General Lu Zhide, determined to protect Lin's Emergency Medi-cal Service Training Centers. He prepared an account of work accom-plished by the training centers, so that the ABMAC Board in New York (and no doubt officials in Chongqing) could see what they were support-ing. This account indicated that the EMSTS had already trained over 7,000 army medical workers, organized the first medical field service training school, initiated field programs to handle triage, delousing, vaccination against waterborne diseases, and also started special dietary programs for hospitals and field stations. The EMSTS organized a vaccine plant, which could supply the entire army if called on, and the only orthopedic service in 1943 in Free China.

The EMSTS schools standardized medical equipment and supplies and trained newly recruited army medical personnel and personnel of certain civilian units.[14] Standardization of medical equipment and supplies, and inclusion of a morphine tablet in each packet of sterilized first aid dress-ings, helped greatly to relieve the pain of wounded soldiers at the battle-front. In fact, under Lin, EMSTS leaders published and circulated manuals covering the entire field of army medicine. This report from Dr. Lu, one of the Nationalist army's most trusted medical leaders, must have reas-sured and impressed the ABMAC directors in New York. Agnes Smedley,

---

[13] Chen Tao (陈韬) (1987), 191–198.
[14] ABMAC box 8, EMSTS 1940–42, Loo to Donald Van Slyke, July 14, 1943. Dr. Lu sent a letter containing much the same information to the UCR Chongqing representative Dwight Edwards (Loo to Edwards, July 12, 1943, in ABMAC box 38, Alfred Kohlberg, cor-respondence folder).

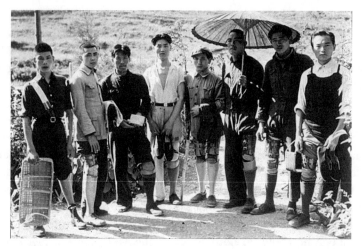

Photograph 5.1: *Beneficiaries of the Main Emergency Medical Service Training*
School's Orthopedic Hospital
The orthopedic hospital rehabilitated military and civilian patients, enabling
them to recover their lives. Among the patients was the ten-year old Xie Xide,
who became a brilliant physicist and President of Fudan University. (*Source:*
ABMAC Archive)

who reported on this work, stated that when she saw wounded soldiers
lying peacefully on their stretchers she felt nothing less than love for Drs.
Lu and Lin. She held that provision of the Army medical service(s) with
"tons" of these dressings was the greatest single factor combatting infection and death from shock.[15] Most striking is the loyalty of EMSTS staff
to Dr. Lin. In noting the turnover in AMA and EMSTS leadership during
1943 Dr. Peng Damou said that it was an "irreparable loss for us to lose
Dr. Lim (Lin)." Dr. Ma Jiaji expressed much the same sentiment when
he said that: "if not for Robert K. S. Lim and what he symbolizes, and
the flimsy thread of personal affection, many of the technical staff would
have left long ago."[16]

But Dr. Lu was getting tired of warding off attacks on Lin by Chinese
and American critics in Chongqing. Around the end of 1943 he resigned as

---

[15] Smedley (1943), 219, 430.
[16] Peng's remark is in his report of January 1–June 30, 1944, Ma's in his report of July
to December 1944. For Dr. Ma see ABMAC, box 9, EMSTS, "Semi-Annual Report, July to
December 1944, Third Branch EMSTS." For Dr. Peng see ibid, Fourth Branch School, fifth
report, January 1–June 30, 1944.

Surgeon General of the Army Medical Administration, stating that he was not getting enough support "from above." In fact Dr. Lu was furious about charges leveled by officers of United China Relief and communicated to the War Ministry, that Americans had no confidence in Lin. That statement was false, he said, and known to be so by UCR's officers,[17] plus it was a blatant interference in China's domestic politics. That combination of interference and falsehood led to a near breakdown in relations between the ABMAC leaders, who steadfastly supported Lin, and the UCR leaders and their Chungking representative Dwight Edwards who did not. But Dr. Lu warned ABMAC's leaders that any attempt to reinstate Lin would only cause further trouble, and he assured them that his successor and former deputy, Dr. Xu Xilin (徐希麟), was in sympathy "with our aims" for EMSTS, and would competently take on its direction.[18]

Although the UCR representative Dwight Edwards abetted Lin's separation from EMSTS it was General He who actually fired him. Lin's status as an internationally recognized physiologist and patriot meant nothing in the politics of Chongqing. General He discounted Lin's patriotism and knowledge of military medicine. Neither the General nor the American NGO representatives accepted Lin's belief that the War of Resistance provided an opportunity to advance China's vital healthcare agendas through military service. Yet Lin continued to enjoy the unwavering support of younger medical patriots as well as of leading public health advocates such as Drs. Liu Ruiheng and John B. Grant.[19] After Lin left the EMSTS in Tuyun'guan, his junior colleagues continued to move these agendas forward.[20] Notably Nurse Zhou Meiyu successfully fought for permission to start up an army nursing school in Guiyang, which became part of the postwar National Defense Medical Center.

---

[17] ABMAC box 38, Alfred Kohlberg, Chinese Army folder, Loo Chih-teh to Kohlberg January 31, 1944.

[18] Ibid. Dr. Xu (b. 1899) was a graduate of Jikei (慈恵) Medical University in Tokyo, an institution that focused on care of the poor and drew its medical philosophy from St. Thomas' Hospital in London. His medical outlook would have been not unlike that of Drs. Lin and Lu. On Jikei see http://www.jikei.ac.jp/eng/our.html. On Dr. Xu see Chinese Ministry of Information (1947), 658.

[19] In his memoir Grant described Lin as "one of the two or three most brilliant all-round men whom I have ever met," also as "probably the best administrator I have ever come up with." Grant Oral History, 350, 354.

[20] Liu Yung-mao, a sanitary engineer who served with Lin during the War of Resistance, recorded a notable story along these lines. See Liu Yung-mao (2008), 20, or Liu Yongmao (1970), 95–98.

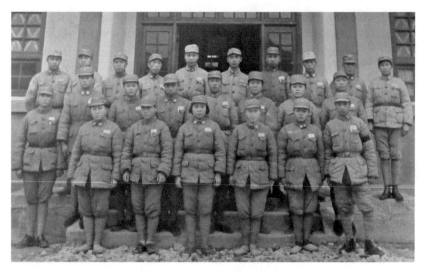

Photograph 5.2: *Army Nursing School Graduation Class*
The Army nursing school was set up in 1943 by Nurse Zhou Meiyu, a graduate of Peking Union Medical College and colleague of Dr. Lin's. The school attracted volunteers from several provinces in West and East China. The distinguished Modern China historian Chang Peng-yuan graduated with this class and is in this photo. (*Source*: ABMAC Archive)

EMSTS, X Force and US Medical Services of Supply:
How Lin's Organizations Continued His Work

Just when the efforts of Drs. Lin and Lu were at low ebb, a new initiative revealed ways to improve China's army medical services. This was Stilwell's establishment of the X Force at Ramgarh (莱姆加, around two hundred miles northwest of Calcutta). X Force was to be a Chinese army that would drive the Japanese out of Northern Burma and redeem the 1942 defeat by the Japanese military. The force would need well-trained and equipped Chinese medical services. Having seen Lin in action during the retreat from Burma, Stilwell's medical aide, Colonel Robert P. Williams, approached Dr. Lu with a request to send an EMSTS team to Ramgarh.[21] In a few days the team was ready. Led by Lt. Colonel Ma Anquan

---

[21] Miscellaneous notes, in ABMAC box 38, Alfred Kohlberg, miscellaneous folder. See also Xue Qingyu (薛庆煜) (1987), 46.

(马安权, an overseas Chinese born in Australia and educated at St. John's University Medical School, Shanghai), and Engineer Dai Genfa (戴根法, 1914–1991, a graduate of Jiaotong University), and consisting of twelve officers and three NCOs trained in surgery, sanitary engineering and triage, the team left Guiyang on December 8, 1942 and arrived in Ramgarh on December 24. There were already two Chinese divisions at Ramgarh. A third arrived in early 1943; two more were flown in during spring 1944.[22]

During the first half of 1943 the EMSTS team provided five training courses for divisional medical personnel on first aid, sanitation, personal hygiene, field nursing, litter bearing, and "related military subjects." A six-week refresher course for medical officers was extended to a six-month course designed to produce junior medical officers from amongst volunteer junior high graduates. Regimental officers went through a one-week first aid and field sanitation course.

In June and July 1944 a branch unit was set up in Ledo (利多), near the Burma border. Here the EMSTS group taught students how to live in the jungle, limit equipment to bare necessities, and assemble regimental aid posts and field hospitals quickly using jungle materials. Clinical teaching took place at a nearby American evacuation hospital. Beyond these duties the EMSTS team showed movies to soldiers on personal hygiene, venereal disease control, malaria control, and delousing. The team also ran a clinic and a delousing station. Its members provided typhoid, cholera and typhus inoculations and smallpox vaccines to recruits.

So much for training; what about battlefield results? A report from the front line by Colonel Xu Yingkui (许英魁, PUMC, 1934 and chief Surgeon for the First Army of the Chinese forces in India),[23] states that once the X Force engaged in battle with the Japanese troops (in October 1943), battalion aid posts were usually no more than 100–200 yards behind the line of contact. Frontline aid posts handled cleaning and binding wounds with sterile dressings, controlling bleeding and pain, and providing splints

---

[22] Information on the training program comes principally from reports by Lt. Colonel [Rolland B.] Sigafoos (U.S. medical officer at the Ramgarh Training Camp) and Colonel Wang Kaixi (汪凯熙, M.D., PUMC, 1934 and Commanding Officer of the Chinese Medical Training Unit after November 1944), in ABMAC box 8, EMSTS (Sigafoos report), and box 9, Ramgarh unit (Wang report). For Dai Genfa see Chen Tao (陈韬) (1987), 196. Dai's wife, Li Zongling, a graduate of the National Central Nursing School, joined the Red Cross as a nursing leader. See http://tc.wangchao.net.cn/baike/detail_2016296.html.
[23] Attached to Report #16 forwarded by Dr. Lin Kesheng in ABMAC Box 2, AMA. Xu's report covers the period October 1943 to March 1945.

for fractures. Regimental aid posts were one or two miles behind, and surgical care was available four to eight miles behind the firing line. These conditions were a huge improvement over those in central China during the first five years of war with Japan. The U.S. army handled hospitalization, but Chinese staff took care of invalided and sick patients. Divisional medical units handled evacuation within divisional combat areas.

Dr. Xu noted that the ratio of wounded to killed-in-action was roughly two to one. Chinese and American medical units treated around 13,000 X Force cases, of whom sixty to seventy percent returned fit to their units. Only around five percent were permanently disabled. He concluded that: "Everything that medical science could do was done to save lives, ease pain and hasten recovery."[24]

The ability of the US military supply system to provide medical equipment and supplies during the X Force campaign to recover North Burma was a major support for Chinese military medical units and the soldiers they served. The official US medical administration history for this period notes that Colonel Williams, while stationed in Chongqing, had almost weekly conferences with Drs. Lu Zhide and Jin Baoshan, Director of the National Health Administration; he also met with Madame Chiang, who served as her husband's medical adviser. They discussed lend lease medical supply and medical training and hospitalization. By midyear 1944 it was clear that the medical resources of the Chinese forces fighting the Japanese in Burma were inadequate to provide evacuation and hospitalization beyond the regimental rear boundary. The U.S. army provided field and evacuation hospitals for the combat zone and rear base hospitals operated by U.S. services of supply. When additional divisions were transferred from Yunnan to the X force, bringing it from around 57,000 troops to around 83,000 by the end of 1944, Williams made a special visit to Washington D.C. to obtain 4,300 more beds for X theater hospitals.[25]

EMSTS, Y Force, and the ABMAC Blood Bank

Chinese and U.S. authorities also collaborated over the organization of a Y Force (Yoke, also Chinese Expeditionary Force), based at Heilinpu near Kunming. Stilwell's tenacity brought this unit into being in the face of stiff opposition from British and Chinese military leaders. The Y force also

[24] Report #16 (see note 21).
[25] Armfield (1963), 196.

needed medical training to maximize its effectiveness. Again the medical team was drawn from the EMSTS. A group of six instructors, eleven assistant instructors, and one hundred and fourteen litter-bearers, under the direction of Colonel Yang Wenda (杨文达, M.D. PUMC 1937) and Dr. Lin, left Guiyang on April 12, 1943, four days after the first medical training class began in Kunming with American instructors.[26]

The Heilinpu center organized a six-week medical class on first aid, preventive medicine and medical field tactics, with a new class enrolled every other week. By the end of July 1943 six classes had graduated and another three were in session, accounting for three hundred and thirty-eight students. The medical unit was responsible for the physical examination and health of all entrants to the training school. The clinic saw around one hundred and seventy to two hundred patients per day, suffering mainly from infectious and nutritional disorders.[27]

In early 1944 the Chinese AMA and the EMSTS assigned another twenty-eight units to the Y Force.[28] As at Ramgarh, American military forces in the China Burma India Theater provided logistical and training support. Beginning in March 1944 the U.S. Army medical supply system provided the Y Force with thirty medical maintenance units per month, flown over the "Hump" air delivery route.[29] Each medical maintenance unit contained seven to nine hundred medical items designed to support 10,000 men for thirty days.[30]

During this period a portable blood bank, equipped and staffed by ABMAC, arrived in Kunming. This was the first blood bank established in China (see cover photo).[31] Under the guidance of ABMAC directors Drs. Frank L. Meleny and John Scudder of Columbia University Medical Center,

---

[26] ABMAC box 38, Alfred Kohlberg, EMSTS folder, "Report on the Work of the Kunming Medical Training Unit of the EMSTS, April–July 1943." Yang signed up with Dr. Lin, his former teacher, shortly after graduating from PUMC. He served in a training unit in Yunnan and worked at the American 27th field hospital, learning how to deal with foreigners ignorant of Chinese customs. See Hsiung (1991), 34.

[27] ABMAC box 38, EMSTS folder, "Report on the work of the Kunming Medical Training Unit of the EMSTS, April to July 1943."

[28] ABMAC box 2: Army Medical Administration, R. Lin report #1, with accompanying letter from Dr. Lin dated November 1, 1944.

[29] Heaton (1968), chapter 15.

[30] Heaton (1968), chapter 5, "Storage and Distribution of Medical Supplies."

[31] Yan Yiwei (颜宜葳) and Zhang Daqing (张大庆) (2006). A briefer account of how the blood bank came into being is in the ARC archive, RG160, Army Service Forces, International Division, folder 440, China volume I, beginning with a letter from Colonel R. P. Williams dated November 6, 1943. The file includes photographs of the Chinese Blood Bank staff.

ABMAC organized a training program to prepare staff to manage the blood bank program in China. They included Drs. Yi Jianlong (易见龙), Fan Qingsheng (樊庆笙) and Helena Wong (Huang Ruozhen 黄若珍). Dr. Wong returned to China in 1942 to locate a placement for the blood bank and joined Dr. Lin's EMSTS work, while ABMAC continued to train other staff.[32] ABMAC established a blood bank center in New York's Chinatown and began collecting blood, plasma, and other materials. With the help of the ARC, the equipment was shipped to India by the U. S. War Department early in 1944.

The bank opened in Kunming on July 12, 1944, with Dr. Yi as director. Scores of people, including local college students, volunteered to give blood, and after three months the unit registered over eight hundred donors.[33] But in wartime Kunming it proved difficult to maintain the equipment in sterilized condition,[34] or to draw a full dose from anemic soldiers and recruits available to donate blood. Yi had sufficient blood for immediate needs, but was unsuccessful in recruiting army donors, so Dr. Lin organized an army blood donor clinic under General Zheng Jiren (M. B. Gibraltar Naval Medical School, Ph.D. in Bacteriology, Edinburgh University), who was attached to Kunming defense HQ with access to troops commanded by General Du Yuming (杜聿明). Zheng had already done a study tour, arranged by Dr. Grant, at the blood bank in Calcutta.[35] Lin also engaged Colonel John T. Tripp, a biologist, to review the functioning of the blood bank. Tripp found that a filter was plugged with coagulated protein and had been improperly assembled during sterilization. He noted that some of the procedures taught in New York were not being carried out.[36]

---

[32] Yan Yiwei and Zhang Daqing (2006). It has not been possible to find biographical data on Dr. Wong. Another member of the staff was Lin Rusi (林如斯), daughter of the distinguished writer and educator Lin Yutang, who had previously worked as Dr. Lin Kesheng's English language secretary. For her participation see Yan and Zhang (2006).

[33] "ABMAC's Chinese Blood Bank" (1944), 218, 304.

[34] Yan and Zhang (2006) discuss the details.

[35] ABMAC box 2, AMA, R. Lim reports 1–10, Lin report #2, dated October 29, 1944. This is the only source found in this research for information about Dr. Zheng Jiren. There is no Gibraltar Naval Medical School on record, but there was a naval hospital in Gibraltar and a naval Medical School in the U.K.

[36] Ibid., Lin report #9, dated January 4, 1945, and sent from the Blood Bank location. Colonel Tripp later published a memoir (*An American Biologist in China*). He was Director of the division of Biologic Products of Michigan State Department of Health Laboratories and a fellow of the American Public Health Association. He spent 18 months in China under a Department of State Cultural Cooperation program helping to set up a central

Despite these problems, the blood bank proved its value during the siege of Japanese forces in Tengchong, a walled city in Yunnan just west of the Salween River, from early July till September 14, 1944. A field report indicated that in cases where plasma was administered to patients at the portable surgical unit, the death rate was only one to two percent. The reputation of the plasma was so great among the Chinese soldiers at the front that the wounded begged for it on arrival at the surgical unit.[37] Buoyed by these results Colonel Tripp and Dr. Zhu Zhanggeng (director of the National Health Administration's National Institute of Health) set about organizing three or more mobile units. By March 1945 Lin reported that the management of the blood bank was improving. He added that another blood bank had been set up in Chongqing with help from the Xiangya Medical College physician Dr. William Pettis.[38]

Some army leaders saw the value of the blood bank. Those who came in to donate blood included Generals Cheves and Lu Zuo, heads of the Chinese Services of Supply; numerous other military notables gave blood. Dr. Wong informed the press that the mobile unit would travel wherever enough donors could be found.[39] As its godfather, Dr. Scudder visited China during March–May 1945 to observe the blood bank in action and visit army medical hospitals.[40]

EMSTS Work in Central China

As noted in chapter 4, under Dr. Lin the original EMSTS set up five regional centers between 1939 and 1942 (see map 4.1). Lin had ambitious ideas for these schools, which he regarded as war area medical centers. They were to act as regional centers for modern medicine, carry out anti-epidemic work, help with post war reconstruction and continue serving the people and the state.[41] Brief descriptions follow of centers three, four and five.[42]

---

laboratory in China for the standardization of biological products. See "News from the Field," *American Journal of Public Health,* 26, April 1946, 435.

[37] Ibid., Appendix B to report #4, dated November 19.

[38] ABMAC Box 2, AMA, R. Lim reports 11–16, Lin report #14, dated March 22, 1945.

[39] Reported in *The China Lantern* (1945).

[40] ABMAC box 2, AMA, R. Lim reports 11–16. For Dr. Scudder's travels in China see Lin reports #14 and 16. For biography, see his entry in Wikipedia and that for his ancestor Dr. John Scudder.

[41] Cf. notes 108 and 109, chapter 4.

[42] No records were found for the Second Center, and those for the first were less informative than those for Centers 3, 4 and 5.

The third center, in Hubei, had two central goals: conserving personnel and annihilating disease. The director, Dr. Ma Jiaji (马家骥, PUMC 1935), carried out a survey of front line units and found them self-sufficient in vegetables and firewood. Smallpox vaccinations and typhoid and cholera inoculations were carried out regularly, however delousing happened rarely because of lack of fuel to boil contaminated clothing, and disposal of dysentery stools was neglected. Disease data were unreliable because diagnostic ability was poor and laboratory tests out of the question. Fuel for boiling water was another problem, and only one field hospital provided a special diet for dysentery patients. An army preventive health unit was doing good work, but evacuation of sick and wounded was compromised by high turnover of stretcher-bearers. In the Center's teaching program course standards had to be set below junior high level in order to qualify sufficient numbers for admission.[43]

Bad as they were, these problems paled by comparison with the indifference of Nationalist army leaders to the logistics of wartime medical care. In October 1944 the Third Center had received direct evidence of this complacency, and its morale was sagging. But it continued operating and in December reported it had trained almost 1,200 army medical men, forty-two of whom had received further training. Then the tables turned. Dr. Lin's return to military medical service that same month as AMA Deputy Surgeon General (discussed below) brought him back into the picture and produced a "wave of excitement." Dr. Ma informed Lin that the third center was well supported by the influential General Li Zongren (李宗仁), commander of the Fifth war area, and his chief of staff. Center staff had converted many people to the idea of scientific medicine and had substantially raised the status of army medicine in the field. But he admitted to a sense of isolation by concluding: "We would welcome your visit to the Gobi Desert!"[44]

The fourth center (in Jianjiang, Southeast Sichuan) combined political orthodoxy with medical and social innovation. Situated in five weather-beaten temples, it had a staff of over one hundred people, eleven microscopes and two x-ray machines. Through its classes it had graduated 523 students by June 30, 1944, of whom the majority was nurses. In late June it initiated a one-year training course for medical assistants. Sixty-nine

[43] ABMAC, box 9, Financial Reports, EMSTS, "Semi-Annual Report, July to December 1944, Third Branch EMSTS."

[44] ABMAC box 2, Lin correspondence, attachment to report #12.

entered the first class, and another ninety were scheduled to begin in September. At the request of General Sun Lianzhong (孙连仲), Commander of the Sixth War area and one of Nationalist China's leading generals, the center organized a mobile surgical unit to serve on the Western Hubei front. It had two old charcoal-fueled trucks to bring in medical equipment and supplies from Guiyang and Chongqing.

This center emphasized moral and Nationalist political education. Staff drilled one hour every Monday morning. In January 1944 the center inaugurated a political training class. This taught party principles, war songs, and political thought; it sought to "institute ideas of racial awakening and national consciousness" in students and staff and draw eighty percent of staff into the Guomindang.

The center had a training hospital in an old temple with room for one hundred patients. In May 1944 (during or after a visit by AMA Surgeon General Xu Xiling) the AMA broke up its 80th army hospital and turned two hundred beds over to the center. This is reported to have improved administration of the hospital and its cooperation with the center. A few months earlier the AMA authorized Dr. Peng Damou, the Center's director, to make a three-month study of Chinese, British and American medical establishments in India. No doubt he used his findings to request a change in the center's hospital facilities and upgrade clinical training. The center also undertook a few epidemiological studies. From July 1943 to June 1944 it recorded 10,760 cases of dysentery and 24,160 cases of malaria among troops in the Sixth war area. The total number of cases for twelve reportable diseases was 38,500.[45]

The fifth center put into practice the ideals of public healthcare; it also suffered the worst consequences of war. The Ninth War Area medical director, General Feng Zixin, requested its establishment, even though a Nationalist Army Medical College field unit was already in the area.[46] The team was assembled in September 1942 and Dr. Lin Jingcheng (林竟成, Tongji Medical College 1933, no relation of Lin Kesheng) went ahead to Dongan in southwest Hunan to make arrangements.[47]

---

[45] ABMAC box 9, EMSTS (Directorate of AMS), information obtained from reports July 1–December 31, 1943, January 1–June 30, 1944, and July 1–December 31, 1944.

[46] ABMAC box 38, Alfred Kohlberg, Originals and Mimeo Copies folder, Kohlberg manuscript report on EMSTS, dated September 27, 1943, with summary of his visit to the Fifth Branch EMSTS; ABMAC Box 38, EMSTS folder, C. C. Lin, Report on Development and Work of Fifth Branch School since its Establishment.

[47] Dr. Lin had previously served as leader of the MRC's 4th Group unit (第四中队部) and was familiar with the incidence of disease in central China. See ABMAC box 20,

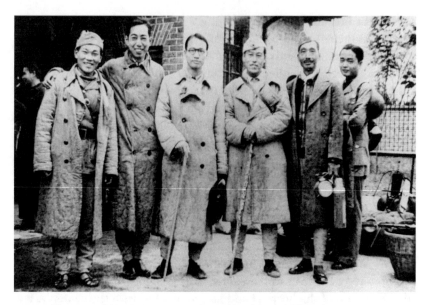

Photograph 5.3: *Dr. Lin Jingcheng (third from left) and Colleagues*
A graduate of Tongji Medical College, Dr. Lin's energy and patriotism attracted
Dr. Lin Kesheng, who appointed him to lead a Medical Relief Corps team and
later to direct the Fifth Emergency Medical Service Training School in Dongan.
His memoir of the retreat from that school is compelling reading. (*Source*: ABMAC
Archive)

The team arrived in November, moved into a neglected Confucian temple
compound and converted the buildings into an assembly hall, three lecture rooms and three dormitories. An army base hospital served as training hospital. Center personnel were equipped to do laboratory analysis.
They organized a sanitary area with five latrines and places for laundry,
mouth washing and bathing. Grease traps and fly controls were used to
demonstrate sanitary teaching.

The center had a staff of seventy-two people. It began its first training
program in March 1943 with eighty trainees. In June it opened a free outpatient department for civilians, which served on average one hundred
sick or wounded local people daily. The staff went into schools and an
orphanage to promote hygiene. They encouraged ball games, track and

National Health Administration, General, Report to MRC Headquarters of June 10, 1942,
covering conditions from 1940–1941.

field athletics, and swimming. Lin Jingcheng gained the approval of the local county magistrate to improve public sanitation and epidemic work through controlling pests, sanitizing latrines and cleaning grounds. The staff organized an anti-cholera campaign and provided over 1,500 vaccinations. They set up an orthopedic program to train disabled soldiers and had on staff a specialist in artificial limbs. For disabled soldiers they opened classes in sock weaving, sewing, spinning and umbrella making. Center personnel cultivated vegetables, cotton, tung trees, castor oil plants, and an insect-preventing chrysanthemum.[48]

Notes from ABMAC Director Alfred Kohlberg's visit to the Ninth war area in March 1943 indicate that the center impressed the Ninth war area medical leaders. According to General Feng Zixin medical personnel started attending the center's programs once they were set up. Before then medical personnel attended a short course run by the AMC's branch school in Shaoyang (central Hunan). But General Feng and his staff regarded the EMSTS course as more practical.[49] Dr. Lin Jingcheng was also director of fifteen Red Cross MRC units still operating in the Ninth war area, two of which were stationed at his center. He reported to Kohlberg that morale of front line medical personnel was better than that of personnel in the rear. Field hospitals were better run, sanitary conditions were better, and inflation was less important because the economy at the front was less monetized. Bathing had reduced incidence of scabies (疥疮) from ninety percent to ten percent per detachment.[50]

Campaign Ichigo, Refugee Crisis, and Disease

In the early summer of 1944 The Japanese military launched their last great campaign in China, to provide a communications link from north China to the South China sea and to disrupt General Chennault's air operations. This onslaught unleashed a huge refugee and disease crisis and

---

[48] ABMAC box 38, Alfred Kohlberg, EMSTS folder, C. C. Lin, "Report on Development and Work of 5th Branch School Since (its) Establishment" and Statistics of the Work of the 5th EMSTS, March–June 1943.

[49] ABMAC box 38, Alfred Kohlberg, A. Kohlberg Reports folder, "Travelogue of Trip to Ninth War Area, August 8–16, 1943."

[50] Ibid., Report by Dr. C. C. Lin.

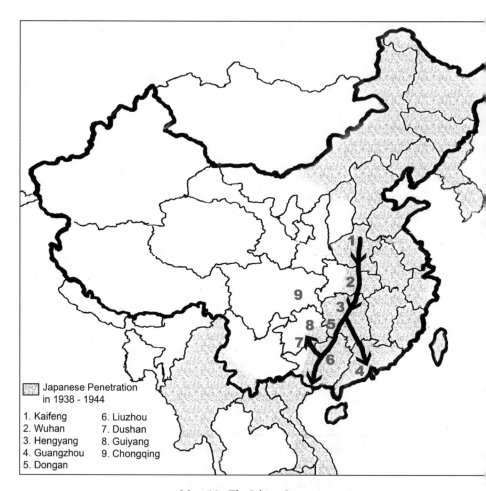

Map 5.1: *The Ichigo Campaign*

In May 1944 the Japanese military, already holding northeast China and much of the north, ea
and southeast, launched their last big China campaign. Its goals were to open an overland rou
from Kaifeng, in Henan province, to the South China Sea and to wipe out Flying Tiger bases
southwest China. The route went through Dongan, forcing evacuation of the Fifth Emergen
Medical Service Training School. A Japanese division advanced toward Guiyang, forcing se
eral more medical agencies to retreat hastily to Chongqing. As winter drew on, unknown tho
sands of refugees were felled by disease and cold. It was a nightmare for healthcare worke
(*Source*: J.R. and A.S. Watt.)

abruptly shut down the fifth EMSTS Center causing the hasty evacuation of medical facilities so arduously developed in Guiyang.[51]

As the military maneuvers have been widely discussed elsewhere this account will summarize them. A preliminary campaign took place in Henan during which the Japanese military, in the words of Theodore White, cut through the Chinese lines "the way a butcher knife cuts through butter."[52] The Chinese armies in Hunan put up a fight, but again in White's words they had "no support, no guns, no directions." By the time the Japanese army approached Guilin the Chinese forces had disintegrated, and in mid-November 1944 "the entire defense gave way."[53]

The combination of Japanese military aggression and Chinese military meltdown resulted in a huge exodus of refugees. Unfortunately the Fifth Emergency Medical Service Training Center was situated right in the way of the Japanese military drive toward Guangxi province. The staff had to give up their innovative rural public healthcare work, thus once again a valuable contribution to China's rural healthcare was aborted by foreign aggression. The staff and students joined thousands of villagers and soldiers retreating southwest through Liuzhou and up towards Dushan and Guiyang.

In a much later memoir Dr. Lin Jingcheng recalled the grievous circumstances of this journey.[54] As they approached the small town of Jinchengjiang (northwest of Liuzhou), a scene of desolation unfolded. Rain had been falling for days, the roads were churned with mud, the river was raging, and there were refugees everywhere. Toilets were overflowing with excrement. Swarms of flies were buzzing over food, and cholera and dysentery were killing off large numbers of refugees, especially the old, the sick and children. Dr. Lin and his companions provided aid where they could, but enemy planes dropped bombs during the day, and in the evening an arsenal blew up, unleashing a firestorm and sending howling people scattering in all directions. It was a searing catastrophe, one that Dr. Lin could never forget.[55]

---

[51] Campaign Ichigo is *"Ichi-go Sakusen"* (一号作战) in Japanese; "Hubei, Hunan, Guangxi Campaign" (豫湘桂会战) in Chinese.

[52] White and Jacoby (1946), 178.

[53] White and Jacoby (1946), 188, 190, 194.

[54] Lin Jingcheng (1987), 73–75.

[55] A brief account of the Jinchengjiang catastrophe is in a memo from Robert M. Drummond, American Red Cross representative in Guiyang, to John D. Nichols, the ARC director in Chongqing, dated October 9, 1944, (letter CK 25, in the American Red Cross China Archive). In late September Drummond was travelling along the road from Nandan to

After negotiating further crises, seventy-five students and two hundred and twenty-five staff and family members reached Tuyun'guan in the middle of December and were greeted by an anxious Dr. Lin Kesheng. The journey had lasted six months, and they walked most of the five hundred miles.

At the end of November elements of the Japanese 11th army, apparently on their own initiative, advanced into Guizhou province. On December 5, one Japanese force penetrated Dushan, directly threatening Guiyang, which led to the evacuation of its major medical organizations. At that nerve-wracking moment a counterattack led by General Tang Enbo (汤恩伯) aided by bitterly cold weather drove the Japanese forces, still clad in summer uniforms and poorly supplied, back into Guangxi province. But by then the demand for medical relief was overwhelming. Typhus, relapsing fever, and severe cold had killed around forty percent of refugees who made it as far as Guiyang. Thousands more were desperately weak, sanitation nonexistent, and it was impossible to bury the dead.[56]

Returning from Kunming to find these appalling conditions, the American military surgeon Colonel Powell joined with the British Red Cross surgeon Dr. Wilfred Flowers to carry out "wholesale amputations of frost bitten extremities." Entire staffs of National Guiyang Medical College and local hospitals worked with them "wholeheartedly." In his correspondence Flowers noted on November 18 that a few weeks earlier he had prepared a report on the refugee situation in the Guangxi-Guizhou region. Among 200,000 refugees huddling in mat sheds normally housing four thousand, cholera had abated due to cold weather, but dysentery and malaria were paramount. The Chinese Red Cross and the NHA had placed personnel, supplies and premises at Flowers' disposal. On December 15 he wrote

---

Yishan (in northwest Guangxi province). He was in Jinchengjiang for about an hour on the morning of September 30th. The explosion occurred on the 25th. Drummond got his information from the railway police and the city magistrate. According to these sources, not much more than one hundred people were killed by the explosion, most of whom were military guards. Two to three hundred were killed getting out of town. The provincial health station was among the buildings destroyed. Given that there were, according to Drummond, as many as 80,000 people jammed together in a town half a mile long, two hundred yards wide, devoid of sanitary facilities, and packed with disease-ridden and unknown refugees, the official casualty record is unlikely to be accurate. Dr. Lin's eyewitness account is much more compelling.

56 i) Lyle Stephenson Powell (1946); ii) Hsu Long-hsuen and Chang Ming-kai (1971); iii) Condition of Japanese soldiers from Lim correspondence, Report #8, in ABMAC, box 2, R. Lim reports 1–10; iv) Composition of Japanese attack forces from Romanus and Sutherland (1959), chapter 2, 64. According to the latter source, p. 165, the Japanese forces claimed that they turned back because their supplies had run out.

from Guiyang that he was establishing a health station at Guiding (some 30 miles east of Guiyang) with nurses picked up on the road from Changsha. Nine days later he recorded that there were twenty-seven camps in or around Guiyang housing 30,000 refugees. National Guiyang Medical College hospital, with a good team of nurses, was treating seventy-five of them. But refugees were still arriving at a rate of 500 a day.[57] Many had continued on towards Kunming or Chongqing and had reportedly died en route.[58] In short, ad hoc army and civilian medical units had taken on, as best as they could, the principal frontline relief for a huge civilian and military catastrophe.

Z Force and American Medical Aid

Through the work of the Z Force medical service one can see how a Chinese army medical unit reinvented itself to respond to a daunting military and civilian crisis. The initial task of the Z Force was to protect General Claire Chennault's Fourteenth Air Force. From late 1943 till July 1944 this medical unit graduated 535 Chinese army medical officers, twenty-four pharmacy officers (who received dental training), four hundred and twelve veterinary officers, and enlisted technicians and men in charge of horseshoeing. Because of the advance of Campaign Ichigo southward into Hunan, the training school was closed on July 25, 1944 after only eight months. Meanwhile the U.S. Army began in July to deliver two medical maintenance units per month flown into Kunming. But by October the Japanese onslaught ended further deliveries. After General Wedemeyer took over Stilwell's responsibilities in China late in October, he regrouped the Y and Z staffs into a Chinese training and combat command, effective November 17, 1944.[59]

Colonel Lyle S. Powell, an American medical officer with a keen interest in Chinese army medical services, was one of six U.S. medical colonels assigned to the Z force at Guilin. After three months he set out with a liaison team to the Chinese 46th army corps, which had just been transferred from the Fourth to the Ninth war area to reinforce the defense of Guilin.

---

[57] W. S. Flowers (1946).
[58] Powell (1946), chapter 7. According to Powell, Flowers estimated that forty percent of the refugees died.
[59] From Armfield (1963). For Wedemeyer's intervention see Romanus (1959), chapter 2.

Powell made a "firm and lasting friendship" with Colonel Duan (段 tuan), the surgeon in charge of the 46th Corps medical services. Although he found great inefficiencies, he recalled that American army medical services had been not much better until after World War I. The 46th Corps had no fully trained physician; Duan, an eager learner, was a graduate only of a "short term medical school." Battle casualties were tremendous, and victims had to be carried, sometimes for long distances, by the weakest men in the division.

Powell and his team began selecting medical soldiers and providing them with improved nutrition and first aid training. In the middle of June the 46th Corps arrived in Guilin, and Powell and his team moved into the recently abandoned American Red Cross building. They had around two and a half months during which they intensified the training of medical personnel. They also worked out a plan with Colonel Duan for medical care and evacuation, establishment of first aid posts, and battalion, regimental and divisional dressing stations. During a visit by the AMA Surgeon General Dr. Xu Xilin they persuaded him to place two Chinese field hospitals ten miles downriver to take evacuees from divisional medical stations. The British Red Cross surgeon Dr. Flowers set up an orthopedic service at a location between Guilin and Liuzhou.

As the Japanese neared Guilin Powell was appointed American Chief Surgeon to all the Z forces. He found a local warehouse full of medical supplies and got them released to support the hard-pressed Chinese troops. But the Japanese forces continued their relentless advance, capturing Guilin after heavy fighting on November 11. The Chinese forces, along with many thousands of refugees, fell back to Liuzhou, Yishan, and thence to Guiyang. Fortunately Powell arrived in time to help with the refugee crisis enveloping that city.

The Alpha Plan Triggers Changes in Military Medical Policy, and Lin Kesheng Returns to Office

A few days after the Japanese capture of Guilin, and barely two weeks after arriving in Chongqing, General Wedemeyer and his staff met with Nationalist military leaders.[60] The goal of Wedemeyer's group was to

---

[60] Wedemeyer honed his strategic thinking during two years of intensive study at the Kriegsakademie in Berlin. He developed diplomatic skills during a year's service at the Allied Southeast Asian Command in New Delhi.

overcome what they saw as a dangerously apathetic response by the Nationalist high command to the military and refugee crisis in southwest China. On November 21, 1944, Wedemeyer presented Chiang Kaishek and his advisers with a plan code-named ALPHA. It called for consolidation of armed forces to defend the vital Kunming air corridor and counterattack Japanese armies in Southwest China. It proposed a centralized field command, a thorough training program, deployment of key divisions and up to 270,000 troops, and a unified service of supply (SOS) system.[61]

Negotiation of the plan took extensive discussion, but Chiang settled on He Yingqin as field commander of the Chinese Alpha forces. General He was not Wedemeyer's first choice. Wedemeyer and his chief of staff, Major General Robert Battey McClure, were particularly concerned about the lack of food for Chinese soldiers. Wedemeyer informed General Marshall in Washington, in a memo dated December 10, 1944, that Chinese soldiers were starving by the hundreds, and that neither Chiang nor his advisers understood supply problems. The Chinese SOS, he warned, was "terrifyingly inefficient." But Wedemeyer wisely knew he had to act within the realities of Chinese politics. After several queries he accepted He's appointment but got McClure to be his deputy. Other American officers were assigned to work with He's staff.[62]

In addition the Chongqing government, prodded by Wedemeyer, ordered the conscription of all final year medical students, all medical college graduates from 1942 to 1944, thirty to fifty percent of medical practitioners, and ten percent of medical college, hospital and NHA staff. This addressed the reluctance by medical college graduates to enter military service that concerned Dr. Lin Kesheng for years and that also bothered American military observers. To prepare for these new conscripts Lin and a group of colleagues translated training materials that he obtained

---

[61] Frank McLynn (2011) treats Wedemeyer as a person of overweening ambition, who succeeded in displacing Stilwell as commander of U.S. forces in China, only to become embroiled in the same devious maneuverings that had characterized Chiang Kaishek's relations with Stilwell. McLynn's biggest criticisms are aimed at Roosevelt, who throughout the war supported Chiang, often against the advice of leading American officials such as Marshall and Stimson. When the Nationalists lost the Civil War, American supporters of Chiang lauded Wedemeyer, reviled Stilwell and General Marshall, and made their views known through such organizations as the Committee of One Million and the Shanghai Tiffin Club. F. W. Mote (2010) presents a much more favorable reading of Wedemeyer than McLynn's. I am grateful to Michael Gasster for sending me a copy of this work.

[62] Romanus and Sutherland (1959), chapter 5. An abbreviated text of Wedemeyer's memo of December 10, 1944, is in Eiler (1987), 83–89. General McClure had served in Tianjin and was fluent in Chinese.

while visiting the U.S. Army's medical field training program at Carlisle, PA in 1944.[63]

In late October the government decided to raise a volunteer army from student groups and government employees, which would apply lessons learned from the X and Y campaigns. Medically these lessons included organization of portable surgical hospitals and field training with cooperation from U.S. army medical personnel.[64] A month later an EMSTS unit arrived in Chongqing to train the first group of medical students enrolled in the new volunteer army.[65] The students were from the AMC, the National Shanghai, Tongji and Jiangsu Medical Colleges, the West China and Qilu Medical Colleges, and the National Pharmacy College. The first course took four weeks and included two hundred and one students, of whom twelve were discharged because of having tuberculosis. Graduates were sent to localities in western China. A second course was scheduled to begin on January 15 and continue for six weeks.[66]

Among bright spots for the AMA, the number of annual graduates from EMSTS programs rose to 3,916 in 1944. This was a thousand more than in any previous year and brought the combined total of EMSTS graduates to 13,848.[67] The replacement of General He by General Chen Cheng (陈诚) as Minister of War on December 1, 1944, and of Chen Lifu by Dr. Zhu Jiahua (朱家骅) as Minister of Education in November was good news for Dr. Lin, as both were his medical patients and supporters. But Lin continued to struggle with a lack of support from his civilian colleagues in Chongqing, both Chinese and American.[68]

To deal with the medical emergency created by Campaign Ichigo, the army asked every medical college and government hospital to take over the army hospitals between Guiyang and Chongqing.[69] National Guiyang,

---

[63] ABMAC Box 2, AMA, Lim reports 1–10, Lin report #4, dated November 19, 1944.

[64] Ibid., Lin report #2, dated October 29, 1944.

[65] Ibid., Lin report #5, dated November 26, 1944. The medical recruits had arrived a day earlier.

[66] ABMAC box 2, AMA, Lim reports 11–16, Report on Training of Medical Section, OTC, Military Council, Central EMSTS Training Unit, Chungking, December 4–31, 1944, attachment to report #12.

[67] ABMAC box 2, Report #4 dated November 19, 1944, Appendix F to Lin correspondence.

[68] Ibid., Lim report #5. Generals Chen Cheng and He Yingqin had very different military backgrounds and were strong rivals. General Chen was preferred by the American military leaders.

[69] "The army," as used in Lin's report #7, presumably refers to the Central Military Commission.

Xiangya and Shanghai Medical Colleges and the central hospitals of Guiyang and Chongqing staffed five army hospitals. Similar arrangements were made to staff army hospitals between Guiyang and Kunming and Chongqing and Chengdu. All Guiyang medical practitioners were drafted, and thirty percent of Chongqing practitioners were drafted for two years. In a report dated December 10 Lin wrote that he had been appointed Acting Deputy AMA Surgeon General to deal with training, equipment, supply of new forces, and liaison with allied forces. The British Red Cross funded ten portable surgical field hospitals and their equipment and supplies.[70]

On December 12, Drs. Xu and Lin and four colleagues, including the National Health Administration's Deputy Director Dr. Shen Kefei, set off on a five-day journey to Guiyang to review the situation and move the medical relief and training agenda forward. They made their way past multitudes of refugees perched on heavily loaded trucks as well as soldiers and students trudging away from the danger zone. They brought with them badly needed rice and money to buy food.

While they were on the way, Colonel Powell and Dr. Lu Zhide prepared the training center and hospital at the EMSTS campus at Tuyun'guan to handle hundreds of sick soldiers and casualties from battles in Hunan and Guangxi. Dr. Lu was short of personnel, so Powell proposed to bring in an American unit to help serve the hospital. Training plans included increasing the number of women nurses and setting up a medical demonstration company.

Meanwhile the provincial government in Guiyang ordered civilian medical institutions and civilians in the EMSTS medical complex at Tuyun'guan to retreat. Medical college personnel were given two months pay and ordered to disperse and await instructions. Students walked north to Zunyi, where some obtained truck transport. Soldiers moved into the abandoned buildings and used wooden furniture to make fires to keep themselves from freezing. It was assumed that this would deny the use of the furniture and buildings to the enemy. The governor, Wu Dingchang (吴鼎昌), remained in the city and restored order before serious damage occurred. Central hospital nurses and nursing students evacuated by truck to Zunyi, but part of the staff remained and, in Dr. Lin's words, held together splendidly. Most Red Cross personnel and families retreated by

---

[70] ABMAC box 2, Lim report #7, dated December 10, 1944. Lin's appointment came very soon after General Chen Cheng's appointment as Minister of War.

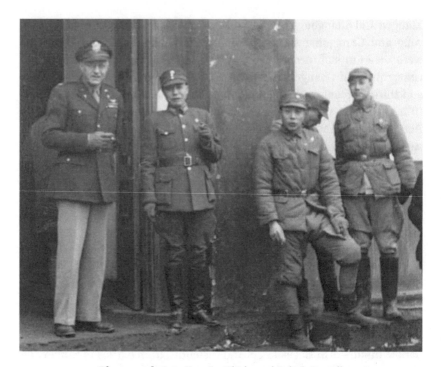

Photograph 5.4: *Drs. Lu Zhide and Lyle S. Powell*
A graduate of PUMC and close colleague of Lin Kesheng, Dr. Lu was chosen by
Liu Ruiheng to help modernize China's backward military medical services. He
did all he could to advance this agenda while at the same time supporting Lin
wholeheartedly. Dr. Powell was a senior American physician who served with
China's armies in 1944 and 1945. Dr. Lu, second from left; Dr. Zhou Shoukai, third
from left. (*Source*: ABMAC Archive)

truck to Zunyi and points beyond, while the director and a small staff
remained. At the central EMSTS campus around one hundred and seventy
women and children moved out at the last moment in five old trucks,
only one of which made it to a discarded horse and mule cart station. The
occupants kept alive under straw bedding while lighting fires, oblivious to
the danger of incineration.[71]

After two days in Guiyang, Lin left for Kunming to set up a Surgeon's
office for the combined Chinese-American command of military forces
of the Southwest. The AMA Surgeon General Dr. Xu Xilin and Dr. Lin as
Deputy Surgeon were to work closely with the American China Theater

---

[71] ABMAC box 2, AMA, Lim report #8 dated December 22, 1944 in Lim reports 1–10.

Surgeon Colonel George Armstrong.[72] The medical leaders put together a front-line force of medical units attached to divisions and armies, and a back-up force of hospitals, depots and medical transit units staffed by conscripted physicians and senior-year medical students. U.S. Army personnel would help train front-line medical workers, while EMSTS would train both front-line and support forces.

Lin reported that the available medical personnel were mostly young and inexperienced and as such good for front-line units but not for hospital work without supervision. The AMA called on the National Health Administration, the Medical Colleges and the CRC to organize a special staff under the veteran hospital administrator and NHA Vice Director Dr. Shen Kefei and Dr. Ni Baochun (倪葆春, P. C. Nyi, 1899–1997, M.D. Johns Hopkins), deputy director of the Red Cross MRC, to ensure that the evacuation and army base hospitals were properly operated. The Red Cross units, under Dr. Nyi, were to staff Chinese-run portable surgical field hospitals.[73]

A lull in war operations due to the Japanese retreat from Guizhou did not last long. Fortunately the opening in January 1945 of the new "Stilwell Road" through Burma to southwest China permitted movement of considerable quantities of war materials into China.[74] Other improvements included better equipment for medical units and further conscription of medically trained personnel. Tents and other mobile equipment replaced the old system of siting hospitals in temples, schools or warehouses. Essential requirements such as bedding and bedpans were stockpiled. All final year medical and nursing students were called up to serve in the medical units of combat troops.[75]

Most significantly the Chongqing government combined the field units of the EMSTS, the AMC and the Medical Reserve Training Corps under one authority. This provided coordinated medical field training at Guiyang

---

[72] A eulogy for Dr. Lin by Dr. Armstrong is in John R. Watt (2008), chapter 3. Dr. Armstrong later became US army surgeon general, vice president for medical affairs at New York University, director of the New York University Bellevue Medical Center, and president of ABMAC.

[73] ABMAC box 2, AMA, Lim reports 1–10, Lim report #9, January 4, 1945. Dr. Nyi did his undergraduate work at the University of Chicago. He was on the faculty of St. John's University Medical School before joining the Red Cross in 1941. See zh.wikipedia.org/wiki/倪葆春.

[74] For construction of the Ledo connection to the old Burma Road, see McLynn (2011), 232–233, 434. The first convoy to Kunming left Ledo on January 12, 1945.

[75] It may be noted that when World War One broke out in 1914 it took two years before universal conscription was legislated in the UK.

and at various army training centers and special army hospitals. Training corps could carry out battlefield medical training at army training centers and SOS training at special army hospitals. The AMC in Anshun (Guizhou) continued to provide undergraduate education.[76] These initiatives indicate the extent to which the experience of working with American military medical systems at the X, Y, and Z training centers was incorporated into China's military medical planning.

Effects of the Alpha Plan on Nationalist Army Medical Field Commands

The Alpha plan ensured further cooperation between American and Chinese military medical leaders during this critical time. When the plan started, one of the six command areas lacked adequate food supplies and two divisions in another were in a "deplorable state of nutrition." In a third division, ninety percent of the men had scabies. The Central Command had the benefit of the Central EMSTS training school and its almost completed hospital, both supervised by Dr. Lu Zhide. These facilities played an important role in the relief of soldiers wounded during the Campaign Ichigo drive through Hunan and Guangxi. The Command was led by General Tang Enbo and supported medically by Colonel Powell. Early in January 1945 a unit of the U.S. 27th field hospital arrived at the EMSTS campus at Tuyun'guan. A little later the field hospital's commanding officer, Colonel [George A?] Sywassink, arrived with a second unit. The EMSTS hospital had two operating theaters, and both were now constantly in use. American ward tents were set up for those not critically ill, and patients were provided with a supervised diet of three meals per day.

In addition, a four-week training class was set up for personnel of the 13th army corps. The first class included twenty officers from Chinese SOS medical installations.[77] General Tang attended the graduation ceremonies, where the brief but vibrant will of Dr. Sun Yat-sen was read aloud. "For forty years," it declares, "I have devoted myself to the cause of the National Revolution with but one end in view, the elevation of China to a position of freedom and equality among the nations." General Tang told the graduates that good medical service was perhaps the greatest single factor contributing to good morale in a modern army.[78]

---

[76] ABMAC box 2, AMA, Lim reports 11–16, Lin report #12.

[77] Powell identifies these forces as the 13th army; this refers to the 13th army corps.

[78] The contrast between Tang's views and those of the Board of Supply and Transport, discussed earlier, is striking.

While the Central Command was well set up, much of the Eastern Command covered a roadless area where transport depended on coolies. Although the mission of the American liaison team was to supervise training and equipment, American training personnel were not sent out until April 1, 1945. By then the Japanese military had signaled their intention to attack and destroy the major Zhijiang airfield. They launched a general advance on April 13. Despite having to deploy partially trained or untrained troops, the Chinese forces were adequately supplied and were able to contain this Japanese attack. The Japanese retreated on June 7.[79]

This victory was costly but decisive. The Japanese lost 1,500 killed and 5,000 wounded. Chinese losses were over 6,800 killed and over 11,700 wounded. The presence of four portable American hospitals and three platoons of the 21st field hospital in the Zhijiang area helped prevent further losses. By the middle of July the Eastern Command was reported to have eight base and six evacuation hospitals along with several medical detachments—a sharp improvement over the pre-battle arrangement.[80]

Food, the Key to Military Health and Performance

It did not take General Wedemeyer long to realize that food was vital to the performance of the Chinese armies. In fact he came to believe that the Chinese troops needed food more than guns. Officially a soldier was allotted 24 ounces of rice or 26 ounces of wheat per person per day "besides beans, vegetables and meat." These materials plus a food allowance were supplied by the Ministry of Food and distributed through the Army Food Bureau to divisions or "commissaries" for allocation to each soldier.[81] This system had provided considerable opportunity for malfeasance. To make matters worse, during the previous two years, growing inflation had caused the old cash allowances for food other than rice to lag considerably behind the cost of living. This had enabled divisional commanders to reduce the number of mouths to be fed while continuing to report full enrolments; soldiers had to forage at the expense of local communities.[82]

---

[79] The campaign that took place is known in Chinese as 湘西会战 (Battle of West Hunan) or 芷江作战 (Zhijiang Campaign).

[80] The campaign is described in detail in Romanus and Sutherland (1959), chapter 9 (Meeting the First Test in China). The overall (two month) campaign casualties on both sides were considerably greater, but figures vary according to source.

[81] Ministry of Information (1944), 324, 650–653.

[82] Details of the new ration scale are in Lim correspondence, Report #12, dated February 27, 1945.

As a consequence, long-continuing malnutrition made too many soldiers too weak to march. Flowers reported as early as December 1942 that soldiers were falling by the wayside, physically incapable of dragging their bodies any further and dying of accumulated days of malnutrition and disease.[83] During the Guizhou campaign late in 1944 General McClure informed the Generalissimo that the troops were "rife with desertion" because of starvation. Lacking sufficient rations, soldiers of the 24th army group were looting villages. In discussions during late November and December the American generals urged the Generalissimo to develop a coherent food provisioning plan.[84]

An interesting aside on diet and military service is provided by Dr. Lin. He noted that the stomachs and colons of peasant soldiers had been enlarged to handle a primarily rice diet. They could work very hard on such a diet but had little bodily reserve with which to handle convalescence. Thus wounded and malarial soldiers commonly developed anemia. Anemia or malnutrition was encountered in almost one third of the cases in army base hospitals—a staggering drain on military efficiency. In addition ten percent of hospital and twenty percent of dispensary cases had tuberculosis. For that reason Lin had insisted that the CRCMRC provided a special diet in army hospitals from 1939.[85]

A basic problem was the tenuous nourishment in the standard army diet. According to Drs. Leon Kamieniecki and George Schoen the average daily ration consisted of 24 ounces of rice, reduced in most divisions to 20 ounces along with pickled vegetables and salted red pepper. This amounted to seven bowls of rice (five if in hospital), in short, nothing but carbohydrates. The vegetable protein and vitamins were destroyed in the two to three year old rice and pickled vegetables issued, exposing soldiers and recruits to the dangers of anemia. This "food" cost the soldier half his monthly pay, and the few dollars left over were useless due to the galloping inflation.[86]

---

[83] Flowers (1946), Changsha, December 13, 1942.

[84] Romanus and Sutherland (1959), chapters 2 and 5.

[85] ABMAC Box 2, Army Medical Administration, Paper on Convalescence and Rehabilitation in China, presented by Lt. Gen. Robert K. S. Lim at New York Academy of Medicine, April 26, 1944.

[86] ABMAC box 38, A. Kohlberg Reports folder, "Report on the Living and Health conditions in the Twelfth Group Armies at the I-Chang front, Chungking, January 8, 1943." An article by K. Chang and H. T. Ch'in (January 1943) reported that the brine in which pickled vegetables were packed was a fruitful source of ascaris eggs, which could survive in brine solution even after a thirty-day immersion. Barbara Tuchman provides virtually the same information on food quality in Tuchman (1970), 264–65.

According to his December 10, 1944 memo to General Marshall, Wedemeyer repeatedly informed the Generalissimo that the Chinese soldiers could not be expected to fight effectively without an improvement in diet, whereas if they were fed well desertions would drop materially and men would even be eager to join the military. He reported that "we have evolved a plan for feeding the men." Their diet would include vitamins and dehydrated foods and would be managed under American supervision to eliminate graft and ensure better and ample food—for the men of the Alpha divisions. The American staff would even make food available during troop movements.[87]

Despite Wedemeyer's considerable diplomatic skills, execution of plans that involved such a shift in existing military practice proved easier said than done. In the early spring of 1945 the food situation in southwest China became critical and great numbers of soldiers, according to Colonel Powell, starved to the point of collapse. Because their bodies cannibalized their red blood cells for protein, the troops contracted critical anemia, and starvation diarrhea further weakened them. Many were already infected with malaria and dysentery; and due to lice infestation, typhus and relapsing fever were widespread. The Chinese hospitals were overcrowded and many sick soldiers could not be admitted. Hospitals also had a big food problem, with the result that hundreds of patients died, and nutritional diseases were more and more prevalent. Faced with this emergency, the medical units divided soldiers into three groups: men fit for combat, men who could be quickly healed, and those needing long convalescence. Looking back on this traumatic period Powell wrote that his memories seemed like

> a nightmare of successive groups of these half-dead soldiers, of truckloads of them being moved from this point to that, gradually making their way back to the zone of communications and a better food supply. The mortality was high, the morbidity something to shudder at.[88]

It happened that Stilwell anticipated the food problem and commissioned a study of China's military nutrition by Colonel Paul P. Logan, Deputy Director of the Subsistence Division of the U.S. Office of Quartermaster General. Logan submitted his findings to Wedemeyer in January 1945. He stated that there was enough food available for troops in the Southwest area of China; the main problem lay in distributing it. He proposed that all

---

[87] Eiler (1987), 85–86.
[88] Powell (1946), chapter 9.

rations be issued in kind; a central procurement agency be set up within the SOS system to plan, purchase, transport, store, and distribute rations to divisions; a food service program be set up in each division; and a specially trained nutrition officer be assigned to each army to report. After high-level conferencing, a modified Logan ration was approved on February 28 and planning completed by mid March.[89] According to Lin, this consisted of 25 ounces of rice, small allotments of soybeans, peanuts, leafy and root vegetables, salt and a multivitamin capsule. It would require setting up new food procurement policies and organizations.[90]

To get a food delivery system into gear to support the 36 divisions and 270,000 men of the Alpha Plan American liaison teams went into the countryside to find supplies. One group discovered that soldiers of the Chinese 13th army were unable to make a short march "without men falling out wholesale and many dying from utter starvation." Nevertheless between April 11 and June 15 five food purchasing commissions went to Guiyang, Zhanyi, Kunming, Zhijiang (in Western Hunan), and Bose (in Western Guangxi), to get the job done.[91] General Tang Enbo was one of the first field commanders to reform food distribution for Chinese armies, long a means for exerting squeeze by junior officers. With Powell's advice he authorized a system of food committees, in which newly drafted university students participated, and a training program was devised for committee members. The system was set up in the third week of February 1945 and (as noted above) a modified version later adopted for all Chinese armies. "Skin and bones" recruits were transported to convalescent camps at Zunyi (Guizhou) and Datung (Yunnan?) for rehabilitation. According to Powell, General Tang "became more and more enthusiastic about our medical program."[92] Thus by the end of the war army rations for ordinary soldiers were at last beginning to improve, but only in Southwest China. Altogether in late March there were five and a half million soldiers in Nationalist China's armies, of whom, according to Lin, two million were in poor condition[93]—and unlikely to benefit from the food reforms.

---

[89] Romanus and Sutherland (1959), chapter 8, "Food for Alpha Soldiers."
[90] ABMAC box 2, AMA, Robert Lim Reports 11–16, Report #12, dated February 27, 1945.
[91] Romanus and Sutherland (1959), chapter 8, "Carrying out the Food Program."
[92] Powell (1946), chapter 8.
[93] ABMAC Box 2, AMA, Robert Lim Reports, Report #14, dated March 22, 1945.

Lin Aids in Upgrading China's Medical Services of Supply (SOS)

Plans to reform the food requisitioning and delivery system threw the spotlight on China's existing military services of supply (SOS). One of the factors that had in the past crippled the performance of the Nationalist armed forces, as well as its medical relief operations, had been the lack of coherent services of supply. As we have seen, this had become a matter of intense concern for Wedemeyer. He organized a new rear echelon at Kunming, headed by Major General Gilbert X. Cheves, the American China Theater SOS Commander and also Theater Deputy Chief of Staff. Cheves was in charge of coordinating logistics and administration, including the all-important requisitioning of lend lease supplies flown over the Hump air route from India. At that time the support of the American SOS ensured that certain Chinese ground forces would receive a steady flow of food, ammunition, and medical supplies.

During January 1945 Wedemeyer was able to bring about a new organization of U.S. liaison services to the Alpha forces commanded by General He Yingqin. To the extent that the Chinese combat command forces depended on Cheves' SOS operation to resist and repulse the Japanese invader, U.S. liaison staff now could exert influence through denial of weapons and essential equipment to any non-cooperating units. Such hardball in management of supplies was nothing new to the Chinese military. Chiang Kaishek himself used it to control the flow of supplies to the hard-pressed Ninth War Area armies of the Cantonese General Xue Yue during the Ichigo campaign of 1944. But the continuing threat of Japanese military attack in southwest China gave the American SOS personnel some leverage, which increased with the reopening of the Burma Road in January 1945.

On February 9, 1945, General Cheves was authorized by Chiang Kaishek to take charge over the Chinese SOS for the 36 Alpha divisions, with General Lu Zuo as deputy commander. Eight departments were set up for planning, headquarters, personnel, administration, signal and transport, quartermaster, food, ordance and medical. At an opening ceremony General Lu noted that Cheves had abundant experience organizing supply functions. "Now our national army is ready to take the offensive," he declared as Cheves pledged to "keep faith with the Chinese soldier and give him what he needs."[94]

---

[94] Information on departments and opening ceremony from *China Command Post*, February 23, 1945.

Certain efficiencies resulted from this development. U.S. liaison teams in the combat command units were instructed to keep comprehensive statistical data covering strength reports, situation reports, training reports, and personnel data. By that time the U.S. SOS had four complete sets of division equipment and enough infantry weapons to supply ten more divisions. Cheves was now in charge of all ammunition, food, clothing, bedding and pay for the Alpha troops, with the rank of Lieutenant General in the Chinese army. Under his command the Chinese SOS headquarters was situated in Kunming, and seven SOS area commands were placed under the direction of Chinese front line generals.[95]

In his communications with ABMAC Dr. Lin reported on the reorganization of the Chinese SOS under General Cheves and noted that the Chinese SOS medical office and the Alpha command medical office had been combined. He had been placed in charge, with General Zhao Zou (formerly Surgeon to the Chinese Expeditionary Force in Burma) as deputy surgeon. On March 23 they had a conference with General Cheves, in which Cheves told them that if the number of physicians conscripted did not meet requirements they should let him know so that he could secure "more rigid enforcement." Cheves also expressed his intention to visit Alpha command hospitals once a week and insisted on their scrupulous cleanliness. In short, Cheves did not neglect the medical responsibilities of SOS.[96]

Unsolved Problems of Army Conscription

Conscription had long been a problem in Nationalist China, for reasons discussed in often brutal detail in Western sources.[97] In an attempt to

---

[95] Information principally from Romanus and Sutherland (1959), chapters 5 and 8.

[96] ABMAC Box 2, AMA, Robert Lim Reports, Reports no. #14, March 22, 1945, and 15, April 4, 1945. Note: Cheves' name is sometimes spelled Cheeves, but Cheves is the correct spelling.

[97] White and Jacoby (1946), 132–3, 273–6, provide a blistering account of the oppressiveness and cruelty of the conscription system. Powell's account (1946, chapter 9) is more restrained but equally gruesome. Flowers, in letter #31 (4/23/1944), describes having to turn new recruits away from his hospital because they were not permitted to be admitted. "We give them the necessary injection and turn our heads away as they stagger back into the ranks...I met a company of them leaving our place the other day, and I have seen few more agonizing spectacles in my time..." The most detailed and chilling account seen by this writer is in Romanus and Sutherland (1959), chapter 12 (The End of Wedemeyer's Experiment), 368–373. This is an abbreviated copy of a report sent to Wedemeyer's headquarters. Because it makes use of medical metaphors, as well as dilating on diseases contracted by conscripts, it may have come from one of Wedemeyer's medical staff. In any

improve recruiting, the Guomindong Government belatedly established a Ministry of Conscription in November 1944. According to an official government publication the Ministry was to be responsible for "the welfare of the recruits both in training and in transfer. Besides the establishment of hospitals and clinics to look after the men's health and meet their medical needs, barracks and service stations have been built along the highways and routes along which the recruits move. Recently arrangements have been made with the American Army authorities to move recruits by air."[98]

Unfortunately a gap remained between descriptions on paper and reality on the ground. Colonel Powell and Dr. Lu paid a surprise visit to a Guiyang a camp for recruits at a time when its commanding officer was not present.[99] They entered the hospital dispensary. It was a long earthen-floored and thatched-roof hut, the sides of which had been dismantled to provide firewood. They found 70 to 80 men lying on boards, almost all dressed only in shirt and trousers, with bare feet or clad in straw sandals. The men were lying as close as possible to keep warm. As those who were too sick were unable to get up, the foulness was "beyond belief." The two physicians counted several dead and others near death.

According to Powell, Dr. Lu had been trying to correct this situation. He and Dr. Lin had drawn up plans for proper selection of recruits and a system for provisioning way-stations along their route. But conflict and inertia stalled these efforts. Although the conscription system was upgraded to ministerial status, it lacked qualified medical manpower, facilities or training capability. Judging by other accounts of the conscription system, the dispensary visited by Drs. Powell and Lu cannot have been an exception to the norm. Wedemeyer bluntly informed General Marshall that for the Chinese peasantry famine, flood and drought were to conscription as chickenpox to plague. By the time they arrived at their destination the conscripted recruits were ready for the general hospital rather than the general reserve.[100]

---

case, Wedemeyer sent it on to the Generalissimo on Aug 5, 1945, with the comment that the report had been "carefully verified and I believe contains much factual data that will assist you and myself in our many intricate problems." A briefer version of this memo is in Young (1963), 358–359.

[98] Chinese Ministry of Information (1947), 287.

[99] Powell (1946), Chapter 9. The date of this visit is uncertain, but in view of the positions of various individuals mentioned in the text it cannot have been earlier than November 1944.

[100] Romanus and Sutherland (1959), chapter 2, 67.

The Alpha plan called for 270,000 combat ready men in 36 divisions by April 1, 1945. This would require detailed examining of existing manpower in those divisions, weeding out injured and sick soldiers and replacing them with healthy and trained conscripts. The Ministry of Conscription was so advised. But could it deliver? Apparently urged on by "highest authority", the Ministry approached the American Chongqing representatives of United China Relief for aid to improve the health of conscripts. Commenting on this, Dr. Lin wrote that the Ministry surely needed help, but it would have to come from the AMA or the NHA. Such robbing of Peter to pay Paul worried Lin. He urged his ABMAC supporters to screen any request from the Ministry and ensure that any plan to provide aid be discussed first with the U.S. Army Theater Surgeon Colonel Armstrong and the AMA. He noted that the U.S. Army was indeed flying recruits to reduce travelling time and liability to sickness from long marches. U.S. authorities were also concerned with the medical care and feeding of recruits. What about drawing on civilian medical personnel in lucrative private practice? Lin said he would be glad to see any scheme that put more civilian doctors into the army under the Conscription Ministry. But creation of another soup kitchen for "our poor soldiers" and provision of a non-army charitable medical service would be demoralizing for the army and another means for medical personnel to evade military service.[101]

Part of Lin's guardedness had to do with the Ministry's approach to United China Relief. He was already having difficulties with the "UCR gods in Chongqing" regarding the attempt by the latter to set up a new committee to handle requests for funds proposing to aid soldiers. On January 8th he had received a letter from Lennig Sweet, the UCR representative in Chongqing replacing Dwight Edwards, assuring him that the new Committee for Aid to Soldiers was not intended to review AMA requests. Instead it would deal with such matters as special services for the Educated Youth Army requested by the Ministry of Education, and the programs of such organizations as Friends of the Wounded, The National Christian Council, The New Life Movement for Service in Camps, Aid to Soldiers and Conscripts in Transit, and Service to Soldiers' Families. Needless to say, all such initiatives designed to support auxiliary organizations with American charitable funds raised warning signals for Dr. Lin.[102]

---

[101] ABMAC Box 2, Robert Lim Reports, Report #11, January 27, 1945, from Kunming.

[102] Ibid., Report #10, January 15, 1945 and letter from Lennig Sweet to Lin January 8, 1945.

In effect the Nationalist government was still trying to raise recruits with methods flourishing at the time when the Great Tang dynasty poet Du Fu (712–770) wrote a scathing poem about recruitment.[103] Forced levies (compulsory enlistment) of ignorant and helpless rural men were the standard method in Imperial China for providing manpower for armies and public works. As long as there were unlimited numbers of peasantry to serve in the ranks, why would the manpower needs for twentieth century warfare be any different? Wedemeyer and Lin knew the answer to that question. The Chinese armies were swelled with manpower, but much of it was unable to function in combat because the soldiers were untrained and because the Chinese economy lacked the means to support large aggregations of human beings. Both knew that a much smaller army, properly fed, trained, armed and medically supported, could perform credibly.

But such an army would need replenishing with properly fed, trained, armed and medically supported recruits. That problem proved insoluble under existing conditions. National and provincial health organizations offered some care of recruits,[104] The educated youth recruitment was designed to make conscription more equitable. But the educated youth were favored with better rations, and there was no intention to send them to the front lines. Once again Wedemeyer had to intervene with the advice that what the front line armies badly needed was the leadership of educated youth serving alongside the "poor man's son."[105] In June 1945 he went so far as to call for a reorganization of the Ministry of Conscription, to insure proper treatment of all conscripts and preclude induction of men mentally defective or physically unfit for military service.[106] Two months later, just as the Pacific war was nearing the end, he sent the Generalissimo an angry report concluding that nothing had changed:

> As they march along they turn into skeletons; they develop signs of beri-beri, their legs swell and their bellies protrude ... Dysentery and typhoid are always with them. They carry cholera from place to place (also louse-borne diseases). Leaving behind them a wake of the sick and the dying, they are

---

[103] See "The Conscription Officer at Stone Channel," also "Song of the War-Carts," in Hinton (2008).

[104] ABMAC Box 2, AMA, Lim Reports, Report #16, May 19, 1945.

[105] Eiler (1987), 128, memo to Gen. Marshall August 1, 1945.

[106] Eiler (1987), 98–99, memo to the Generalissimo June 18, 1945.

still performing the most important function of a citizen of Free China: to be a source of income for officials.[107]

1945: Reorganization of the AMA

During the early days of the Zhijiang campaign Dr. Xu Xilin resigned as Army Medical Administration Surgeon General, and on or around April 17, 1945 Chiang Kaishek ordered Lin Kesheng to take his place.[108] The fact that Lin was able to gain this appointment after his eclipse in 1943 reflects the growing importance of American military advice and resources in the conduct of the war in southwest China, as well as the premium placed on Lin's war experience by the Ichigo crisis and by his relationship with General Chen Cheng.

Lin wanted the medical aspects of Services of Supply built into Chinese military practice. He was determined to make the civilian medical world face up to its duties at this time of national crisis. He knew that American military physicians could help move his agendas forward. He also knew the strongest base for military medical reform was in the Southwest, where many of his former students and colleagues were serving. Senior government ministers who came into power late in 1944 added to those who saw Lin and his work as an asset.

Sometime in 1945 the Nationalist government consolidated management of the army central medical services under the leadership of the AMA. The Board of Supplies and Transportation and the Central Wounded Soldiers Administration were abolished. The AMA was to have "general charge of all army medical and rehabilitation services."[109] Branch EMSTS centers, long under AMA management, were reorganized into army hospitals and training units, following the Alpha model. The Army Medical Field Training School (formerly the Central EMSTS in Guiyang) now had an American team on site, "lending energy and hope." Americans provided fuel so that the hospital had electricity through most hours of the day and night. Two American officers helped run a medical field service course, and provide clinical instruction. In addition, National Xiangya and Shanghai Medical Colleges agreed to sponsor army hospitals by supplying

---

[107] Romanus and Sutherland (1959), chapter 12 (The End of Wedemeyer's Experiment), 368–373.

[108] Powell places this appointment in early March; the date that Lin gives in his report of May 19 is likely to be more accurate.

[109] Chinese Ministry of Information (1947), 502.

physicians and nurses, while the AMA provided administrative personnel and orderlies. National Guiyang Medical College lost many staff during the evacuation from Guiyang, but its president, Dr. Li Zongen (李宗恩 C. U. Lee), still hoped to sponsor a base hospital in the Guiyang area.[110]

By the end of the war Drs. Lin and Lu were the dominant army medical leaders serving the Nationalist government. Lin was the sole AMA Surgeon General and Lu was Commandant of the newly named Army Medical Field Service School. Lu was appointed special delegate of the Ministry of War, with responsibility to take over Japanese medical establishments and supplies in east, north, and central China. Other leading EMSTS personnel were appointed superintendents of Japanese army hospitals and members of special commissions, including one to plan a future army medical center. A Conference took place in February 1946 in Shanghai, at which plans were made to establish an Army Medical Center in Jiangwan, Shanghai. EMSTS Branch centers were assigned new duties. The Second center survived the war and was charged to form an Army Medical Hospital in Nanchang. A school of army medicine was formed combining EMSTS and AMC personnel, and the nursing school founded by Zhou Meiyu (周美玉) in Guiyang in 1943 was incorporated into the Jiangwan Center.[111]

None of this was plain sailing. The EMSTS and AMC medical communities were not natural allies. Getting them together required negotiation and arm-twisting, the latter supplied by General Chen Cheng.[112] Much to his credit the AMC dean, Dr. Zhang Jian, agreed to the plan and accepted appointment as co-vice Director of the new organization[113] (*Guofang Yixueyuan* 国防医学院 in Chinese, National Defense Medical Center in English), with Lu as the other vice director. Dr. Lin assumed overall charge.[114]

---

[110] ABMAC, box 2, AMA, Report #16, May 19, 1945.

[111] ABMAC, box 8, EMSTS, 1944–46. Report of Army Medical Field Service School for 1945, August 1945–March 1946.

[112] The details are in Watt (2008), "The National Defense Medical Center: The first Fifteen Years," 47–61.

[113] Although he studied in Berlin, Zhang was respected by leaders in the Anglo-American medical world. Dr. Liu Ruiheng recommended him as someone who "puts his heart and soul into his work;" his problems resulted from "inability to make good men work for him." See ABMAC, box 15, Liu, J. Heng, January-June 1947, Liu to Helen Kennedy Stevens, June 17, 1947. Dr. Wang Kaixi described Zhang as a "very quiet and humble person," who cooperated with Lin because he recognized that Lin was more capable. (Personal interview, August 27, 1987.)

[114] The difference in titles was a compromise between the Chinese name for the College and Lin's plan for the joint enterprise to function as a medical center.

There is no knowing how long this formula would have worked. As it was, Civil War between the Nationalists and the Communists erupted in full force in 1947. In November 1948 the National Defense Medical Center received orders to prepare to move to Taiwan. Approximately two-thirds of the its personnel did so between February to May 1949, including the top leaders Drs. Lin, Lu, and Zhang, many staff who had joined the Nationalist party, others trained at PUMC or at other colleges oriented to the Anglo-American medical education system, and many of the rank and file soldiers. Various others, including Dr. Lin, eventually dispersed to the U.S. and Australia.[115]

Other prominent individuals in the EMSTS, the CRCMRC, and the army hospitals in Guiyang and Chongqing, chose to stay. They included Drs. Rong Dushan (荣独山, hospital vice director), Zhou Shoukai (周寿恺, chair of internal medicine), Tu Kaiyuan (屠开元, orthopedics chair), and five other departmental chairs.[116] Many of the younger hospital staff who stayed later rose to senior positions in medical institutions throughout Communist China. Yang Xishou (杨锡寿), who is the source of this information, attributes this record of leadership to the high standards of patriotism and professionalism demanded of the hospital staff and the example set by Dr. Lin on both these counts. While Lin may have set the standards, the fact that half the hospital's top leaders came from PUMC and most of the rest from National Tongji Medical College also helped put high standards into effect.[117]

Conclusion: Unsolvable Problems

Nationalist China's Army medical services were in better shape in 1945 than when the war began eight years earlier. The AMA had been simplified and strengthened. Services of Supply had improved in units participating

---

[115] A list of the dispersal and whereabouts (where known) of former Red Cross and EMSTS staff is in Xue Qingyu (1987), 48–55. Hospital staff who went to Taiwan included Superintendent Yang Wenda, Chief of Surgery Zhang Xianlin 张先林, and Chief of Nursing Zhou Meiyu 周美玉.

[116] Dr. Zhou met his death in 1970 during the Cultural Revolution. Twenty years later, in a ceremony honoring his life and work, his younger brother and daughter delivered impassioned speeches in his memory. See http://goodteachernet.cn/shownewsjb.asp?newsid=16286126.

[117] Yang Xishou (杨锡寿) (1987), 167–176. See especially 170 for the hospital's impact on the medical world in China.

in the Alpha Plan. The importance of medical work in sustaining army morale had become clear to several of Nationalist China's most effective military field commanders. Other elements of the Nationalist leadership, including its civilian medical agencies, were forced by Campaign Ichigo to see that the army was the only barrier averting a collapse of Nationalist government. Finally a more rigorously enforced conscription of medically trained people took place.

Another important development, initiated by Dr. Lin and continued by Dr. Lu, was the training of thousands of individuals serving as army medical assistants in basic triage, primary medical care, and sanitary services. In its 1946 report the Army Medical Field Service School (formerly EMSTS) stated that its units had trained 15,931 individuals, including 1,158 during 1945.

Unfortunately the influence of the Red Cross Medical Relief Corps units rapidly declined after August 1942, and as late as spring 1945 emergencies could still send the fragile state of health of Nationalist China's soldiers and recruits into free fall. For that to happen we should recall the unsparing efforts by army and civilian leaders during 1942–1943 to disparage the work of Lin and his lieutenants, undermine Lin's reputation and drive him out of office. Second is the widespread corruption in the Nationalist army Services of Supplies and among regimental officers, resulting in delivery of abysmal army rations to front line soldiers; and third is the complacency of the army logistics leadership towards military and conscript health care, reflecting a dangerous incapacity to understand the impact of disease and malnutrition on army performance.[118]

One might thus conclude that the only feasible job of the MRC and even the EMSTS was to respond to medical emergency. But that is not how the EMSTS leaders and their ABMAC friends in New York saw it. In early 1943 Dr. Frank Co Tui asked his fellow directors to think of ABMAC not as a temporary relief organization but as an integrator of the willing energies of American scientists with the energies and vision of the medical statesmen of China in a threefold task: 1) build a modern medical service for the Chinese army; 2) build a public health structure for a

---

[118] Recent publications on the great Chinese famine of 1958–1962, which illustrate how the malfeasance of central, regional and local party officials contributed to the starvation and death of country people, provide insight into how Nationalist China's front line soldiers could be starved in 1943–1945 even though food was available.

new-born nation of 450 million people; 3) help provide medical personnel to carry out the first two tasks.[119]

The first task was the immediate focus of Lin and his colleagues and the second was their long-term agenda. They saw that their first challenge was to apply medical science to save lives and raise army morale and capability. All Dr. Lin's junior colleagues who spoke highly of his patriotism had his commitment to these goals in mind.[120] They also knew that the rural soldiers trained as medical aides could become emissaries of public healthcare. Although the work of army medical reformers flagged during 1943 and part of 1944, the arrival of American military medical personnel in southwest China in 1944 brought Dr. Lin Kesheng back into an important leadership role and brought new resources to their work, particularly in the vital logistical areas covered by services of supply.

If only it had succeeded. But last minute reforms by new government leaders, such as simplifying the Army medical hierarchy and appointing Dr. Lin to head it in April 1945 were much too late to have any serious impact. A government at war that couldn't or wouldn't feed its troops properly or understand the importance of a modern army healthcare system could not prevail. Even the best medical reformers—and Drs. Lin and Lu and their colleagues were the best—couldn't alter that fundamental deficit.

It is not good news to see a true patriot brought down by senior military officials conniving with foreigners, especially when that patriot was so eager to save lives and so capable of developing resources to advance that cause. But it is useless to get annoyed with generals, even with He Yingqin, when incompetence of generals and their indifference to military mortality is such a common occurrence.[121] We have to ask rather what was it about Lin's modus operandi that ended up putting him out of action? An explanation offered by ABMAC's representative Zheng Baonan (郑宝南) is that Lin was years ahead of his time.[122] Given the fact that

---

[119] Co Tui to Alfred Kohlberg, April 16, 1943, in ABMAC box 38, Alfred Kohlberg, miscellaneous letters, instructions, reports.

[120] The essay by Lü Yunming (1987) is emblematic of this perspective.

[121] This is the pervasive and shocking theme in Dixon (1994). Dixon's book is about the astonishing incompetence—with rare exceptions—of British generals. The collapse of the Nationalist armies during the Chinese civil war of 1947–1949 reminds one that the same critique applied to some—even many—of Nationalist China's military leaders.

[122] ABMAC box 5, Cheng Pao-nan, Cheng Pao-nan to Frank Co Tui, September 24, 1942. Zheng argued that Lin's thoughts were "some fifty years too advanced for the mediocre and the simpleton."

Chinese society had not yet entered into the epidemiological and demographic transitions when Lin began his reforms, he and his fellow health-care reformers had no alternative other than to advance their medical agendas at a time when the general society—including the leadership and intelligentsia on the one hand and the vast uneducated masses on the other—were unready to embark on that course. The crisis of Japanese invasion in 1937 played into Lin's hands by creating an intolerably large number of wounded and untreated soldiers and refugees. But after 1939 Japanese military pressure on Nationalist China's armies eased off and would not significantly resume until the Ichigo campaign began in spring 1944. During that long interlude the Burma road pipeline was cut off, greatly diminishing fuel supplies in West China, Southeast Asia fell to Japan cutting off aid from overseas Chinese, and inflation in West China soared. These conditions cut the ground out from under Lin's operation and enabled his enemies to get the better of him. It was only when Ichigo bore down on southwest China late in 1944 and He Yingqin was replaced as Minister of War by Chen Cheng that Lin was restored to a position of leadership.

During the long interlude when costs escalated, the air went out of the Medical Relief Corps and medical personnel found themselves relying on the civilian economy to stay afloat.[123] Nationalist China's military logistics personnel came to regard army medical affairs as a sideline. When Ichigo tore down through central China in summer and autumn 1944 creating masses of civilian and military refugees, suddenly Nationalist China's leaders needed Dr. Lin again. By then soldiers were dropping dead from starvation.

This is a sad reflection on bad leadership, indifference to human values, and blindness to real dangers and real resources. China's soldiers deserved better. Dr. Lin also deserved better. But amidst all the military incompetence his work, and that of his colleagues, in improving medical care of China's soldiers under severe wartime conditions stands out like a beacon. The next chapter will discuss how well civilian healthcare functioned under the same severe wartime conditions.

---

[123] This problem will be discussed further in the next chapter, particularly with regard to public health in Sichuan.

CHAPTER SIX

PUBLIC HEALTH AMID THE TURMOIL OF WAR, 1938–1949

Whether the Public Health Movement in this country will be recorded as just a historical event of the past, or as an epoch-making contribution to the modern history of Chinese civilization, is now dependent on whether we can uphold standards before the war is over.[1]

Anonymous, 1943

By the end of 1937 the modern public health movement in China was in crisis. Due to the Japanese military onslaught on Nanjing the whole NHA had to let go of many of its staff and restart in marginal circumstances in southwest China. Once again it became an appendage of the Ministry of the Interior.

Despite these setbacks the NHA kept public health initiatives going during the eight-year War of Resistance against Japan. Led for most of this period by Dr. Jin Baoshan (金宝山), the NHA responded actively to epidemics and against the odds promoted public, preventive healthcare in rural China. Due to sharp inflation and social upheaval these initiatives became increasingly difficult to carry out during the mid 1940s. Yet the public health leaders did not give up.

Did the case for preventive healthcare advance because of their work? Were standards upheld? Or did the bombing, the displacement, the epidemic diseases, the hyperinflation, the loss of staff, or an inherent conservatism, undermine these efforts? The reason for considering such questions is that there has been a tendency over the last sixty years to write off the work of the Nationalist government's NHA as marginal and reactionary, so that the public health movement had to begin again in 1949 under more auspicious leadership. Such an interpretation seemed plausible until it became clear that during 1958–62 the PRC leaders presided over one of the most life-destructive famines in human history, far worse than the famines and health crises suffered during the War of

---

[1] From Anon., "Conservation of Technical Personnel in Important Positions," received in New York February 2, 1943, in ABMAC box 20, NHA General. The report reflects the thinking of Dr. Chen Zhiqian.

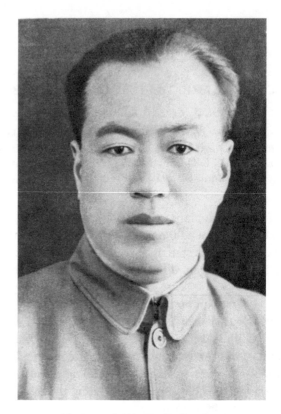

Photograph 6.1: *Dr. Jin Baoshan*
Director General, National Health Administration, 1940–1947. A protégé of the
influential writer Lu Xun and also of Dr. Liu Ruiheng, Dr. Jin studied medicine in
Japan and public health at Johns Hopkins. He was a tireless worker who strove
to promote universal health care under far from positive circumstances. (*Source*:
ABMAC Archive)

Resistance.[2] The lowly but active Nationalist NHA did not preside over
any such disaster; instead its agents moved ahead in unoccupied China
with their preventive rural health strategies. How well did they succeed?

---

[2] See i) Frank Dikotter (2010); ii) Yang Jisheng (2012). These works call for a fundamental reassessment of the relationship between famine and human causation, especially as
regards the famine of 1958–1962.

Setbacks and Recoveries during Early War Years

The eruption of hostilities with the Japanese military in July 1937 forced an immediate change in the work of the NHA. To deal with the crisis caused by Japanese military invasion the government linked the NHA and the AMA into a Combined Health Services Ministry (*Weisheng Qinwubu* 卫生勤务部) under the leadership of Dr. Liu Ruiheng (刘瑞恒). Before long the campaign around Shanghai intensified and Japanese planes were bombing Nanjing. At some point early in this period Japanese bombs struck the buildings of the Ministry of Health and the Central Field Health Station.[3] The Central Military Commission remained in Nanjing to oversee the military campaign, but civilian administrations retreated to West China. By December 1937 the doomed capital was in the hands of the enemy.

The NHA's westward retreat ended the healthcare progress achieved in eastern China during the Nanjing decade. The model districts in Jiangsu province had to be abandoned. Almost half of the NHA employees were sent home and never returned to NHA service.[4] The head office relocated in Chongqing, the wartime capital in Sichuan, while the Central Hospital, the Central Field Health Station, and the Public Health Personnel Training Institute moved to Guiyang, capital of Guizhou province. Guiyang became headquarters of a variety of educational, public and military health agencies. The Central Epidemic Prevention Bureau (中央防疫处) relocated in Kunming,[5] and the pioneer virologist Dr. Tang Feifan (汤飞凡) was its director throughout the War of Resistance.[6]

---

[3] "Control of Epidemics: the Epidemic Commission of the League," (August 1938): 182–189. The text says that the buildings were wrecked "at the beginning of the war," suggesting that it happened around September 1937.

[4] Fu Hui and Deng Zongyu (1989). According to the 1937 diaries of John B. Grant the central government retrenchment had already begun by September 20. See Grant diary 1937–39, September 20, 1937. Rockefeller Foundation archive (RF), RG 12.

[5] Dr. Liu later told Grant that between the Japanese breakthrough across the Suzhou-Jiaxing line and the stabilization of retreat after the capture of Nanjing, the experience had been "almost nightmarish." Almost unbelievable circumstances had occurred, including the looting of Nanjing by mutinous Chinese military forces before their retreat, resulting in an "impossible medical situation." Grant Diary, February 12, 1938, in RF, RG 12.

[6] Dr. Tang was a graduate of the Xiangya Medical College in Changsha with several years advanced study at the Peking University Medical College and Harvard University. He is noted for his studies on the etiology of trachoma, which he carried out while he was in Kunming. There are now several studies of Dr. Tang's life and work, e.g. Liu Junxiang, Tang Feifan, a Medical Scientist, (Beijing, 1999, not seen). He died in 1958 under tragic circumstances.

In January 1938 the Combined Health Services Ministry was broken up. The Army Medical Administration reverted to the Ministry of Defense and the NHA to the Ministry of the Interior, now directed by He Jian (何键), a former army general and governor of Hunan. Dr. Liu Ruiheng was squeezed out by this move, which occurred while he was attending a meeting in Hong Kong with League of Nations representatives. His job as NHA director was turned over to Dr. Yan Fuqing (颜福庆), an older and less activist public health specialist, who made his career principally as a medical college administrator.[7] The removal of Dr. Liu indicated that his agenda and activist leadership was out of line with what Nationalist government leaders regarded as an appropriate role for health policy.[8] Perhaps it was true, as Dr. Grant suggested, that Dr. Liu—when confronted with the nightmarish retreat of the Chinese armed forces from Nanjing—threw up his hands in despair. Yet he was not a quitter. He became involved in the work of China Defense Supplies and served as an advisor to, and later medical director of, ABMAC.[9]

Despite these difficulties, by late 1938 the NHA put together a plan to deal with the war emergency. In response to the epidemic crisis threatened by movements of huge numbers of refugees, it organized an epidemic prevention corps, which grew to twenty-five units with a staff of four hundred physicians and nurses.[10] In 1939 the NHA instituted a series of highway health stations which provided medical support along new highways being urgently constructed in west China. This system grew quite rapidly; by 1942 when there were over 6,000 km of new highways, fifty-seven health stations were in place, modeled on county health stations and providing much the same services.[11]

---

[7] Grant recorded in his diary that after witnessing the collapse of the Nanjing government and the looting carried out by retreating Chinese soldiers, Liu's "general mental condition resulted in a laissez faire attitude, with the consequence that Dr. F. C. Yen (颜福庆) was appointed director." Dr. Liu afterwards held several non-governmental positions; after the initiation of the U.S. Lend Lease program he became Medical Director of China Defense Supplies, the agency set up by Song Ziwen in Washington to administer Lend Lease to China. A biography of Dr. Yan, the founding director of Hunan's Xiangya Medical College, is in Huang Jiasi (1985), 2–15. On He Jian, see Boorman (1967), II, 60–63.

[8] As Ka-che Yip points out, Dr. Liu was investigated in 1936 for questionable practices in financial reporting. The problem was that he lacked sufficient funding to support NHA agendas and had to shuffle accounts to cover the bills. He survived an investigation, but it must have left him weakened and more easily disposable. See Yip (1995), 65.

[9] For an account of Dr. Liu's later career see Watt (1989), 188–205.

[10] The central government authorized the NHA to put together up to one hundred epidemic prevention units. Grant Diary, April 10, 1938, in RF, RG 12.

[11] ABMAC box 20, NHA General, "National Health Administration," November 1942.

The NHA picked up on its public healthcare agenda by supplying senior staff to the fledgling health departments of Sichuan, Guizhou and Yunnan provinces and helping to establish model health stations.[12] In Guizhou province, Guiyang city set up a health demonstration center in May 1938, and within a year the province had eight county health centers and twenty-one health stations open.[13] After the CRCMRC located its emergency medical service training school just outside Guiyang, personnel of the epidemic prevention corps were sent there for training.[14]

Developments in Rural Healthcare in Southwest China

In 1935 the NHA had sent a team of advisers led by Drs. Stampar and Yao Yongzheng (姚永政 also Yao Yung-tsung) to help plan a provincial health bureau and hospital in Yunnan.[15] Dr. Yao Xunyuan (姚寻源), who had worked for NHA's Central Field Health Station and then as provincial health administrator in Ningxia, arrived in Yunnan in March 1936 to serve as provincial director of health, and the bureau opened in July.[16] The National Economic Council provided a subsidy that lasted until October 1937. The new bureau constructed a provincial hospital. It had a provincial nursing and midwifery school, a hygiene laboratory, a school health program in six central primary schools, and as of August 1937 a municipal health station. By the end of 1937 sixty-three counties each had a county

---

[12] ABMAC, box 21, NHA 1940–41, "Health Program of the NHA," undated but internally datable to late 1938 or the beginning of 1939.

[13] Ibid.

[14] In October 1938 Grant reported from Changsha that the epidemic prevention corps' headquarters were now located in the commodious offices of the Emergency Medical Service Training School. By then the corps had twelve hospitals and twenty-five field units, each with four teams, with an additional six isolation hospitals and eighteen field units in process of organization. All personnel passed through the school before assuming field duties. Grant diary, October 8, 1938, in RF, RG 12.

[15] Dr. Yao Yongzheng received an MPH in parasitology from Johns Hopkins in 1930 and undertook advanced research at the London School of Tropical Medicine. He became noted for several publications in this field. See http://www.hudong.com/wiki/姚永政.

[16] Born into a village family, Dr. Yao Xunyuan graduated from PUMC in 1925. He worked for the Peking No. 1 Health Station and was first director of the health program at Dingxian. He received a CPH from Johns Hopkins in 1932. He was chief of the department of medical relief and social medicine at NHA's Central Field Health Station before becoming a provincial health director. See Chinese Medical Directory (1941), and Hayford (1990), 133–134. For personal insight into Yao's background see Bullock (1980), 112.

health worker, but due to lack of funds this rural initiative was only a skeletal operation.[17]

In southwestern Yunnan malaria was a severe problem. A survey in 1935 showed an average of twenty-seven percent of the population in malarial regions to be infected with malaria parasites and fifty percent with enlarged spleens.[18] In 1936, Dr. Yao Yongzheng and two colleagues published articles on the miasma (瘴气 *zhangqi*) found along the borders between Guizhou and Guangxi and Yunnan and Burma and believed by locals to be connected with the heavy incidence of malaria in those regions. The authors discovered that the vast majority of the people, including educated people and officials, did not understand the etiology of the disease. In various places it was associated with eels, toads, butterflies and cholera, while more educated people attributed it to inhalation of poisonous gas emanating from decaying animal and vegetable matter. The authors stated that malaria was responsible for more deaths in Yunnan than all other infectious diseases combined.[19] It incapacitated at least thirty percent of the labor gang coolies working on the Burma Road.[20]

Dr. Yao Xunyuan noted that the government originally had six small health stations in malarial regions in southwest Yunnan, which could be reached only by sedan chair or horse. By 1939 there were 13 health centers, one with four health stations and four substations.[21] The opening in early 1939 of the Burma Road from Kunming to Lashio in Burma created new malarial hazards. The area from the Salween River to the Burmese frontier was severely infested with mosquitos; a temple inscription advised travellers crossing the Salween to the west during the rainy season that there was little chance of their returning alive. The 25th unit of the NHA's anti-epidemic corps was now patrolling the region.[22] In September 1940 the NHA organized a special health department with eight health stations and four mobile units between Tsu-yung (Ch'u-hsiung, west of Kunming) and Wanting (on the border with Burma). During 1941 the NHA operated

---

[17] H. Y. Yao (Yao Hsun-yuan/Xunyuan) (1938), 577–583.

[18] Yao Hsun-yuan, (1939), 63–68.

[19] Y. T. Yao, L. C. Ling, and K. R. Liu (1936): 726–738, 1815–1828. In an effort to control the disease one magistrate employed many people to dig out and remove eels. Ironically the connection of malaria to a mosquito-borne parasite was demonstrated by Robert Ross in India in 1898, and the Japanese colonial regime in Taiwan began examining blood smears of Taiwanese people as early as 1910. See Department of Health (May 1991).

[20] ABMAC box 21, NHA 1940–41, P. Z. King (Jin Baoshan), "The Chinese National Health Administration during the Sino-Japanese Hostilities," Chongqing, June 1940.

[21] Yao Hsun-yuan (1939). Dr. Grant recorded in his diary that the NHA began its malaria prevention program in Yunnan with a $50,000 per annum budget.

[22] Robertson (1940), 57–73.

eight class A, eight class B, and fourteen mobile units on the highway. By 1942 these numbers had increased. The stations operated an outpatient department, small hospitals for serious cases and small diagnostic laboratories. During 1941 they provided 455,000 preventive inoculations, treated 774,000 patients, and carried out health promotion, education and environmental sanitation projects.[23]

The U.S. Public Health Service sent a 16-person mission with malarial expertise to the area. The NHA contributed 155 staff to this mission, including eighteen medical officers and sanitary engineers, six entomologists and the rest sanitary supervisors and inspectors. This task force began working in January 1942, but as a result of the Japanese conquest of Burma its work was suspended in April; and following the termination of traffic on the Yunnan-Burma highway, the health stations on the route were closed in August.[24] Malarial work in southwest Yunnan would have to wait for more peaceable times.

Another important initiative in Yunnan was the development of a health demonstration center at Qujing (曲靖 Kutsing), around 110 km east of Kunming. The NHA, the Yunnan provincial health bureau, and the National Shanghai Medical College were the sponsoring agencies.[25] The center had a staff of forty-three people, including the director and four physicians. It had several interns from the College and four to seven student nurses from the Yunnan Provincial School of Nursing and Midwifery. It served a local population of over 12,000 people. The station began collecting reliable vital statistics. The crude birthrate was 40.4 and crude death rate 18.7 (per 1,000 live people). The infant mortality rate was 165.3 per 1000 live births under one year of age. These rates compare favorably with national crude birth and death rates estimated by rural workers for 1937 as 30, 25, and around 200.[26]

Illiteracy and education were also measured. Male illiteracy rates were fifty-three percent and female, eighty-nine percent. That meant that communication about healthcare would have to be primarily oral. The schools had 1,600 boy and 300 girl students. Sixty-eight percent had trachoma,

[23] ABMAC box 21, NHA, 1942, "The Chinese National Health Administration and its Subsidiary Organizations," May 11, 1942.

[24] ABMAC box 21, NHA, King, P. Z., 1942–43, P. Z. King, "Public Health during 1940–1942;" P. Z. King (1943), 47–54.

[25] Daniel G. Lai (Lai Douyan (赖斗岩) and C. M. Chu (Zhu Jiming 朱既明) (May 1940), 468–475. Dr. Lai was professor of public health and Dr. Zhu an assistant instructor at National Shanghai Medical College. See http://baike.soso.com/v372394.htm for information on Dr. Zhu.

[26] League of Nations Health Organization, (1937).

an indication of how severe that disease was for China's children, and over twenty-five percent suffered from malnutrition. Nearly 12,000 treatments for trachoma were administered, along with 823 smallpox vaccinations and 4,495 cholera inoculations. The school nurse put on health plays and lectures and made home visits. Over 3,000 lbs. of soybean milk with cakes were distributed free to 768 malnourished children. In the clinic the most common cases were ulcers, scabies, trachoma, bronchitis, diarrhea, bacillary dysentery, malaria and typhus. The general population received 4,421 smallpox vaccinations and 8,835 cholera inoculations, over 2,000 of which were secondary doses. Public health nurses made 5,300 visits to 2,300 homes, gave nearly 13,000 health talks, and administered another 4,395 smallpox vaccinations and over 11,000 cholera-typhoid inoculations. Other preventive health work included disinfection of wells and latrines, distribution of boiled water, and inspection of food shops.

Obviously Qujing had in many respects a model health center. There is no mention of a clinical laboratory, and as for aseptic childbirth the results were modest: 179 mothers attending prenatal clinic, 131 deliveries, and 38 babies in a well baby clinic. However a special women's day exhibit on maternal child health drew 500 visitors.

In Guizhou a fascinating example of rural healthcare is provided in a 1943 report from the Guizhu (贵筑) health station in Huaxi (花溪) County, Guizhou province. This station was a field training center for several nearby medical schools and training institutes in Guiyang. The central station and four substations had a staff of approximately thirty and at the time of the report had given a preliminary three-week course to ten village auxiliaries.[27]

The district catered to an eighty-five percent illiterate population. The inhabitants were reportedly steeped in "superstition, folklore and witchcraft" and had little or no exposure to modern medicine. The district set up Maternal Child health (MCH), school health, communicable disease control, and sanitation services. The report acknowledged that MCH services reached only "upper and middle class people" and carried out only one twentieth of total deliveries. Many maternal deaths were reported because the "illiterate classes" were too ignorant or shy to come to the health station. However all school children were given a health examination and vaccinated, and public health nurses taught them good health habits.

---

[27] ABMAC, box 20, NHA, General, "Report of the Kwei-chu Hsien Health Station," 1943.

Communicable disease control was more limited. Less than nine percent of the people accepted smallpox vaccination and ten percent cholera. Thus a midsummer cholera epidemic spreading from Guiyang caused one hundred and seventy-nine deaths and a seventy-nine percent death rate. Despite lack of trained personnel, the center chlorinated 7,530 sanitary buckets and carried out over 2,000 shop and street stall inspections. Apart from widespread malaria, the main diseases were trachoma (沙眼) and malnutrition (营养不良) resulting in chronic ulcers (溃).

The Guizhu program was not typical. The director, Dr. Shi Zhengxin (施正信 Sze Tsung-sing), had a Ph.D. in public health administration from Johns Hopkins and was director of public health at National Guiyang Medical College.[28] It was his job to help students connect with the preliterate, indigenous inhabitants, many belonging to ethnic minorities. Obviously it was one thing to devise a public healthcare system and another to make it happen. Before the War of Resistance one sixteen-bed hospital was the only public healthcare institution in Guizhou. But during the war modern public health came to Guizhou. The leaders of the provincial health bureau and the two national medical colleges in Guiyang were committed to advancing rural healthcare. By 1942 seventy-eight county health stations were in operation, most of them third class stations headed by a qualified nurse. Three stations trained ninety-five health aides. The province had an anti-malaria institute, six mobile anti-epidemic units and a medical vocational school for training nurses, midwives and attendants. In short, a structure for the delivery of public healthcare was in place.[29] Health Demonstration centers were set up at Dingfan (Huishui, 60 km south of Guiyang), Qingzhen (Tsingchen, 25 km west of Guiyang), as well as in Guiyang.[30]

A summary account by the experienced public health official Dr. Huang Zifang (黄子方 Tsefang F. Huang) of the development of health centers

---

[28] A graduate of the University of Hong Kong Medical School, Dr. Shi went on to study at the London School of Tropical Medicine before going to John's Hopkins. He became Guizhou provincial director of health and then spent several years on the staff of the World Health Organization before becoming vice president of the Chinese Medical Association. For his services to local, provincial, national, and international health the University of Hong Kong awarded him a special prize.

[29] ABMAC, box 21, NHA, 1942, "A Brief Account of Kweichow Health Work", by Dr. K. F. Yao, Health Commissioner Guizhou Province, (姚克方 Yao Kefang), with stamped date of November 12, 1942.

[30] ABMAC box 21, NHA, 1940–1941, C. K. Chu (Zhu Zhanggeng), "Training of Public Health Personnel in 1939–1940."

illustrates both the advances as well as continuing hazards.[31] From Dr. Huang's perspective, the U.S. set the pace in health centers by growing from twelve in 1917 to over one thousand by the end of 1926. Yet in Poland and Yugoslavia the health agencies created national systems of modern healthcare. By the end of 1937 Poland had 235 centers with 500 full or part time physicians, 402 nurses, and 90 sanitary inspectors. By 1935 Yugoslavia had 48 district health centers, 120 rural health centers and 111 centers for specific fields, coordinated by nine provincial institutes and a Central Institute of Hygiene.

Two developmental models had emerged, both adopted by China: first, centers such as Qujing and Guizhu demonstrated modern public health work managed by medical college departments of public health; second, modern governmental public health administrative centers such as Bishan (see below) oversaw small local centers. The small centers were run by visiting nurse-midwives and sanitary inspectors and focused on preventive strategies. The larger centers dealt with major infectious diseases not susceptible to vaccination, and provided field education and laboratory analysis. For Dr. Huang the work of public health nurses was especially important because it reached out to individual households.

China had been developing public health centers for 14 years and Dr. Huang was involved in public health work since becoming director of the Beijing first health station and city commissioner of health. After the war with Japan broke out he joined the Shanghai medical college as professor of public health and was instrumental in organizing the Qujing Health Demonstration center. He contracted typhoid fever in December 1939 while making a health inspection of poor homes and died aged forty-two while in transit to Hong Kong.[32] His death raised the awkward question: did China have the professional leadership and committed rank and file necessary to push the rural healthcare model forward? Before leaving China in 1939 Dr. John Grant recorded a conversation with Luo Jialun (罗家伦), President of National Central University, in which Luo argued that the war successfully taught the Chinese government to initiate Chinese social-economic measures in place of previous European-American ones. We have seen this process having a real impact in the once backward provinces of Guizhou and Yunnan. How well did the reformers maintain this initiative as the War of Resistance dragged on?

---

[31] Obituary in CMJ, 57 (1940): 494–496.

[32] Obituary, op. cit., note 31. Another source states that Dr. Huang died of stomach cancer (but no further details). See, e.g., biography of Dr. Zhu Jiming in note 25.

More Crises and Recovery at the NHA

In May 1939 the new Rockefeller Foundation representative Dr. Marshall Balfour arrived in Chongqing. He learned that the NHA director Dr. Yan Fuqing had a narrow escape from Japanese bombing that destroyed the NHA central office building.[33] The NHA was relocated well outside the city, and a city branch office was maintained at the municipal hospital. Unfortunately the NHA staff moved into what one author called "the very center of one of the worst malaria areas" in Sichuan province. Sixty percent of the workers constructing the new NHA building came down with malaria, and NHA personnel were also infected. This was a very serious setback for NHA; however by the spring of 1941 its work was again under way.[34]

The NHA budget for 1939 showed that the epidemic prevention corps had now the largest centrally managed health services budget, with the next largest sums going to the Narcotics Bureau and the highway health station corps.[35] In Guiyang Balfour found no direct head at the once favored Central Field Health Station. "One should not be hypercritical," he commented; the Station's incubators were being run with kerosene lamps and it had no rubber stoppers for vaccine bottles. On the other hand, the Central Hospital, in spite of no electricity or running water, showed a surprising degree of order and cleanliness. All windows and doors were screened. The two hundred and forty beds were wooden forms on trestles covered with a thin mattress. Each case appeared to have as complete a record of examinations as one would find in Beijing or Boston. The out-patient department was active.[36]

Back in Chongqing Dr. Balfour met Dr. Li Tingan (李廷安), former head of the greater Shanghai Department of Health, now working as head of NHA's Epidemic Prevention Corps. Dr. Li stated that the Corps' mobile units were aiding refugees caught between the front lines and the "fixed

---

[33] The Chongqing bombing campaign, described in White and Jacoby (1946), is regarded in China as one of the "Three Great Disasters" (三大惨案 san da can'an) of the War of Resistance.

[34] Winfield (1948), 223. Winfield's conclusion was that despite NHA's excellent record "the national health program has been retarded by decades."

[35] The total 1939 budget for the centrally administered offices was ¥2,944,000, of which the epidemic prevention corps got 588,000, the Narcotics Bureau 360,000 and the Highway Corps 350,000. In the estimated budget for 1940 these figures went up to 4,159,000 for all central departments with twenty-five percent going to the epidemic prevention corps. M. C. Balfour diary, May 22, 1939, in RF, RG 12.

[36] Balfour diary, May 25 and 26, 1939.

civilian administrations." Dr. Yang Chongrui, officially head of the maternal and child health department of the Central Field Health Station in Guiyang, was still spending much of her time working on Mme. Chiang's orphanages.[37] Balfour met with the minister of education, Chen Lifu, who told him that Chinese medicine should be given a thorough opportunity to prove itself. In June, Balfour visited the National Epidemic Prevention Bureau in Kunming and found the staff working twenty-four hours a day mainly producing typhoid and cholera vaccines.[38]

These comments illustrate difficulties the NHA had getting back on its feet. It had again lost its main office due to wartime destruction. The CFHS, the prime engine for promotion of public healthcare, was leaderless. The leader most qualified to promote modern midwife education was busy managing orphans. The minister of education was vigorously advocating for Chinese medicine practitioners. And why not? They existed throughout China's towns. But they were not set up to deal with the epidemics, the physical trauma of masses of refugees, the numerous patients needing hospitalization, or the need for hygienic midwifery, preventive inoculations, and health education, in other words the agenda of public healthcare. By putting the health of China's people in such jeopardy the war demonstrated that a fully functioning NHA was needed to look after the health of China's war-torn people.

Between 1939 and 1940 the NHA underwent further reorganization. Due to the indiscretion of a relative Dr. Yan was forced to resign in April 1940, which precipitated another series of changes in the NHA's status and mission.[39] It was restored to its earlier status directly under the Executive Yuan (executive cabinet).[40] In May Dr. Liu Ruiheng and Dr. Yan were brought back as NHA advisors, and the government adopted a constitution for provincial health departments. With that constitution in place the

---

[37] Dr. Yang Chongrui, 1891–1983, a pioneer in the development of maternal-child health and modern midwifery, graduated from the Peking Union Medical College for Women in 1917. She joined the PUMC Dept of Obstetrics and Gynecology from 1922 to 1926, undertook postgraduate study at Johns Hopkins and in Europe from 1925 to 1927, and then served in the PUMC's Dept. of Public Health and as head of the division of medical services of the Beijing Health Station from 1927 to 1930. She became Director of the first National Midwifery School in Beijing in 1929. Who's Who in China (1936), 269; Wong and Wu (1935), 751–2. For further discussion of her career during the 1930 and 40s see Bullock (1980), 173–178, Johnson (2011), and www.chinabaike.com/article/316/336/2007/2007022582409.html.

[38] Balfour Diary, May 29 and June 2, 1939.

[39] Information from Dr. J. H. Fan (Fan Rixin).

[40] P. Z. King (1940), 198–228.

Executive Yuan issued a document in June formally adopting the county government public healthcare system. Dr. Jin Baoshan (金宝善), who had been NHA deputy director, took over as director general and was permitted to attend Executive Yuan meetings as a nonvoting member. He soon added Dr. Lin Kesheng, an influential advocate of public healthcare, and Dr. Zhu Hengbi, the forceful president of National Shanghai Medical College, as NHA advisors.[41]

Suddenly things looked much better for the NHA. It was authorized to move ahead on the public healthcare system and positioned, in Dr. Jin's words, "to fit into the dual program of meeting both the emergent wartime needs and the permanent public health reconstruction."[42] Dr. Jin Baoshan was the right person to handle this. He had a strong record in epidemic prevention and provincial health work. As Dr. Liu Ruiheng's chief technical director he organized the medical relief corps during the 1931 Yangzi River floods and set up quarantine stations in Hankou and also around Guangzhou. He visited the health services of various European countries, especially Yugoslavia, and with the aid of Dr. Borcic organized the Central Field Health Station, modeling it on a Yugoslav prototype. He was in charge of organizing epidemic prevention bureaus in Lanzhou, Inner Mongolia and Suiyuan and traveled around the country setting up public health departments and laboratories.[43] After the NHA landed in Chongqing, Dr. Jin spent much of the next two years traveling in Hunan, Guangxi and Guizhou provinces helping to organize rescue services for wounded soldiers and refugees.[44] By 1940 he was ready to move forward on both civilian health agendas: emergent wartime needs and permanent public health reconstruction.

Emergent Wartime Needs: Epidemic Prevention and Medical Relief

The NHA was now one of three major government systems concerned with healthcare in time of war, the other two being the AMA and the CRCMRC. In reports issued in 1941 Dr. Jin defined the main NHA wartime role as "preservation of manpower" (civilian lives) through epidemic

---

[41] Fu and Deng (1989). The most informative source for weishengshu appointments is "Guanyu Zhonghua Minguo Zhengfu de Weisheng Jigou" (2011).
[42] P. Z. King (1940), 199.
[43] Li Xiangming (李向明) (1984), 280–286.
[44] Li Xiangming (1984), 281.

prevention, protection of highway health, and medical relief, including health protection for refugee children and medical care for wounded civilians. In the spring of 1940 the NHA set up a department of epidemic prevention in its office outside Chongqing to coordinate epidemic prevention work.[45] This work included production and distribution of vaccines and biologicals, roving epidemic interventions and intelligence collection, and maintenance of highway health stations on routes vulnerable to spread of infections. The mobile epidemic prevention corps now had thirty-five units working in sixty-five localities in sixteen provinces. These units carried out preventive inoculations, built delousing stations to control typhus and relapsing fever, disinfected wells and drinking water, and provided ambulatory treatment. Also the NHA cosponsored the formation of a joint epidemic intelligence service with the AMA and the medical department of the Ministry of Transport and Supplies. Late in 1941 it began issuing epidemiological reports. During 1941 the NHA organized five stations for venereal disease treatment and one hundred and two stations for delousing and treatment of scabies.[46] Backing up these interventions was the production of vaccines and biologicals by the Epidemic Prevention Bureaus in Kunming and Lanzhou.

These developments resulted in a gradual improvement in reporting of epidemic diseases (Table 6.1) and administration of vaccinations (Graph 6.6). Table 6.1 illustrates the very incomplete yet better-than-nothing data on which the NHA relied to mobilize its anti-epidemic resources. NHA leaders were not under the illusion that these figures represented reality. A letter from Dr. Jin Baoshan to the ABMAC representative Dr. George Bachman, dated August 23, 1943, reported 61,952 cholera cases and 29,029 deaths in eleven provinces in 1942. Of the figures for dysentery (and typhoid) Dr. Jin wrote, "One can be sure that this represents only a very small fraction of the actual incidence." It was hardly possible to know the actual incidence of typhoid, he added, because of inadequate diagnostic facilities.[47]

---

[45] ABMAC box 20, NHA General, "Epidemic Prevention and Control Work in China."

[46] In addition to vaccinations, NHA epidemic prevention units deloused 12,000 people and disinfected 270,000 wells (mostly in 1939). See ABMAC box 21, NHA 1940–41, October 1941 report section II, Projects of Public Health Reconstruction. The appointment of the PUMC-trained Dr. Rong Qirong (容启荣 Winston W. Yung) as director of epidemic prevention led to improvements in reporting, as reflected in Table 6.1 and Graph 6.6. See Fu and Deng (1989), 269.

[47] ABMAC, box 21, NHA, King, P. Z. 1942–43.

Table 6.1: Partial Data Collection for Four Major Communicable Diseases Reported to NHA, 1939 to 1947

Year	Cholera 霍乱		Dysentery 痢疾		Smallpox 鼠疫		Malaria 疟疾	
	Sick	Dead	Sick	Dead	Sick	Dead	Sick	Dead
1939					2,786	437		
1940	14,781	1,954	57,855	2,507	2546	288	199,718	—
1941	351	71	101,984	5,049	12,646	1,996	386,360	3,789
1942	23,597*	9,521*	89,740*	3,447	9,772	1,142	336,291	1,858
1943	17,385	6,318	86,621	3,795	6,450	944	363,880	1,751
1944	1,196	350	41,130	861	5,573	724	193,523	623
1945	21,552	5,201	59,163	1,499	5338	671	235,648	945
1946	54,197	15,460	165,550	2,469	20,385	2,533	984,252	3,932
1947	201	23	51,457	304	15,832	2,989	357,934	651

Source: "Guomin zhengfu shiqi gongi zhidu shouxiao shenwei yuanyin tanxi" (2011).

For that reason the inference in the title of the essay reporting this data deserves comment. Certainly the data in the chart is not comprehensive. The data collection service only got off the ground late in 1941; in large areas of China NHA was unable to collect any data at all, it had to rely on physicians not all of whom were familiar with the diagnostic symptoms of the disease categories or who lacked the resources to make the diagnoses, and on data collectors many if not most of whom had no training in data collection. It is also reasonable to assume that under the precarious conditions of communication between east and west China a fair amount of collected data never made it to Chongqing.[48] Why then bother to amass defective evidence? Mainly it was to show that the NHA was developing a data collecting capacity. The graduates of international public health programs who ran China's public health services knew that a public health service must collect data. Developing such a capacity in wartime was far from ideal, but at least collection of data got started.[49]

---

[48] For example, provincial health bureaus existed in Zhejiang, Jiangxi and Fujian, but communications were subject to military interventions.

[49] For 1942 NHA reported additional disease cases as follows: typhoid 25,317; relapsing fever 18,483; typhus 8,016; diphtheria 3,524; scarlet fever 1,949; meningitis 1,154. For plague it reported 2,847 cases and 2,382 deaths in five eastern and southern provinces and just under 700 deaths in northwestern provinces. Whereas the cholera data was reported from 338 districts, the malaria data came from 746 districts, equivalent to 95 percent of the 783 districts enrolled in the county healthcare system in 1942. To collect data from 746 counties during wartime when only 783 had any public healthcare staffing is a reasonable start.

The NHA had help from several international specialists in epidemic diseases to assist with control of outbreaks. The treatment of a cholera outbreak in southwest China during 1939–1940 illustrates how rapid application of basic interventions was able to do much to keep this epidemic under control. According to Dr. Fan Rixin (范日新), the epidemic was precipitated by an influx of overseas Chinese returning from Hong Kong, Singapore and Burma; it was very severe in Guiyang. Fortunately the NHA's consultant epidemiologist Dr. Robert H. Pollitzer was on hand. Following his advice Chinese Red Cross and International Red Cross teams carried out four vital control procedures: 1) all food for sale was to be covered by fly-proof screens, and no cut fruit or melons were allowed in open stalls; 2) public trench latrines were built, provided with ample supplies of chloride of lime, and supervised; 3) all drinking water was supervised by boy scouts and armed soldiers and provided with a thimbleful of chloride of lime emulsion for every five gallon kerosene can of water; 4) the entire population was vaccinated by means of six tons of cholera vaccine obtained from the French government in Indochina. The vaccine was unloaded into beer bottles and administered by high school students. Following these procedures six million people were vaccinated in three weeks and the epidemic was stopped. The Canadian missionary physician Dr. Robert B. McClure (no relation to General Robert B. McClure), who is the source of this information, commented that through his responses to outbreaks of cholera and plague "the rare Dr. Pollitzer saved the lives of millions in a dedicated, low profile life of great scientific but humble service."[50]

A vital element in the NHA's overall plan included provision of drugs, vaccines and medical supplies by the Central and Northwest Epidemic Prevention Bureaus. The biologist Dr. Yang Yongnian (杨永年) directed the Northwest Bureau (西北防疫处) in Lanzhou. Dr. Yang persuaded a good number of other biologists to join him in this enterprise at what was then widely regarded as a border town on the edge of the desert.[51] Under

---

[50] i) J. H. Fan, "Resume of my academic training, professional public health services and relevant bibliography regarding problems of cholera in China." ii) Robert B. McLure, "Dr. Robert Pollitzer, 1885–1968." These documents were obtained from Drs. Fan and McClure and are in the possession of the writer.

[51] For Dr. Yang see Fu and Deng (1989), 270 and biography at http://blog.sina.com .cn/s/blog_676014580100ibfl.html. For other Lanzhou agencies see Fu and Deng (1989). A medical college was opened in Lanzhou in August 1942, and a nursing school in Novem-

the leadership of Drs. Tang and Yang the bureaus produced a substantial amount of vaccines, sera and other biological products, as indicated in Graphs 6.1 and 6.2.[52] In 1942, the Central Bureau opened a branch laboratory in Guiyang; the Northwest Bureau had three branch laboratories in Pingliang (east Gansu), Xian and Chengdu.

A Central Pharmaceutical Manufacturing Company was set up in May 1940 to handle large-scale production of therapeutic agents other than quinine (anti-malarial), sulfonamides (for treating gonorrhea) and arsenicals (for treating syphilis), which could not yet be produced in China. It had factories in Chongqing and Chengdu. In 1941 NHA's Narcotics Bureau was enlarged and charged with production of non-narcotic drugs. It produced Dover's powder (used for colds and fever), Brown's mixture (an expectorant), Blaud's pills (a ferrous carbonate for treatment of anemia), and aspirin, as well as sodium sulphate, morphine, codeine, and strychnine (presumably used as a pesticide). The NHA also encouraged large-scale production of drugs by private factories.[53]

NHA's remedial services included central hospital facilities, subsidies to private and mission hospitals, and supervision of public provincial and municipal hospitals. By 1939 there were four central hospitals, two reporting directly to NHA in Chongqing and Guiyang, and two regional hospitals in Xi'an and Lanzhou reporting to the NHA regional commissioner's office in Xi'an. These hospitals catered to wounded soldiers and civilians.[54] The NHA also operated four isolation hospitals (in Chongqing, Jiangxi, Sichuan and Yunnan).[55] Since 1938 the NHA obtained funds to help 220 private and missionary hospitals care for wounded patients. Seventy of these hospitals were in occupied China and received subsidies through the China Medical Association.

---

ber 1943 (for details see CMB box 96, folder 687). The epidemic prevention bureaus in Mongolia and Suiyuan took over treatment of veterinary diseases.

[52] By August 1943 Dr. Jin could write that the two bureaus had the capacity to meet "a large part of the required needs" of China provided that materials essential for biological production could be procured in large quantities (e.g. through ABMAC or the American Red Cross). ABMAC box 21, NHA, King, P. Z., 1942–43, King to Bachman, August 23, 1943.

[53] ABMAC box 21, NHA, King, P. Z., 1942–1943, P. Z. King, "Public Health During 1940–1942."

[54] ABMAC box 21, NHA 1940–1941, "An Abridgement of the Annual Report of the NHA," (May 1940–April 1941 but including information dated June 1940).

[55] ABMAC box 21, NHA 1942, "National Health Administration of the ROC, November 1942."

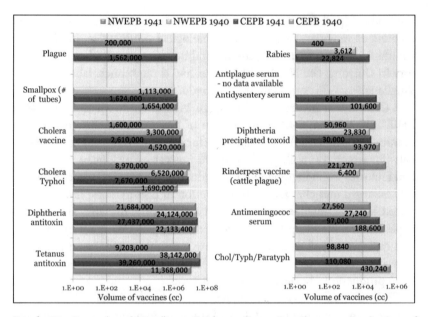

Graph 6.1: *Central and Northwest Epidemic Prevention Bureaus: Production of Vaccines, Sera, and Antitoxins, 1940 and 1941* (*Source:* ABMAC Archive, box 21 NHA, P. Z. King, 1942–43, P. Z. King, "Public Health During 1940–42." *Note:* E+ represents units of the power of 10. E+02 represents units of the power of 100; E+04 represents units of the power of 10,000.)

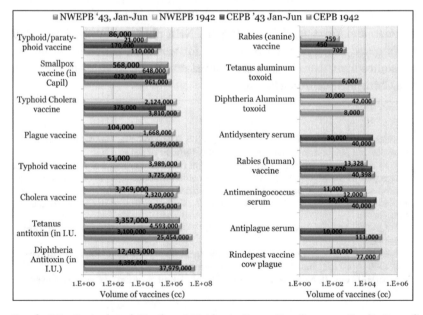

Graph 6.2: *Central and Northwest Epidemic Prevention Bureaus: Production of Vaccines, Sera, and Antitoxins, January 1942 to June 1943* (*Source:* ABMAC box 20, NHA General, "Report of Anti-Epidemic Activities, NHA, January 1, 1942–June 30, 1943." *Note:* E+ represents units of the power of 10. E+02 represents units of the power of 100; E+04 represents units of the power of 10,000.)

Around the middle of 1941 the main central hospital in Guiyang moved to Chongqing, leaving a branch hospital in Guiyang. The hospital in Chongqing acquired a 220–bed capacity, while the hospital in Guiyang had 200 beds. This move brought the Central Hospital director Dr. Shen Kefei (沈克非) to Chongqing, where given his seniority he should have been all along. At that time the problem of food supply had become quite acute, and at the battlefront disease casualties exceeded wounds. The most prevalent diseases were malaria, scabies, dysentery and leg ulcers, the last two related to nutritional problems. Since NHA's health units all provided outpatient and inpatient services, treatment of disease became a priority, comparable to disease prevention.

Consequently in November 1941 Dr. Shen took on the position of NHA deputy director general, agreeing to stay in it until the war was over. As part of the agreement he spent three days a week at NHA HQ and three as superintendent of the Central Hospital. A graduate Western Reserve University Medical School in Ohio and a protégé of Dr. Liu Ruiheng, Shen had been chief of surgery and Superintendent of the Central Hospital in Nanjing, where he initiated clinical and public health training programs. After the War of Resistance began, he opened the central hospital wards to wounded soldiers (it then had 1,200 beds). In retreat from Nanjing he led the central hospital to Changsha, Guiyang and eventually Chongqing, at each stop opening its wards to clinical teaching for medical students. His passion for clinical education and his administrative experience were needed to enable NHA to manage its curative work.[56]

Almost certainly as a result of Dr. Shen's leadership, a survey was done of clinical work in 3 central hospitals, 22 provincial and municipal hospitals, highway health stations and anti-epidemic corps centers during 1942 (see Graph 6.3 for main findings).

---

[56] Huang Jiasi (1985), 114–117.

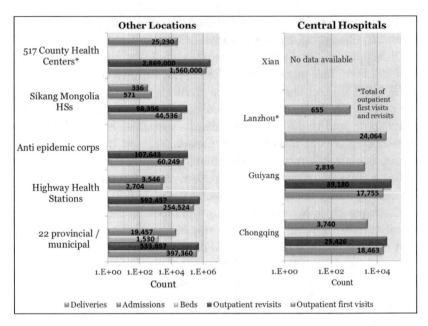

Graph 6.3: *National Health Administration: Clinical Treatment Data 1942* (*Source*: Statistical summary in "Organization of the National Heath Administration and its Subsidiary Organizations," ABMAC box 21, National Health Administration: King, P. Z. 1942–43. *Not all the returns from the 517 reporting health centers were received. Around 850 county health centers were in operation at the time. *Note*: E+ represents powers of 10. E+02 represents units of the power of 100, E+4 powers of 10,000.)

This graph provides a relatively clear impression of clinical treatment work going on in NHA organizations. It is more accurate at the Central Hospital level and less so at the county health center level; thus we are getting an impression rather than a report of the actual number of patient visits. Although no data was available for private and mission hospitals, the figures nonetheless provide a uniquely informative picture of curative work carried on by public healthcare agencies during one year in the long war with Japan. It says a good deal about the standards set by Dr. Shen that he was able to report such information about the commitment of China's healthcare workers to the wellbeing of China's people. Six and a half million recorded patient visits in one year indicate clearly that work was going on.

Public Health Reconstruction: The Public Healthcare System

Public health reconstruction required the development of a system to deliver low-cost yet effective preventive healthcare to the 350 million or more people living in rural areas. The seeds for this initiative were sown in the 1930s in the experimental counties (discussed in chapter 2). It was now up to the reformers to develop a system that would carry public preventive healthcare in China into a postwar era.

The system that evolved had three basic elements: a policy function at the center; a supervisory function at the provincial level; and an executive function at the county (*xian*) level, along with a county substructure to incorporate China's hundreds and thousands of villages into the system. This model followed the traditional system for diffusion of government from the center to the microcosm. In the 1930s that system, although fragmented by warlord rule, was still functioning in China. What the healthcare reformers did was to insert a healthcare function into the governmental process. The Nationalist government's adoption of the public healthcare system in April 1940 gave the NHA authority to move forward with this initiative.

As indicated in Graph 6.4, there were fifteen provincial bureaus in 1940 (fourteen in an earlier source) and an annual budget of $1.2 million to spend on provincial medical services. Six hundred and ninety-one counties, representing over fifty percent of the counties in the designated provinces, had health centers (*weishengyuan*).[57] In principle, if not in fact, there would be a health subcenter (*weisheng fenyuan*) in each subdistrict (*qu*), a health station for each town or group of villages (*xiang*), and a health aide for each hundredth (*bao*, a rural security unit averaging 100 families). The county center was to include a 20 to 40–bed hospital, a small diagnostic laboratory and a mobile clinic. The NHA sent forty-two senior medical officers and medical supplies to assist the provincial health bureaus in installing such services.[58]

The adoption of the county health system gave new impetus to the Public Health Personnel Training Institute, which since August 1939 had been under the direction of Dr. Zhu Zhanggeng (朱章庚). The Institute offered postgraduate courses on public health, supplementary public

---

[57] ABMAC box 21, NHA 1940–1941, National Health Administration, May 1941.
[58] ABMAC box 21, NHA 1940–41, P. Z. King, "The Chinese NHA during the Sino-Japanese Hostilities," Chongqing June 1940.

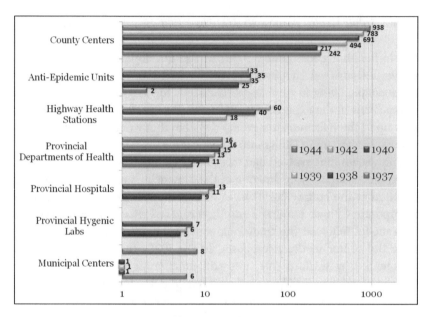

Graph 6.4: *Development of Public Healthcare Agencies in Nationalist China, 1937–1944* (*Sources*: *1937*: China Medical Board Archive, IV, 2, B9, box 22, folder 157, Report of UNRRA Committee on Health and Medical Care to the Committee on Investigation and Planning of Relief and Rehabilitation of the Executive Yuan, July 1, 1944. That source reports 242 Xian county health enters in 1937, but due to the Japanese invasion that number is meaningless as a base line figure for wartime work. Source for 2 anti-epidemic units: P. Z. King: ABMAC, box 21, NHA, 1940–41, "The Chinese NHA during the Sino-Japanese Hostilities." *1938–1940*: all units except AEUs and HHS: ABMAC box 21, NHA 1940–41, P. Z. King, "The Chinese NHA during the Sino-Japanese Hostilities," Chongqing, June 1940. *1938*: AEUs: ABMAC box 21, NHA, 1940–41, Health Program of NHA, undated document but around 1939. *1939*: AEUs and HHS: ABMAC box 21, King, P. Z. 1942–43, P. Z. King, "Public Health During 1942." *1940*: AEUs and HHS: ABMAC box 21, NHA, 1940–41, National Health Administration (May 1941). *1942*: "National Health Administration," November 1942, in ABMAC box 20, NHA General. *1944*: UNRRA Committee report, as in 1937. * According to NHA report of May 10–11, 1942 in ABMAC box 21, NHA, 1942, there were 60 highway health stations. ** In 1942 Guizhou had 77 county health stations divided into 10 first grade, 10 second grade and 58 third grade. The first grade had at least 3 physicians and 5–8 nurses; the second 1 physician and 3–5 nurses, the third grade one nurse. Only three counties had health aides. See K. F. Yao "A Brief Account of Kweichow Health Work," carrying November 12, 1942, date, in ABMAC box 21, NHA 1942. Such detailed breakdowns are not generally available in ABMAC documents.)

health training for graduates of medical, nursing and midwifery colleges, and demonstrations on how to teach undergraduate public health courses and train junior public health personnel. The latter were the health aides, auxiliaries and assistants needed to staff the local health services, for whom no systematic training yet existed. Under Dr. Zhu's plan, aides would be individuals with six years elementary school training. They would receive one month's training and be stationed in villages or communes. Auxiliaries (attendants, dressers, lab attendants) would be junior middle school graduates, receiving one year's training. Assistants would include clinical and public health nurses, midwives and sanitary inspectors. They would also be junior middle school graduates but receive four years of technical or vocational training, including six months to one year in public health work.

To provide such training the Institute organized nine teaching departments with field work in municipal and rural demonstration centers and a vital statistics program to carry out a general census.[59] It was anticipated that the public healthcare system would require a growing number of special consultants and technical officers, such as sanitary engineers and inspectors, public health nurses and nurse-midwives, to fulfill the needs of a strategy focused on prevention of disease. China still had few sanitary specialists, far fewer physicians, nurses and midwives than were needed, and no system for training sanitary inspectors or village health aides.[60] Thus, a greater focus on training was needed.

In April 1941, the NHA merged the Central Field Health Station and the Public Health Personnel Training Institute into a National Institute of Health (NIH *Zhongyang weisheng shiyanyuan* 中央卫生实验院). This was located outside Chongqing on a "bare farming field" at Keleshan adjoining the Central Hospital and the National Shanghai Medical College.[61] The experienced Dr. Li Tingan was appointed director and Dr. Zhu Zhanggeng vice director. A report published at the time indicates that the NIH program concentrated its training on physicians, sanitary engineers, nurses and midwifes, with the latter group predominating. It did not include training of local assistants and auxiliaries.[62] The training institute

---

[59] ABMAC, Box 21, NHA, 1940–1941, "Training of Public Health Personnel in 1939–40," by Dr. C. K. Chu.

[60] Ibid.

[61] ABMAC box 21, NHA 1942, Quote from "National Institute of Health in 1942: An Annual Report," by C. K. Chu.

[62] RF, RG5, Series 3 Reports, Routine, Box 218, "Public Health Personnel Training Work," April–August 1941; also in ABMAC box 21, NHA 1940–41.

at Guiyang continued to function, albeit on a smaller scale, and another regional training institute was set up at Lanzhou.

In collaboration with the Sichuan provincial health bureau the NIH established a demonstration teaching area in nearby Bishan County, a community of 520,000 people on the road towards Chengdu. In early 1941, Bishan had a clinic, a fifteen-bed ward, a simple diagnostic laboratory, a minor operating room, a delousing station, three substations, and thirty village health agents. A year later its hospital had thirty beds, forty-eight village health aides, and a maternal service averaging twenty-five deliveries per month.[63] NIH had another teaching field in Xinqiao-Shapingba, now part of downtown Chongqing. During 1942 the clinic received 22,982 outpatient visits and performed 7,084 diagnostic tests. The hospital began admitting in October 1942. A third demonstration program opened up at Shazi in September 1942. This community included three market towns with a population of around 120,000 people. The program covered family health, maternal-child health, school health, industrial health, and preventive dentistry. The clinic received 7,614 outpatient visits during September through December 1942.[64]

During its first two years NIH promoted the development of regional and provincial training centers. It reported that during 1940–42 provincial training centers were set up in Sichuan, Yunnan, Guangxi, Shaanxi, Hunan, Jiangxi and Fujian. It also announced that in the seven years since the founding of the first training institute in 1935 1,641 health professionals had graduated from its program, mostly medical officers, public health nurses (the largest category) and sanitary inspectors.[65] This finding made it clear that lack of adequately trained public health personnel had become the most pressing problem in public health administration.[66]

The NIH also functioned as NHA's research center. It took over parasitology and bacteriology laboratories previously used by a League of Nation's epidemic prevention unit. Its department of Chemistry undertook studies of human vitamin C nutrition and wartime dietary surveys. The department of sanitary engineering carried out malaria surveys in the

---

[63] For 1941, ABMAC box 21, NHA 1940–41, "The Initial Year of the NIH, April 1 to December 31, 1941;" for 1942, ABMAC box 21, NHA 1942, C. K. Chu, "NIH in 1942: an Annual Report." The ABMAC archive contains a set of photographs illustrating the work of the Bishan health center.

[64] See "NIH in 1942: an Annual Report" in note 63.

[65] Ibid.

[66] ABMAC box 21, NHA 1942, "The National Health Administration of the ROC," November 1942.

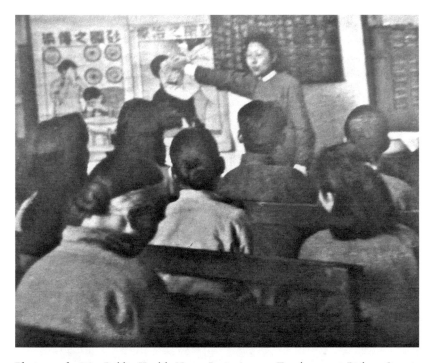

Photograph 6.2: *Public Health Nurse Lecturing on Trachoma at Bishan County Health Center.*
A public health nurse is teaching ordinary, not well educated, parents on how to control an eye disease rampant among children during the 1930s and 1940s. (*Source*: ABMAC Archive.)

immediate Xinqiao area and started planning an area waterworks. The department of health education compiled twelve textbooks on health for elementary children.[67]

A measure of progress can be assessed from 1942 data, that year being the most productive in delivery of quantitative material available to this research. The total budget for 15 reporting provinces and the Chongqing municipality was ¥44,022,016. Yunnan was the biggest beneficiary with ¥8,683,100; Ningxia the lowest with ¥91,500. At the county level, one finds 848 county health centers with a total staff of 6,419. The highest staff ratios were in Fujian (averaging 16.4 per center), the lowest were among Guizhou's 78 reporting county centers, which averaged only 2.6 per center.

---

[67] ABMAC, box 21, NHA, 1940–41, "The Initial Year of the National Institute of Health," April 1–December 31, 1941.

Obviously these centers could not staff beyond the county town level. Nevertheless 517 reporting counties administered 5.891 million smallpox vaccinations, 2.153 million cholera inoculations and 1.356 million cholera-typhoid inoculations in addition to the curative work noted in Graph 6.3.[68]

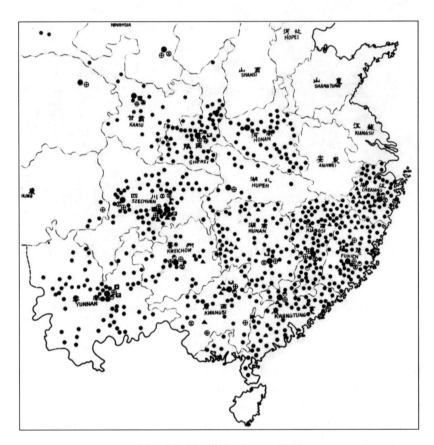

Map 6.1: *Health Stations in 1942*

1942 was a high point for the National Health Administration. Local health stations were increasing in number, distributed widely through south and central China, and engaging in preventive healthcare. Data collection of preventive health work, morbidity and mortality improved. In 1943–1944 these advances were set back by hyperinflation and the Ichigo Campaign. But in 1942 one can begin to see what the public health advocates could achieve if given a chance. (*Source*: ABMAC Archive)

---

[68] ABMAC box 21, NHA, King, P. Z., 1942–43, Statistical summaries accompanying "Organization of NHA and its subsidiary organizations," December 31, 1942. Quantitative reports on county hospital admissions, school and home visits, and numbers and health of children examined are not available in this data series.

The reports of this era identify problems that the NHA and NIH would face during the remaining war years. In the training field there were very few sanitary engineers.[69] Enrollment of physicians and midwives was below what the circumstances required.[70] Outreach of laboratories was limited to their immediate surrounding area, except in special circumstances such as the outbreak of plague at Changde in Hunan in November 1941. This latter event called for professional investigation because bacterial warfare was correctly suspected as the cause of the outbreak.[71] The principle of relying on demonstration stations to model local public health services depended on availability of transportation, roads and tuition funds, without which students could not attend the classes. As for medical reporting, readers familiar with medical reporting systems in other countries will be aware from the data in Tables 6.1 and 6.2 that epidemic reporting was in its infancy in China in the 1940s.[72] Nevertheless examination of Table 6.1 and Graph 6.7 indicates that the principle of reporting had been established, Graph 6.6 gives a sense of the gradual increase in reporting capacity, and Table 6.2 indicates that the NHA leadership was well aware of the scope and challenges of infectious disease in China.

Lastly, NHA's public healthcare system required protection from economic and military pressures if it was to take root in the country's underdeveloped southwest and northwest regions. That would prove a huge challenge.

---

[69] During 1935 to 1940 the Training Institute graduated thirty sanitary engineers in six classes and 214 sanitary inspectors in eight classes. In 1941 it had three students in its Eighth class and five sanitary overseers in a two-year college course.

[70] In 1941 the NIH placed seven physicians in provincial health administrations, three in the epidemic prevention corps and one in the Army medical service, and twelve midwives in a total of seven units. Placement of nurses was somewhat better at forty-three in eighteen units. See RF, RG5 Series 3, Box 218, Reports, Routine, "Recent Assignments" in "Public Health Personnel Training Work April-August, 1941."

[71] See ABMAC, box 21, NHA Reports, 1940–41, Epidemiological Report #1. The plague expert Dr. Robert H. Pollitzer wrote, "Circumstantial evidence strongly suggests that the plague outbreak in Changteh was caused by enemy action." Reports on plague in wartime China in Zhejiang were also connected with Japanese military bacterial warfare. See P. Z. King (1943), 47–48. Reports on plague outbreaks in Fujian, Suiyuan and Shaanxi were not apparently connected at the time with Japanese military action. Dr. Jin produced a report on "Japanese Attempt at Bacterial Warfare in China," dated March 12, 1942. This must be the report referenced in note 80 below.

[72] The immense quantities of data available for study of state medicine in Nineteenth century India did not exist in 1940s China. For India see Arnold (1993).

Hyperinflation and Survival during the Later War Years

By summer 1942 China was entering the sixth year of the War of Resistance with no clear end in sight. As Japanese military power had blocked off all sea-lanes, the Chongqing government had to rely on the perilous 'air hump' over Burma to transport aid to China's forces.[73]

In June 1942 the NHA director Dr. Jin Baoshan wrote to Dr. John Grant saying that an urgent need had come up to renew China's national health program, strengthen its public health services and pave the way for post war reconstruction. Could he visit and give advice? In response to this request from the service he personally helped to shape, Grant returned to west China for three weeks during July and August 1942.

In the three years since his previous visit Chongqing had become the "most expensive city today in the world." The cost of living was up over 30 times that of July 1937, but salaries and rice subsidies had risen only three or four times. Senior NHA officials were selling all nonessentials. The NHA was housed in temporary buildings that were "merely thatched bamboo huts, generally with earthen floors." The midsummer weather was drenching. The economic pressures on low paid public healthcare workers were mounting.

Another problem was the decline of trucking in west China resulting from the shutdown of gasoline supplies up the Burma Road. Individuals and administrative units were becoming isolated. Intellectual life suffered from loss of current publications. Grant approved reorganization of the NHA if that enabled it to develop "along quality lines" but was guarded about changes in healthcare training, seeing neither personnel nor facilities in unoccupied China for more than one good training program in any one field.[74]

Some of these problems were pointed out in contemporary reports. In a 1942 report Dr. Zhu Zhanggeng, now NIH director, said that eighty percent of administrative effort was spent on provision of rice, coal, housing and other life essentials. Due to high prices NIH had overspent in six months its entire annual budget for office expenses. As for program, NIH had scaled down training goals for numbers of medical officers, nurses

---

[73] Koenig (1972). Sevareid (1978), 245–309, provides a dramatic account of an abortive journey heading across the Hump in August 1943, which he survived, followed by a successful crossing to Kunming and Chongqing.

[74] RF, RG 12, Grant diaries, July 15 to August 6, 1942.

and midwives to staff the state medical service (Graph 6.5). Instead it focused on village health aides, who could be trained locally. The job of village aides was defined in 1940 as smallpox vaccination, first aid, reports of births and deaths, supervision of general cleanliness, and propaganda work, in short, the basic minimum in preventive health care.[75]

By the end of 1942 NHA goals boiled down to dealing with emergency needs and planning postwar reconstruction. The production of drugs was very urgent, wrote Dr. Jin in a letter to the ABMAC Chongqing representative Dr. George Bachman.[76] Epidemic diseases were on the upsurge. Following the Japanese occupation of Hong Kong and Burma and the return of overseas Chinese to unoccupied (i.e., West) China, cholera had spread rapidly along the communication routes, from Mandalay to Xiaguan to Kunming and Guizhou, and from Guangdong northwest into Guangxi and Guizhou. In November 1942 the NHA tabulated 11,951 cases with 4,576 deaths reported by the end of September.[77] A report on anti-epidemic activities, covering the period from January 1, 1942, to June 30, 1943, reported 41,613 cases and 21,691 deaths due to cholera in Yunnan.[78] These cases are now known to be due to Japanese military bacterial warfare.[79]

NHA officials were aware of Japanese bacterial warfare but only had solid evidence of outbreaks of plague. In an essay on bacterial warfare Dr. Jin listed six cases in which there was either laboratory-tested or strong circumstantial evidence to indicate that plague-infested materials had been dropped by Japanese planes over Ningbo, Zhuxian and Jinhua,

[75] ABMAC, box 21, NHA 1942, "The National Institute of Health in 1942: an Annual Report," by C. K. Chu, Director, NIH.

[76] ABMAC box 21, P. Z. King correspondence, letter dated December 16, 1942.

[77] ABMAC, box 21, NHA, 1942, Information from "The National Health Administration of the Republic of China, November 1942." The figures are at odds with the estimates of cholera deaths resulting from the Japanese military bacterial warfare campaign in Yunnan in 1942. Even so, these figures indicate that a cholera epidemic had occurred.

[78] ABMAC, box 20, NHA General, information from "Report of Anti-Epidemic Activities for 1942–43." This report from the Central Epidemic Prevention Bureau in Kunming, gives total figures for cholera as 61,952 cases and 29,029 mortalities. In Yunnan the disease appeared in fifty-five counties out of a hundred and six; in Guangxi in fifty-eight out of seventy-two; in Hunan in fifty-three out of eighty-five; and in Guizhou in thirty-two out of seventy. In Guangdong, which may have been the site of another outbreak, cholera appeared in fifty-four counties out of ninety-four, resulting in 2,663 reported cases and 895 deaths. The Bureau was aware of reporting limitations, noting that 89,740 cases of dysentery reported in 1942 were *only a very small fraction of actual incidence*." (Emphasis added).

[79] Xie Benshu (谢本书) (November 2010); Barenblatt (2004), 163–168. Prof. Xie is at the Yunnan Minority Nationality University, Kunming.

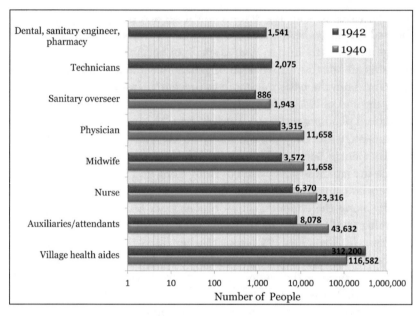

Graph 6.5: *Adjustments in National Institute of Health (NIH) Goals for Training County Health Staff between 1940 and 1942* (*Sources*: 1940: ABMAC box 21, NHA 1940–1941, C. K. Chu, "Training of Public Health Personnel in 1939–1940;" 1942: ABMAC box 21, NHA 1942, C. K. Chu, "National Institute of Health in 1942: an Annual Report.")

Zhangde, Suiyuan, Ningxia and Shaanxi provinces, and Nanyang.[80] Most of these cases were noted in the China Handbook for 1937–1944.[81] There is no indication that NHA personnel were aware of the Japanese military's use of other bacterial materials, including cholera vibrios, in their heavily camouflaged bacterial warfare campaigns (discussed in chapter 7).

In any case the NHA had other epidemics to deal with. Malaria was endemic in southeast and southwest China. The fall of Burma interrupted the government's malaria research and control programs. Dysentery was "perhaps the most important but least heeded" communicable disease in China. It was a major cause of infant mortality and adult debility and too common to attract statistical attention. Plague and diphtheria had broken out in northwest China.[82] An American Red Cross report dated end of

---

[80] P. Z. King (Jin Baoshan) statement on bacterial warfare released on April 9, 1942, and published in Chinese Ministry of Information (1943), 679–682.

[81] Chinese Ministry of Information (1944).

[82] ABMAC, box 21, NHA 1942, "The National Health Administration of the Republic of China," November 1942; and ABMAC box 21, 1942–1943 folder, King, P. Z., "Public Health During 1940–42," by P. Z. King (in very faint typescript).

March 1942 spoke of tremendous destruction in Kunming and Chongqing and an influx into all parts of unoccupied China of millions of refugees and escapees.[83] These destitute people threatened renewed outbreaks of louse-borne typhus and relapsing fever. Normally such outbreaks could be controlled by DBS stations, of which the NHA had set up over 50.[84] But according to one observer they were not functioning because there was no money for fuel.[85]

The NHA's epidemic prevention agencies by now lacked the personnel or resources to handle such widespread epidemics. The efforts of public health agencies to control the diseases, said one report, "had been taxed to the utmost." The need for medical equipment, drugs and personnel had become increasingly acute as supplies from Burma to Kunming dwindled.[86] Nevertheless the NHA's Highway health stations administered 197,000 smallpox vaccinations and over 350,000 cholera inoculations, and the epidemic prevention corps administered 221,000 vaccinations and 276,000 cholera inoculations (see Graph 6.6).[87] Allowing for under-reporting, the evidence is that the NHA pursued this vital preventive health function at least through 1942. The fact that there is no data for 1943 in this data series and little for 1944 (none from the county health centers) is indicative of a breakdown in the data collecting function, for which hyper inflation must bear some responsibility. Specifically, medical personnel were drifting into "lucrative private practice" because of the marginal salaries in public health service.[88]

Loss of Burma aggravated the NHA's problems. A request for fifty million atabrine tablets urgently needed to treat civilian malaria cases had to

---

[83] ARC, Box 1394, China: Reports, Statistics, Surveys and Studies, 1942–43, Report for period ending March 31, 1942, by Albert Evans. A communication in the same file from Arnold Vaught of the Canadian Mission, Chongqing, received in July 1942, warned that "Emergency battle zone needs (are) now greater than last two years because vast population again being displaced creating hundreds thousands refugees..."

[84] Dr. Jin's report on "Public Health During 1940–42," in ABMAC box 21, NHA, King, P. Z., 1942–43, says that fifty DBS stations had been set up, which between October 1941 and August 1842 deloused 46,736 people, gave scabies treatments to 24,676 and deloused 97,076 articles of clothing. Another report dated May 1942, in ABMAC, box 21, NHA 1942, speaks of fifty-eight DBS stations in places where the population was concentrated. For the latter, see "The Chinese NHA and its Subsidiary Organization."

[85] ABMAC, box 3, Bachman, George W., 1942, George Bachman to Helen Kennedy Stevens, #9, dated June 17, 1942.

[86] "The Chinese NHA and its Subsidiary Organizations" (see note 84).

[87] "Public Health during 1940–42," by P. Z. King (see note 84).

[88] ABMAC Box 21, National Health Administration, 1942, "The Chinese NHA and its Subsidiary Organizations," dated May 1942.

be deferred.[89] During the middle of 1942 the American Red Cross managed to bring in twenty-five tons of supplies per month by air. But by
October nearly all air traffic had been commandeered for military use,
leaving only three planes to carry civilian supplies.[90] By the end of 1942
lack of medical supplies and continuing malnutrition were bearing down
on the military and led the Nationalist government reportedly to order a
one-third reduction in the size of its armed services.[91]

The NHA was far from total dependence on foreign sources for medical
supplies. Its Epidemic Prevention Bureaus were reported to have made
unoccupied China "almost self-sufficient" in production of vaccines and
other immunological products.[92] Graph 6.7 shows the range of biological
products that Chinese agencies were able to produce by 1943 for local
epidemiological work.

In April 1942 the government held a drug-manufacturing exhibit in
Chongqing using local materials and attended by over 30,000 people.[93]
But according to an NHA report received in September 1942, "Of the many
drug factories now operating there are ... few worthy of the name."[94] In
August, Dr. Jin wrote to the Lend Lease administrator Lauchlin Currie
requesting US experts to assist in the production of vaccines, sera and
drugs.[95]

Comparable efforts were made to enlarge the pool of registered medical
personnel. In 1940 the NHA decided that qualified applicants serving six
months in designated public health or army medical organizations could
register, if a special committee approved their qualifications. In two years
this produced over one thousand applicants, of whom four hundred and
eighty were registered to practice, while three hundred and ten remained
on probation. Authority to register Chinese medicine practitioners was
left to local administrations, but since 1939 the NHA registered five hundred and thirteen to help meet war exigencies. This decision reversed the
negative policies pursued by NHA towards Chinese medicine practitioners

---

[89] National Archive, Washington, DC, RG160, Army Service Forces, box 360, folder
440A, Ralph G. Hubbell (ARC) to Col. Herbert L. Shaftoe, June 11, 1942. Only two months
previously Dr. Jin had written to Song Ziwen in Washington, DC, urgently requesting drugs
by plane. See ABMAC, box 21, P. Z. King correspondence, April 13, 1942.

[90] ARC archive, box 1394, Dr. Phillips F. Greene, Director's Report of Operations,
March 1, 1942–March 1, 1943.

[91] ARC archive, box 1394 China War Relief, Vol. 1, p. 35, Phillips F. Greene to R. F. Allen,
letter number 195, December 21, 1942.

[92] "The Chinese NHA and its Subsidiary Organizations," see note 88.

[93] Ibid.

[94] ABMAC, box 21, NHA, 1942, "Report on the Drug Situation in China," received on
September 7, 1942.

[95] ABMAC box 21, King Pao-zan correspondence, P. Z. King, letter of August 4, 1942,
to Laughlin Currie.

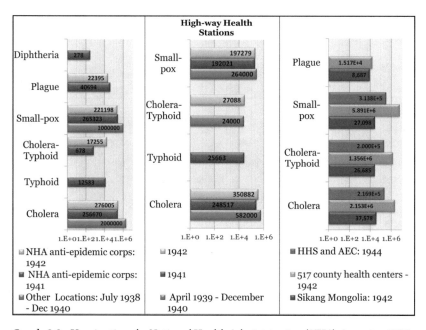

Graph 6.6: *Vaccinations by National Health Administration (NHA) Agencies, 1938–1944 (Sources: 1938–40*: ABMAC box 21, NHA, 1940–41, P. Z. King, "The Chinese NHA during the Sino-Japanese Hostilities," revised October 1941. (Not all highway health station inoculations were recorded). *1941*: for anti-epidemic corps, P. Z. King, (January–March, 1943), Table 2, p. 53; for highway health stations "National Health Administration," (1943): 75–84. *1942*: for anti-epidemic, HH stations, Sikang-Mgl, ABMAC box 21, NHA, King, P. Z., 1942–43, "Organization of NHA and Its Subsidiary Organizations," December 31, 1942, in; for 517 county health center reporting, see same report. *1944*: Chinese Ministry of Information (1947), 494, 501. (These figures are likely to be underreported). *Note*: E+ represents units of the power of ten. Thus 5.891E+6 represents 5.891 million. E+5 represents units of 100,000; E+4 represents units of 10,000. HHS=Highway Health Stations, AEC=Anti Epidemic Corps.)

during the 1930s. Conscription of physicians and pharmacists began in 1940 and was extended in 1941 to dentists and nurses and in 1942 to midwives. By October 1942 the government had registered altogether 12,018 physicians, 793 pharmacists, 5,796 nurses and 5,003 midwives.[96]

The problem lay in persuading registrants to enter public service. Trained individuals were needed to promote postwar public health; as

---

[96] ABMAC box 21, National Health Administration, King, P. Z., 1942–1943, Data from P. Z. King, "Public Health During 1940–1942." By comparison, Japan recorded 58,511 physicians, of whom 53,376 were in practice, and 59,560 midwives by the end of 1936, and 16,857 nurses by the end of 1935. 12,494 physicians and 20,746 midwives were working in villages. Around 5,000 public health nurses were working in schools, factories and child welfare centers. See League of Nations Health Organization (1937b), found in Library of New York Academy of Medicine.

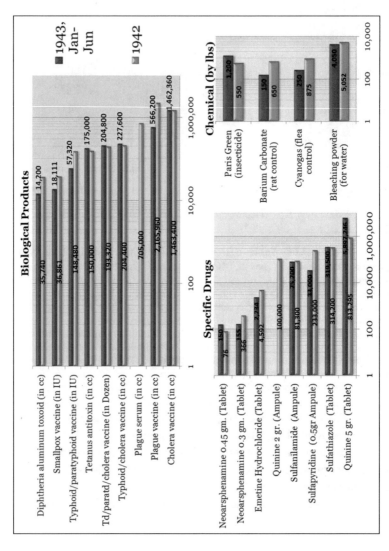

Graph 6.7: *Biological Supplies for Local Epidemic Control, January 1942 to June 1943 (Source:* ABMAC, box 21, NHA, King, P. Z., 1942–43, P. Z. King to George Bachman, August 23, 1943.)

Dr. Jin wrote to ABMAC, "We have to start to make due preparations for... reconstruction work on public health after our victory."[97] The NHA calculated it would need around 25,500 personnel above the village health aide level to maintain current state public health and medical services. As of December 1942 it had trained only 1,641.[98] Five hundred of the latter had been trained since 1940 and another three hundred and forty-five were in training in five NHA centers.[99]

As the war dragged on options for relief and reconstruction narrowed. Due to the relentless inflation, the Executive Yuan in March 1943 ordered all central government organizations to reduce their staff by twenty-five percent as soon as possible. The NHA was forced to hand over its regional training institute in Guiyang to the provincial health bureau. In Chongqing public health courses for physicians and nurses were postponed because very few graduates passed the qualifying examinations.[100] In the spring of 1943 Brian Dyer, now a Rockefeller Foundation sanitary engineer, reported that NIH's health education department was doing three exhibits a year but no extension (i.e. no work in schools). The nursing department had no students. The engineering department had seventeen engineers who were mainly boys just out of school. They had little training, no practical experience, and were thinking of "big jobs and big money." No courses were planned for 1943 except for six sanitary overseers. The epidemic prevention corps was well organized but doing little because of lack of transportation.[101]

During 1942–1943 famine gripped Henan province, sending millions of starving refugees westward in search of food. Cannibalism broke out there and also in Guangdong province.[102] It was up to the government's National Relief Commission to respond to these disasters. Even so the NHA, beset by declining staff and inadequate funding, did what it could to help by sending three epidemic prevention teams to Henan, along with

---

[97] ABMAC, Box 21, National Health Administration, King, P. Z., 1942–43, P. Z. King to Van Slyke, April 21, 1942.

[98] Ibid., Figures in King to Bachman, December 4, 1942; the target figures are taken from the NIH 1942 report in ABMAC Box 21, NHA 1942.

[99] Ibid.

[100] RF, RG5, Box 218, Semi-Annual Report of the NIH, January to June 1943.

[101] RF, RG1, Series 601, box 3, folder 33, Dyer, Brian R, "Visit to China," April 12 to May 26, 1943.

[102] Cf. White and Jacoby (1946), and Munroe Scott (1977), chapter 31. Other data are from ARC archive, China War Relief, Vol. I, Appendix, p 29a ff, and 42e–f (covering conditions in 1943). According to Balfour's 1943 diary (entry for August 30) in the Rockefeller archives, several million deaths were reported.

mobile laboratory and sanitation units. Its budget had no funds for such an emergency; the costs were covered from American financial aid.[103]

In 1944, Dr. John Grant again visited the NHA. He found that relations with the Ministry of Education were distant, leaving the NHA with little influence over educational policies. The director, Dr. Jin, received ninety percent of his orders from the Generalissimo but had no opportunity to meet with him to discuss problems. Inflation was demoralizing the staff and emasculating the budget, of which almost one-third depended on foreign aid. Meanwhile the Ministry of Social Welfare was rapidly extending its own network of health services despite having no technical ability in this field.

The disconnect between Dr. Jin and Chiang Kaishek points to a continuing lack of consensus among top government officials as to the political and social significance of public health. Control continued to be hierarchical, with Chiang transmitting orders through Kong Xiangxi (孔祥熙), the vice president of the Executive Yuan and Chiang's brother-in-law. There is no clear indication as to the nature of these orders, but one can assume that they were either ad hoc or geared to non-public health priorities. As Grant pointed out, China was long overdue for public health legislation if not a public health act.[104] In the absence of such an act, there was no clear guidance regarding healthcare policy, and no assurance that the chief political executive and those responsible for healthcare policy were on the same page.

At the National Institute of Health a recently established government central planning board had produced a preliminary medical and public health framework for postwar UNRRA assistance, but hadn't found out what funds might be available nor assessed overall objectives and personnel needs.[105] Dr. Zhu Zhanggeng tried without success to get the China Medical Board interested in a loan program to help get public health staff through the current financial crisis without abandoning government

---

[103] ABMAC, box 38, Chinese Army folder, P. Z. King notes. Primary responsibility for dealing with disaster and refugee relief rested with the National Relief Commission. According to official records the Commission had in operation at the end of 1942 twenty-nine clinics and twelve circuit medical corps; in 1943 this was changed to twenty clinics and thirteen medical corps and in 1944 to thirteen clinics and twenty-four medical corps. The Commission also subsidized hospitals, clinics and medical corps of other organizations. See Chinese Ministry of Information 1937–1944 (November 1944), chapter 19. The writer is indebted to Dr. Pan Shu-jen for a copy of this source.

[104] RF, RG 12, John B. Grant diary, 1944–1945.

[105] Ibid., Grant diary, 1944–1945.

service for the private sector.[106] Later that year he reported that a simple waterworks put up at the Bishan demonstration center had been poorly designed and would have to be improved so as not to lose the confidence of the common people.[107] An annual training report for 1945 admitted to difficulty in maintaining staff morale during two years of inflation and agreed that the work of one of the demonstration centers had "not been very fruitful."[108]

A glance at Table 6.2 provides a reminder of the daunting health problems that China still faced. These numbers were the orders of magnitude with which China's health authorities believed they were dealing. By 1944 there was little chance of reducing this level of infection until the war was over. The NHA could only plan for the future and conserve its modest existing resources.

Despite such problems, the NHA continued to contribute to war relief and health improvement. In 1944 it initiated an industrial health demonstration service in the Chongqing area with the aid of American funds. In response to the wave of refugees created by the Japanese military onslaught into South and Southwest China in summer and autumn 1944, the NHA concentrated its field services along a few important highways in the war theater. After UNRRA announced a $900 million appropriation to aid relief and rehabilitation in China, the NHA called for over 30,000 health workers to staff the public healthcare service. To assist the direct war work it sent six mobile surgery units to serve the Chinese expeditionary forces in the Burma-Yunnan area (the Y force) and provided the U.S. Army theater surgeon with medical information.[109]

At NIH the epidemic research institute undertook several parasite surveys of workers and children. The department of maternal and child

---

[106] CMB archive, box 95, folder 682, C. K. Chu to Claude E. Forkner, February 29, 1944, and Forkner to Chu, June 7, 1944. The idea was picked up by Dr. Jin Baoshan in a letter of July 6, 1944, to Drs. Van Slyke and Co Tui of ABMAC, see ABMAC box 21, National Health Administration, King, P. Z., 1944.

[107] In RF, RG5, Series 3, box 218, Progress Note (from C. K. Chu), January to June 1944, NIH, China.

[108] RF, RG5, Section 3, box 218, Reports—Routine, China Health, Training of Personnel, Annual Report 194. It was morale problems that had led Dr. Zhu to suggest the loan program to Dr. Forkner.

[109] ABMAC box 21, data from P. Z. King correspondence file; i) letter to Dr. Van Slyke of September 8, 1944; ii) Emergency Wartime Medical Relief Program, sent out on February 3, 1945; iii) Emergency Training Program for UNRRA Medical and Health Personnel, sent out same date; and iv) letter of May 2, 1945, to Dr. J. H. Liu (Liu Ruiheng). Dr. Jin was resentful of any imputation that the NHA was not doing its part to help the war effort and wrote Dr. Liu specifically on this topic.

Table 6.2: United Nations Relief and Rehabilitation Agency (UNRRA)
Estimates of Communicable Disease Infection in China, July 1944

Disease		Annual Estimate	Percent of population*
Cholera	霍乱	Variable; expect up to 200,000 during liberation	
Plague	鼠疫	Variable	1.5
Dysentery	痢疾	6 million (90% bacillary)	0.175
Typhoid fever	伤寒	Probably over 700,000	0.125
Smallpox	天花	Probably 500,000	5.32
Malaria	疟疾	Around 21.3 million	
Tuberculosis	结核	Nearly 100% tuberculin positive at age 20	
TB mortality	死亡率	300 per 100,000	0.252
Typhus	斑疹伤寒	Wartime incidence probably around 80,000**	0.02
Relapsing fever	回归热	Wartime incidence probably c. 350,000**	0.087
Hookworm	钩虫病	Around 10 million	2.5
Schistosomiasis	血吸虫病	At least 10 million	2.5
Kala-azar	黑热病	Around 225,000	0.052
Syphilis	梅毒	(Around 20 million)	5.0***
Gonorrhea	淋病	(Over 20 million)	5.0 plus***
Diphtheria, scarlet fever, meningitis	白喉, 猩红热, 脑膜炎	(No estimates)	—

Source: CMB archive IV, 2, B9, box 22, folder 157, "Report of Committee on Health and Medical Care, submitted to the Commission on Investigation and Planning of Relief and Rehabilitation of the Executive Yuan," July 1, 1944, Chungking.

* Based on estimated population of 400 million.

** Projected from reported cases for 1943; typhus estimate is low.

*** Estimated as a percentage.

health promoted MCH services in Sichuan, Guizhou, and Lanchow and the northwest (see chapter 7 for discussion of MCH in the northwest). It organized an UNRRA-sponsored training program for thirty-four senior students of the National Central School of Midwifery and published several booklets on family health. The department of health education put on a conference to organize a national postwar school health rehabilitation program and a five-year plan for rural and municipal school health units. It put out filmstrips, monthly health posters and a quarterly bulletin. The department of nursing organized a thirteen-week course on nursing aid, which was taken by one hundred and ninety-five volunteers from the recently established Youth army (see chapter 5). In 1945 the public health nursing service in one of the county demonstration centers made over 12,000 home visits. Later in 1945 NIH enrolled over two hundred and fifty students in a variety of short and medium term courses, including one hundred and ten unlicensed medical practitioners in a nine-month course.[110]

Heights and Depths of Rural Healthcare in Sichuan

The most ambitious attempt to create a province-wide public healthcare service occurred in Sichuan, led by Dr. Chen Zhiqian (陈志潜). When he became the first Health Commissioner in 1939, there was no provincial health service. By 1945 the province had one hundred and thirty-one county health centers and one hundred and thirty-nine sub-county health stations serving over ninety-five percent of the province's one hundred and thirty-nine counties. Health budgets had risen from 0.14 to 1.3 percent of total county budgets. A provincial Institute for Infectious Diseases provided field and diagnostic laboratories for investigation of epidemics, and a provincial Public Health Training Institute provided technical courses for public health professionals and introductory courses for health assistants.[111]

---

[110] RF, RG 5, Series 3, box 218, information from NIH reports for 1944 and 1945.

[111] RF, RG 5, series 3, reports 600/601, "A Review of Government Health Service in Szechuan, China, for the Period 1939–1945." Researchers should note that RF has two depositories for Sichuan provincial health administration documents: i) RF, RG 1, series 601, China, box 18, folders 161–162, contains miscellaneous correspondence, etc, and annual reports; ii) RG5 International Health Board, series 3, box 218 contains annual reports from 1941 to 1944 plus a review of service from 1939 to 1945.

The motivation for all this development was Dr. Chen's belief that the "fundamental function" of the provincial health administration was "the gradual development of county health centers of good professional standard."[112] After assuming leadership Chen started a two-month training program for health assistants, to which 150 high school students applied. Physicians and nurses were trained in public health work.[113] By 1943 the province had ninety-six county health centers, of which half were under the direction of medical school graduates.[114] The provincial health bureau held conferences to keep directors in touch with developments in primary health care, and beginning in 1941 distributed a monthly bulletin. Dr. Chen and his associates covered thousands of kilometers each year to visit the health stations. Maternal child health, school health, and sanitation services were added as and when staff became available. In 1942 county health centers reported that six hundred wells were improved or remodeled and over 1,000 public latrines rebuilt. During the cholera epidemic of that summer nearly 5,000 wells were regularly inspected.[115]

Some of this work, Dr. Chen noted, "made a profound impression on the authorities." In January 1941 the entire sanitary corps was sent to Xinjin (Sintsing 新津, near Chengdu) where 100,000 farmers had been conscripted to work on an airfield. The corps dug 2,000 pit latrines and disinfected water in wooden tubs each day with bleaching powder, thereby preventing acute gastro-intestinal infections. The corps deloused hundreds of workers who had contact with relapsing fever. In 1944 it spent five months providing sanitary services in airfields around Chengdu, saving around 500,000 airport laborers from dysentery, typhoid fever, pneumonia, smallpox, and tetanus. Only three hundred and fourteen laborers died during the whole period. The authorities were again "educated," and Dr. Chen received a medal.[116]

Despite this vigorous leadership, Sichuan's health service had problems. Public health work was unprofitable and depended on public commitment. Once inflation set in, the underpaid health workers began looking around for more remunerative work, and it became hard to attract new

---

[112] RF, RG1, series 601, box 18, folder 161, "First Report of Szechuan Provincial Health Administration, May-December 1939."

[113] Ibid.

[114] "A Review of Government Health Service in Szechuan . . . 1939–1945," (see note 111).

[115] ABMAC, box 3, B-BI, George Bachman 1942 folder, "Report of the Szechuan Provincial Health Administration for the Year 1942."

[116] i) RF, RG 5, IHBD, series 3, box 218, folders 600/601, Szechuan Provincial Health Administration, "First Semi Annual report for 1941;" ii) RG1, series 601, box 18, folder 162, "The Annual Report of the Szechuan Provincial Health Administration for the Year 1944."

workers. According to Dr. Chen's 1942 report, the purchasing power of the Chinese yuan had dropped over the previous two and a half years from 1 to 0.16, while health budgets had only doubled or tripled. Surveys of county health centers found that roughly a quarter were struggling for a bare existence, and in some cases the physician was either holding additional positions or engaged in private practice.[117] Half of the chiefs were found unfit for the job because of inadequate training or demoralization. As a result Dr. Chen closed two centers, replaced nine chiefs and had one imprisoned for misconduct.[118]

Subsequent reports were hardly more encouraging. By the end of 1943 public health service was "struggling for existence."[119] 1944 brought "worse inflation, worse morale and approaching collapse." "Public health is such an intellectual and idealistic enterprise," wrote Dr. Chen, "that in the past year every thinking man began to doubt its practicability in the China of this generation."[120] By the end of the war Chen's pessimism had deepened. Nine years of war had "washed out" a great number of promising health workers. Without a new vigorous group of trained personnel they would not "get far in socialization of medicine in China."[121] But in a generally critical and at times angry report Chen affirmed that, "there is now in this province an intense desire for public health."[122] Dr. Grant remarked that Chen had done "one of the outstanding public health jobs … in any community under such conditions as he confronted."[123] It was a great pity that government-driven inflation got in the way of Dr. Chen's far-sighted leadership.

Postwar Challenges

With the sudden end of the war in August 1945 the Nationalist government had to scramble to regain its authority in southeast and north

---

[117] ABMAC, box 3, B-BI, Bachman 1942 folder, Report of the Szechuan Provincial Health Administration for the Year 1942.

[118] RF, RG1, series 601, box 18, folder 162, "Preliminary Report of Szechuan Provincial Health Administration, December 25, 1942."

[119] RF, RG5, IHBD, series 3, reports, box 218, "Annual Report of the Szechuan Provincial Health Administration for 1943."

[120] RF, RG1, series 601, box 18, folder 162, "Annual Report of the Szechuan Provincial Health Administration for the year 1944."

[121] C. C. Ch'en to J. B. Grant, September 30, 1945, (marked 'personal'). RF, RG1, series 601, box 18, folder 162.

[122] 1939–1945 Report (see note 111).

[123] Columbia University Oral History Archive, John B. Grant, p. 647c.

central China. Because the NHA was not treated as a priority agency, it waited for the limited facilities available to transport its belongings back to Nanjing. A skeleton team returned in 1945 but the main offices were not back in Nanjing until summer 1946 and then only after squeezing the air force out of NHA's office and hospital buildings. After returning to Nanjing the NIH set up branches in Beijing and Lanzhou. The National Central Hospital returned to Nanjing, and branch hospitals were continued or set up in Lanzhou, Tianjin and Guangzhou. The Central Epidemic Prevention Bureau returned to Beijing leaving a branch office in Kunming; other branches were set up in Shanghai and continued in Lanzhou. By the end of 1946 the NHA convened a conference of central government and provincial heads of health agencies to review current conditions and challenges.[124]

That there were serious public health problems was not in doubt. Dr. Borcic, returning to China at the beginning of 1946 to head the UNRRA medical program, found an increase in kala-azar (黑热病 leishmaniasis, a parasitic disease spread by sandflies) from prewar levels of around 200,000 cases to post war levels of two to three million.[125] Scabies (疥疮 *jiechuang*) was everywhere—up to ninety to one hundred percent incidence in some rural areas; schistosomiasis (血吸虫病 a blood fluke disease spread by snails) was up to 400,000 cases. Dr. Borcic found too much emphasis on hospital treatment and too little on prevention. He said, "I still consider hospitals as having practically no influence on the health of China as such." Of the 50,000 beds available for 400 million or more people half were of no use in saving lives because the medical services were inferior.[126] As a result, UNRRA wound up its health program in March 1947 leaving only thirty people behind under the auspices of the World Health Organization (WHO).[127]

---

[124] Fu and Deng (1989).

[125] The National Northwest Institute of Health was sufficiently aware of this problem to run a two-week training course late in 1944 for twenty-seven physicians. The graduates were responsible for setting up kala-azar clinics and mobile units and catching sandflies for study. See ABMAC box 21, NIH, National Northwest Institute of Health, "A Report on the Training Program of Health Personnel, 1941–1945," in. By 1945 twenty-five kala-azar stations were operating.

[126] ABMAC, box 3, B-BI folder, Speech at meeting of ABMAC Executive, February 11, 1947.

[127] Ibid., Borcic speech at meeting of ABMAC Executive on February 11, 1947. At the Conference in June 1946 Dr. Shen had reported that there were then twenty-nine medical schools in operation. Dr. Szeming Sze commented that about ten could be regarded as good colleges.

Many additional problems existed. Tuberculosis registered around 1.4 million annual deaths and fourteen million cases per year. In 1948, when these estimates were compiled, China had only three thousand beds for the care of tuberculosis patients. Studies suggested that by the age of fourteen almost eighty-five percent of children were infected with the tubercle bacillus; by age nineteen the infection rate was ninety-nine percent. The WHO mission dispatched a tuberculosis adviser to assist with preventive measures, plans were made for the National Epidemic Prevention Bureau in Beijing to produce BCG vaccine, and a National Anti-Tuberculosis Association of China was reestablished.[128]

Urban water management was another area of concern for a country susceptible to gastrointestinal diseases. As Dr. Liu Ruiheng (now ABMAC representative in China) wrote in 1948, "Only a few of the largest cities in China have municipal waterworks and even in them, Shanghai included, city water is available only to a fraction of the population. Many large cities with populations of 100,000 to 400,000 have no water except what can be obtained with buckets from rivers, canals or wells."[129] Because of such conditions it is not surprising that gastrointestinal diseases still predominated in UNRRA's epidemiological reports. Apart from cholera, typhoid fever and dysentery continued to be major public health problems, particularly in urban areas.[130]

Chinese health officials returning to their original locations before the war of resistance found scenes of devastation, compounded by a difficult transportation situation and relentless inflation. According to Dr. Shen Kefei, the NHA returned east with five, ten and thirty year plans but found the situation "very fluid," negating the possibility of even a five year plan. So it focused on emergency relief and rehabilitation.[131] Dr. Borcic worried about public health education. An outspoken advocate for preventive medicine, he was under the impression that only the PUMC had engaged seriously in public health training. In fact several of the fifty-two medical

---

[128] ABMAC box 16, J. Heng Liu to Magnus I. Gregersen, October 25, 1948.

[129] Ibid., Liu to Magnus I. Gregersen, February 21, 1948. According to official records, up to June 1948 127 cities had installed water supply and sewage systems. An underground sewage system for Chongqing was completed in June 1947. A survey for a sewage system for Nanjing was completed in June 1948. Other water and sewage systems were planned for Lanzhou, Xining and Changsha, to be carried out with UNRRA assistance. See Chinese Ministry of Information (1950), 699.

[130] J. H. Fan (1945), 495–536; Knud Stowman (1945a), 551–561, and (1945b), 673–686.

[131] ABMAC, box 18, Medical Conference June 1946, Shen Kefei (James Shen), remarks at "Conference on the Present Medical Situation in China," held in New York on June 15, 1946.

colleges had public and rural health training programs (e.g. National Guiyang and Xiangya Medical Colleges), but many did not. When he and Dr. Liu Ruiheng visited Shenyang, capital of Liaoning province, in September 1947, they were appalled by the state of its once flourishing medical college.[132]

Nothing daunted, Dr. Jin Baoshan published an article early in 1946 unequivocally advocating public healthcare. He insisted that state medicine was designed to overcome the defects resulting from medical practice for personal gain. The system of private practice was in Dr. Jin's opinion as out of date as the artisan in the modem machine age. It catered to the rich minority to the utter neglect of the real sufferings of the needy poor. Through state medicine not only the individual but the nation as a whole benefited.[133] Dr. Jin knew that China still had a long way to go to reach healthcare modernity. The American armed forces had reduced their mortality rate by ninety-five percent over that sustained during World War One. "A glance over our own record," he admitted, "emphasizes our weakness." But experience of war convinced him that a public healthcare system addressing the afflictions of poor people was more needed than ever.[134]

In April 1947 the Nationalist government underwent a last ditch reorganization and the NHA was re-upgraded to ministerial status. Zhou Yichun (周诒春, also 周贻春, Y. T. Tsur), an experienced financial administrator with a long established interest in health education, was appointed minister.[135] Dr. Jin was kept on as technical vice-minister. Dr. Zhu Zhanggeng, who had been director of the NIH, was sent to New York as Chinese representative to the World Health Organization.[136] But civil war and public disenchantment with Guomindang leadership preempted further social reconstruction. The new ministry had not long been established before its leadership began to unravel. Dr. Jin left to become head of the department of public health at National Shanghai Medical College

---

[132] ABMAC Box 16, J. Heng Liu, July to December 1947, J. Heng Liu to Helen Kennedy Stevens, September 19, 1947, in. Dr. Liu suspected the drug factory of being in the opium business.

[133] P. Z. King (1946), 3–16.

[134] Ibid.

[135] Fu and Deng (1989); Boorman (1967), vol 1, 413–415, entry for Chou I-ch'un. Mr. Zhou was ten years older than Dr. Jin and already had ministerial status as minister of agriculture.

[136] Fu and Deng (1989); J. Heng Liu to Helen Kennedy Stevens, April 26, 1947. ABMAC, box 15, Liu, J. Heng, January–June 1947.

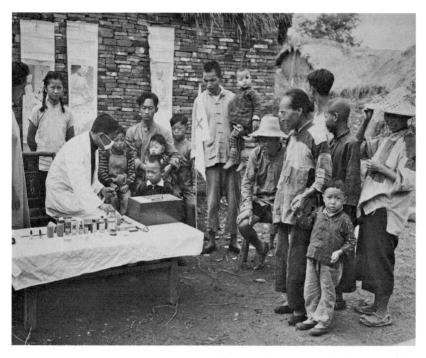

Photograph 6.3: *Postwar Rural Health Clinic Near Nanjing*
This is a postwar example of bringing basic health services to rural people. It is
clear that the type of medicine practiced by this white coated, masked physician
is still unfamiliar to onlookers. (*Source*: ABMAC Archive)

and then took a UNICEF appointment in New York.[137] By November 1948
there was little government left in Nanjing, and in December Mr. Zhou
resigned as minister.[138] Efforts to replace him with Dr. Lin Kesheng and
Dr. Jin failed, but Dr. Zhu Zhanggeng returned from the US to be acting
minister.[139] In 1949 Dr. Zhu left Nanjing on the last army plane before the
city was taken over by Communist forces, leaving eighty NHA employees
in the city. The residual Nationalist government in Guangzhou reassigned

---

[137] Li Xiangming (李向明) (1984), 280–286, biography of Jin Baoshan, states that he
left the Ministry in 1947 because of corruption. See also ABMAC, Box 16, Liu to Gregersen,
October 20, 1948, and October 29, 1948.

[138] Boorman (1967) vol 1, 415.

[139] For approach to Lin see Liu to Gregersen December 30, 1948, and Fu and Deng
(1989). So far as the writer can tell, Fu and Deng are incorrect in stating that Dr. Wang
Zuxiang (王祖祥) took over as director of the remnant NHA in Guangzhou. Late in 1949
Dr. Wang is reported to have come from Chongqing to Taiwan to lead the remnant NIH
group. See Liu to Gregersen November 17, 1949, in ABMAC, box 16.

the health administration to the Ministry of the Interior with Dr. Zhu presiding over a staff of eighty.[140] By October 1949 Dr. Zhu was in Hong Kong writing a history of public health in China,[141] while the remnants of his former NIH group reassembled in Taiwan and desperately sought foreign subsidies.[142] Thus ended the Nationalist Government's National Health Administration on the Chinese mainland.[143]

Postscript

Most NHA staff remained in the mainland, seeing no need to flee a regime consisting of its own compatriots. Available evidence suggests that most found positions in post–1949 health administrations. Dr. Jin accepted an invitation from the new Minister of Public Health and returned to China early in 1950. In 1952, *Da Gongbao* in Hong Kong published his self-criticism attacking his own record as a health administrator. He characterized twenty years of work for the Nationalist Government as window dressing for the reactionary ruling class and foreign imperialists and said that all his efforts for over thirty years had made "no contribution whatever to social progress." The reason for all this wasted effort lay in his purely technical viewpoint, his mistaken assumption that medicine should have a solid scientific foundation, and a failure to base his thinking on a realization of the acute needs of the masses (his 1946 article belies this criticism). Jin reported that in summer 1951 he had participated in land reform, during which he witnessed the cruel exploitation of the landed class and their oppression of farmers. To his amazement he saw doctors united in Chinese and Western medical clinics cooperating to solve rural medical problems. His thought underwent deep changes and he realized he had been "on the wrong trail for several decades."[144]

That statement reflects mandatory Maoist era self-negation. By the late 1980s biographers of this decent and hard-working man took a completely different view of his career. As a youth Dr. Jin was a protégé of the

---

[140] ABMAC, box 6, ABMAC, minutes of Board Meeting, May 24, 1949.

[141] Ibid., ABMAC, Executive Committee minutes, October 13, 1949.

[142] Ibid., ABMAC, Executive Committee minutes, November 22, 1949; Liu to Gregersen, November 7, 1949.

[143] A more detailed analysis of this period would require an examination of the successes and failures of the UNRRA and CNRRA health programs in China. Substantial documentation for such a study exists but has been outside the scope of this research.

[144] ABMAC, box 17, J. Heng Liu January 21, 1952. The article appeared in "early January."

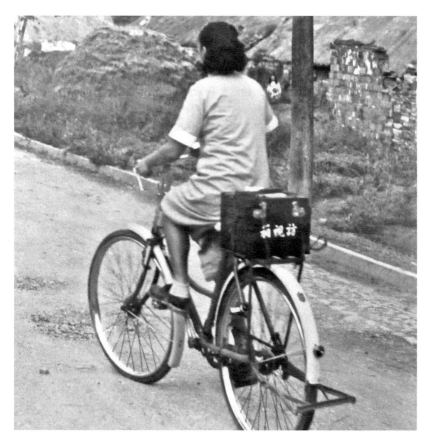

Photograph 6.4: *Visiting Nurse-Midwife on the Road*
This practitioner and the public health nurse in Photograph 6.2 are the frontline workers in the campaign to bring public preventive healthcare into rural and urban communities. (*Source*: ABMAC Archive)

revered writer Lu Xun and through him became involved in revolutionary activities. This may have helped revive his standing; it was also significant that he returned of his own free will to China in 1950. In the field of epidemic prevention he was credited with a decade of work during the 1920s for the Central Epidemic Prevention Bureau as well as for the development of the epidemic prevention corps during the War of Resistance.[145] Such recognition was long overdue. Dr. Jin and his colleagues found new

---

[145] Li Xiangming (1984), 280–286, biography of Jin Baoshan. See also Cui Yueli (催月犁) (1987), 386–388.

ways to define and carry out public healthcare and to enroll national and international experts in contributing to the rise of modern public health in China. In their day their work was internationally recognized. The British medical missionary Dr. Harold Balme wrote in 1939 that; "There was no department of Chinese Government Service which displayed such energy, or achieved so large a measure of success, as the Ministry of Health."[146] Dr. Jin is now recognized in China as "one of the founders of modern public health."[147]

From this perspective we can better appreciate the extent to which the public health movement in the 1930s and 1940s initiated "sustainable Chinese socio-economic measures."

Though deprived of peace and political support, the public health leaders during the Nationalist era launched preventive health services and tested them through the work of model county and provincial healthcare agencies and personnel. They also began the arduous task of collecting data. Even though by 1945 a nationwide rural health service was still a distant goal, it was recognized as the primary objective of the public healthcare movement. Given the wartime conditions, this was no small achievement. Postwar upheavals and all-out civil war were not a friendly setting for resumption of rural health initiatives. But although the central policy agencies fell apart, public health work continued at the grass roots level. The question remained whether a new government could reorganize and give some reasonable priority to public healthcare.

---

[146] Harold Balme (1939): 836–839.
[147] Brief biography at http//:www.hudong.com/wiki/金宝善. After he returned to China he served as chair of the department of public health at Beijing Medical College and as President of the Chinese Medical Association. He died in 1984 at the age of 91.

CHAPTER SEVEN

YAN'AN'S HEALTH SERVICES UNDER MAO ZEDONG'S LEADERSHIP, 1937–1945

The Chinese masses need everything—
food, clothing, housing, education, medical help
                    —Agnes Smedley, September 1937.[1]

Poverty is one of the most pronounced causes of disease....
This is a dark side of present-day hygienic culture
                    —Andrija Stampar, M.D.[2]

Rescue the dying and heal the wounded,
Practice revolutionary humanitarianism

                            —Mao Zedong[3]

The health challenges in northwest China were among the most arduous anywhere in the country. At the time when the Long Marchers arrived, Yan'an was in a region beset by communicable diseases, high maternal child mortality rates, and famine.[4] Although the Nationalist government had set up nominal departments of health in Xi'an and other northwestern provincial cities, in rural areas public health was nonexistent. Even in good times it would have been much harder to initiate modern standards of hygiene and sanitation in the arid and impoverished northwest than in other areas of China.

Revival of the United Front at the end of 1936 provided a brief respite for the Communist forces. Once the War of Resistance broke out, the Japanese military focused as much on destruction of Communism as had the Nationalist government, and it was far better armed. In South Shaanxi a Nationalist army blockaded Yan'an and from 1940 on prevented passage

---

[1] Smedley (1938), 21.
[2] Andrija Stampar, M.D. (August 2006), 1382–1385. Dr. Stampar was a pioneer in the development of rural healthcare and social medicine in post World War One Croatia. He visited China several times in the 1930s as a League of Nations healthcare consultant.
[3] 救死扶伤, 实行人道主义. For an inscription in Mao's hand, see *Yanan Baiqiuen guoji heping yiyuan* (1986), photo 1.
[4] Lillian M. Li (2007) provides a definitive account of this subject.

of much needed medical supplies. Yet because of the strategic vision of
Mao and his leaders, their familiarity with guerrilla warfare, their attrac-
tion of patriotic youth, and international aid from idealistic foreigners, the
Communists managed not only to survive but to develop highly motivated
teams of health workers.

There has been much political and military analysis by scholars on the
Yan'an period. The war led to visits to Yan'an by a number of American
journalists, military and diplomatic personnel, several of whom published
accounts of their observations. In addition, significant support came from
international health workers, among whom Drs. Norman Bethune (Baiqiuen), Ma Haide, D. S. Kotnis (Kedihua), Hans Mueller, the Soviet physician Dr. Orlov (阿洛夫) and the Korean Dr. Bang Wooyong (방우용, in
Chinese 方禹镛) have received special recognition. Two books by Agnes
Smedley provide eyewitness accounts of military healthcare in action in
both the Eighth Route and New Fourth armies.

None of these accounts deal with the overall business of healthcare and
life saving in northwest and north China during the period under review.
Chinese scholars are now studying this pivotal era, during which Communist healthcare workers had to rescue soldiers fighting the Japanese
military, serve an impoverished civilian population, and lead the struggle
against feudal superstition. This chapter describes how military and civilian health workers addressed these tasks, by drawing on a combination
of leadership, training, patriotism, party discipline and international aid.
'Saving lives' provided a rallying cry around which both leaders and fol-
lowers could unite to advance the Chinese Communist revolution.

Confronting Famine and Disease

Northwest China was a land of arid but minerally rich soil, whose people
for years had been battered by famine and communicable disease. During
the great north China drought of 1920–1921 500,000 people were estimated to have died while nearly 20 million were believed to be destitute.
Local people survived off poplar buds, corncobs, sawdust, gaoliang (高粱
sorghum) husks, elm-tree bark and sweet potato vines. Sale of women
and children flourished. Relief was more accessible than during the great
famine of 1876–1879 but did not address underlying problems.[5]

---

[5] Mallory (1926), 2–3, 30. See also Peking United International Famine Relief Committee (1922). This report deals mainly with famine in West Chihli. As the product of a

In describing the northwest China famine of 1928–1930 in *Red Star Over China*, Edgar Snow estimated that it resulted in well over 3 million deaths.[6] Two million people starved in Gansu. Landlords, tax collectors and local militias bought land cheap or squeezed taxes and supplies from surviving cultivators. Dr. Stampar, who seldom minced words, described tax assessment in Shaanxi as "haphazard" and tax collection as "wasteful, brutal and in many cases corrupt."[7] Recent research indicates that the famine caused much internal migration as well as emigration from Shaanxi. Just in Shaanxi alone death and emigration caused a lowering of the recorded population from 11.8 million in 1928 to 8.9 million in 1931. In 1932 bubonic plague infected ten counties, followed by cholera, which spread rapidly through the province.[8] These afflictions opened the door to exploitation of peasants by officials, moneylenders, landlords and bandits. Female babies were disposed of, girls sold, and maternal and child mortality rates became dangerously high. Migration of destitute peasants into towns and cities aggravated existing urban problems.[9]

Epidemic diseases gripped northwest China along with poverty, illiteracy, superstition, and lack of public health. When the war with Japan broke out, smallpox, tuberculosis, cholera and syphilis were widespread.[10] Riding through the countryside from Yan'an to Xi'an, Agnes Smedley found cooks in wayside hovels wiping chopsticks with dishrags "literally

---

non-governmental operation, the report covers immediate crises and responses without addressing more systemic problems.

[6] In his classic work Land and Labor in China, R. H. Tawney cited a report by the Shaanxi-born central government official Yu Youren (于右任 also Yu Yu-jan) that by the beginning of 1931 more than three million people had died of hunger in Shaanxi and that 400,000 women and children had been sold. (Source: Peking and Tientsin Times, January 21, 1931. A tireless supporter of Dr. Sun Yat-sen, Mr. Yu became president of the Control Yuan). Tawney also cited a report by G. Findlay Andrew published in November 1930 that In Gansu one-third of the population had died since 1926 due to famine, civil war, banditry and typhus. (Source: *Manchester Guardian Weekly*, November 21, 1930). See Tawney (1964), 76.

[7] Snow (1961), 214–218.

[8] At the request of Dr. Liu Ruiheng Drs. Heinrich M. Jettmar, Lu Tih-huan and Chan Chin-tao traveled to the region in November 1931. Jettmar reported around 20,000 cases of plague having occurred in the Ordos-Shaanxi-Shanxi region in 1931. City people knew how to control the disease and isolate victims; country people did not know that rat fleas, not rats, were the primary vector, thus the diseases was more contagious and frightening than in the cities. Jettmar reported that rats were encountered everywhere. The disease abated with the onset of winter. Jettmar (April 1932), 429–435.

[9] Li Lixia (李丽霞) (December 2006), 27–30. The author is at the Institute for Social Development at Henan Normal University.

[10] Wang Yuanzhou (王元周), (2009): 59–76. The author of this thoroughly documented work is professor at the Department of History, Beijing University.

black with filth." She saw people wearing rags "dirty and patched beyond description." Dry bread-cakes for sale were covered with flies, and flies had been baked into the dough. In the entire Shaanxi, Gansu and Ningxia (henceforth Shaanganning 陝甘宁) base area at this time there were reportedly only 1,000 Chinese medicine doctors and fifty animal veterinarians as compared with 2,000 witch (i.e. shamanic or charlatan) doctors.[11]

In short, northwest China was beset with political, economic and cultural problems. In Tawney's words, there were counties in which the position of the rural population "is that of a man standing permanently up to the neck in water, so that even a ripple is sufficient to drown him."[12] It was to this precarious region that the Red Armies in 1935–36 made their way.

Significance of Healthcare for Mao Zedong

The organization of health services in Yan'an and surrounding base areas developed despite lack of trained personnel, facilities, equipment, medications and funds, and under the threat of enemy bombardment and scorched earth campaigns. From Mao Zedong's perspective it was essential to develop health services that could perform the tactical function of saving lives while pursuing the long-term strategic function of promoting revolution and political transformation.[13]

To take the latter first, it was in Mao's view the revolutionary task of health workers to undermine the feudal thinking that gripped China's huge rural population and help replace it with the modern rational order represented by Marxist socialism. Specifically it was their task to dethrone Yan Wang (阎王), the Lord of the Underworld and chieftain of the feudal demons that held people's minds in thrall, so that Marx and Marxism could take Yan Wang's place.[14] It is important for us to understand the power of this analysis, which was based on Mao's studies of the mid nineteen-twenties peasant uprisings in Hunan (discussed in chapter 3), as it helps to explain why his talks and speeches were so gripping for his audiences. Health workers, he told them, were the "white coated warriors"

---

[11] The Shaanganning base area included most of northern Shaanxi and part of eastern Gansu and southern Ningxia.

[12] Tawney (1964), 77. Li (2007), 310, also cites this compelling metaphor.

[13] Mao's interest in medical ethics is discussed by Qiu Yunhong (2011). The essay draws on remarks by Mao during the Jiangxi and Yan'an eras.

[14] Huang Shuze (黄树则) (1986), 8.

of the revolution, whose work of social mobilization was just as important in its own context as that of Red Army military units defeating landlord militias, Guomindang armies, or Japanese invaders.

Despite maintaining this strategic stance, Mao was fully aware of the tactical importance of health work. This was expressed most clearly in his enthusiastic response when the Canadian Communist physician Norman Bethune showed up in Yan'an at the end of March 1938. Persuaded by Bethune's claim that front-line mobile medical teams could save seventy-five percent of battle casualties if they were operated on right away, Mao threw his weight behind Bethune's work as did Nie Rongzhen, the French-trained engineer and Jinchaji field commander with whom Bethune worked most closely. After Bethune's heroic achievements and self-sacrificial death, Mao praised him greatly, asserting that he was a greater physician than the legendary post-Han dynasty doctor Hua Tuo (华陀), thus anchoring him in a tradition of exceptional medical service to China's people.[15] Mao also argued that the technical task of medical workers was to establish the precedence of the two "micro" disciplines (*xibao* cells, cytology; and *xijun* bacteria, bacteriology) over the nostrums of witch doctors, in ways that made the world of medical science accessible to China's millions of victims of contagious diseases.[16] In short, medical science and Marxism would march together to overthrow superstition. Not surprisingly, a publication of 784 biographies of north China healthcare workers indicates that virtually all of them joined the Communist party.[17]

Mao's ideas received important support from both Zhou Enlai and Zhu De. Zhou, whose health was vulnerable, came one day to the army rear hospital near Yan'an to get an elbow fracture x-rayed, only to find that the only x-ray machine available in north Shaanxi was on the blink. He delivered a stern lecture to the hospital staff, reminding them that they were scientists and could not treat scientific work in a perfunctory manner. He examined their work and asked questions that reportedly left them tongue-tied. He challenged them to engage in preventive work rather than simply search around for medications. When told that kala-azar and pertussis (whooping cough) were major pediatric diseases, he told them to

---

[15] Wang Xueli (王学礼), Yin Xing (尹醒) (1986), 14. The Canadian missionary nurse Jean Ewen acted as an interpreter during Bethune's one meeting with Mao Zedong on March 31–April 1, 1938.

[16] Huang Shuze (1986), 7.

[17] Yang Lifu (杨立夫) (1988).

teach the laws of hygiene to nursery workers. As for Zhu De, he asserted
that commanders were needed to fight battles but medical workers were
needed to fight diseases. "Without you," he pointed out, "we cannot build
our country."[18] He also held that medical workers were needed not only
to heal people but even more to heal China.[19]

Thus Yan'an's leaders did not neglect political training and logistical
service as part of the overall organization of medical workers. Political
training was a given for workers who were already members of the Communist party or youth league or committed to service with the Eighth
Route Army. Logistics, however, had not been a strong point of traditional
army organization. Early in 1939 the Yan'an Military Commission established an army Rear Service Command (*houqinbu* 后勤部), consisting of
three divisions managing political, logistic, and healthcare work. Zhang
Lingbin (张令彬), a survivor of the Hunan autumn harvest uprisings of
1927, headed the logistical division. Zhang had known deprivation all his
life, joined the Communist Party in 1926, and served the Red Army from
1927. He was one of many veterans of Red Army struggle who served for
the most part out of the limelight, but whose work was part of the reason
for its success.[20]

Setting up Central Medical Services and Strengthening Party Medical Policy

The Communist party leaders needed a central facility to improve health
services for the rapidly expanding population of Yan'an, provide back
up for the field health services, and firm up the political importance of
medical work. After the Border Area Hospital was moved out of Yan'an
in autumn 1938 to escape Japanese bombing, Dr. Fu Lianzhang (傅连暲),
who played a key role in maintaining the health of Mao Zedong and other
party leaders, was asked to plan a new hospital, organize a central health
department and serve as its director. In 1939 the new hospital was set
up in a residential cave area of Yan'an, which enjoyed protection from
bombing raids.[21]

---

[18] Huang Shuze (1986a).
[19] Yi Ming (佚名) (2007), 7.
[20] For a biography of Zhang see Feng Caizhang and Li Baoding (1991), 39–46.
[21] "Dong Ping" (东平) and Wang Fan (王凡) (2007–9), "Zhonggong Lingxiu yu Yan'an
Zhongyang Yiyuan Wangshi."

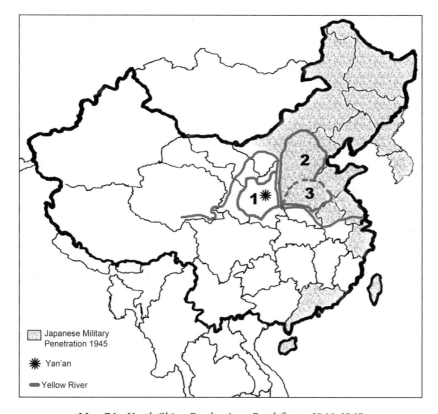

Map 7.1: *North China Border Area Battlefronts 1944–1945*
1. Shaanganning, west of the Yellow river, served as the main base area for the Yan'an Communist government and location for its main base hospitals.
2. Jinchaji is a largely mountainous area, where Drs. Bethune, Kotnis and colleagues carried out battlefield surgery under adverse conditions, often on the move.
3. Jinchaji and Jinjiluyu were locations where the savage Japanese military scorched earth campaigns (san guang 'three alls') took place. (*Source*: J. R. and A. S. Watt)

Not long after the hospital opened, Mao Zedong and Zhu De organized a dinner meeting with two of its senior staff, Drs. Jin Maoyue (金茂岳) and Wei Yizhai (魏一斋), both graduates of the missionary Qilu Medical College in Shandong with advanced study at the Peking Union Medical College hospital in Beijing, to discuss medicine and politics. The two physicians were high-level intellectuals who made the decision to stay in Yan'an and join the revolution. Mao told them that doing medicine did not mean disregarding politics, especially since in their work they would come across many difficulties. It was vital for them to strengthen their political study and their ability to change the world. "You can only go calmly about your work," he maintained, "if you have a firm political stand."

At a more practical level Zhou Enlai and the hospital vice director He Mu (何穆, a pulmonary physician with a degree from the University of Toulouse), combed Chongqing for medical workers and equipment to send to the Yan'an central hospital, and Zhou even returned with samples of typhoid and paratyphoid bacteria for hospital staff to study. The Marxist educator Ai Siqi (艾思奇) was enlisted to give lectures on Marxism to the medical staff, and party organization leaders Chen Yun (陈云) and Li Fuchun (李富春) evaluated progress and enrolled medical workers as party members. As a result of these efforts, many central hospital high-level intellectuals joined the party.[22] Chen Yun also mobilized students from the Central Party School to study medicine at the Central Hospital.[23]

The central health system provided a central clinic and a convalescent hospital.[24] The former First Front Army medical school was combined with the medical school personnel of the Second and Fourth Front armies and became the Medical Science University in Yan'an. The noted surgeon Wang Bin (王斌 1909–1992) became its principal, succeeding He Cheng (贺诚), who was sent to Moscow to get his health back. Urged on by Zhou Enlai, the school was able by July 1937 to graduate three classes totaling sixty-eight students.[25]

One way in which the northwest Communist health services differed from those of the Jiangxi Soviet was in attracting international support. The China Defense League and its vigorous leader, Mme. Sun Yat-sen (Song Qingling 宋庆龄), provided the Central Communist Party and Eighth Route Army health services with significant material support and advocacy. Meanwhile, the American and Swiss trained physician Dr. Ma Haide (马海德, formerly George Hatem) in Yan'an facilitated contacts with the League of Nations and other international friends. Ma was born in Buffalo and grew up in the U.S.; but as a professional physician he devoted his energies to the Chinese Communist revolution and served as medical adviser to top leaders. He arrived in Northern Shaanxi in 1936

---

[22] Yi Ming (2007).

[23] Ibid.

[24] The idea of organizing health services by systems is taken from Zhang Qi'an (张启安) (2001), 57. The author is at the College of Humanities, Jiaotong University, Xi'an.

[25] Zhang Ruguang (1989), 236. Wang Bin was one of the physicians who took care of Zhou during the Long March. Dr. He Cheng did not return to China until after the war was over.

along with Edgar Snow, and then spent four months on the front lines with the Eighth Route Army, noting the medical services and writing up a report for Mao and the Party Central Committee. Based on this report, Dr. Ma was invited to stay on as adviser to the Central Health Department.[26]

In a January 1940 report to the China Defense League Dr. Ma surveyed accomplishments during the previous four years. The Central Health Department had set up six hospitals (one for convalescent soldiers), with a capacity of 2,000–2,500 beds. To staff these hospitals there were fourteen qualified physicians, twenty-one medical assistants, and around 200 nursing aides with an average age of 16–18, of whom one-third had some training and the rest were local volunteers. There were also twenty pharmacists and dispensers. The Central Medical Department had two Western-trained physicians. It organized a Chinese pharmaceutical section with four Chinese medicine doctors, who prepared medicines from herbs gathered locally. A fifth Chinese medicine doctor undertook research work. A blacksmith made surgical instruments.[27]

The central hospital, with 150 beds, provided an obstetrics and gynecology service to help reduce the high rate of infant mortality in the region. Dr. Jin Maoyue was its director. Several offspring of party leaders were born at the hospital, including Li Na (李讷 also Li Ne), daughter of Mao and Jiang Qing (江青). But Mao was adamant that the hospital should serve the people and not just the political elite. Hospital data show that the obstetrical staff delivered over 2,750 infants between 1939 and 1945, and altogether 3,814 by April 1949. 1945 was the peak year with 714 deliveries; during the civil war the numbers for obvious reasons dropped considerably.[28]

In November 1940 He Mu took over as director of the Central Hospital. With the aid of the Soviet physician Dr. Orlov (阿洛夫), he developed an integrated management system ensuring that employees knew what their jobs entailed. In addition to departments of internal medicine, surgery and obstetrics and gynecology, the hospital added departments for pediatrics, tuberculosis, and infectious diseases; by 1945 it had over 200 beds. Between September 1939 and June 1946 it treated 13,886 patients, of whom 13,423 were cured, representing a recovery rate of 96.67 percent. It was especially successful in treating women in childbirth, losing only

---

[26] For Dr. Ma see Porter (1997).
[27] Information is from Ma Hai-teh (Haide) "Medical work in the Northwest Border Region, Yenan January 21, 1940," in ABMAC archive, box 5.
[28] Yi Ming (2007).

two who had been mishandled by traditional midwives. Hospital department heads carried out regular schedules of clinical teaching, and the hospital invited outside experts to give lectures. Thus despite difficulties in acquiring equipment and medications the hospital reportedly achieved impressive comparative results in patient care. Whereas overall Chinese hospital mortality rates for pediatric enteritis, pediatric bronchial pneumonia or adult pneumonia were reportedly twenty percent or more, the central hospital's mortality rates for these afflictions were only eight percent, five percent, and 3.7 percent respectively.[29]

These results reflected the emphasis of party and medical leaders on preventive health. Thus in 1941, when a typhoid epidemic hit Yan'an, Mao Zedong urged the central health department to strengthen preventive work. As medications were not available, the central hospital experimented with supplementary diets, particularly soymilk and cow's milk, to strengthen patient immune systems. In 1943 it formed a roving medical team to help treat people living near Yan'an and also to propagate preventive health knowledge. In 1944 the central health department and the central hospital put on a new year's festival play, which entertained the public and received plaudits from Mao Zedong.[30]

Mao continued to emphasize the connections between backward culture, illiteracy and ill health. In a report given in October 1944 at a conference of cultural workers of the Shaanganning border area (region of Shaanxi, Gansu and Ningxia provinces north and northwest of Yan'an), he complained that among the 1.5 million border-area population there were still one million illiterates, 2,000 witch doctors and pervasive superstitious thinking. These mental enemies, he argued, were greater obstacles than Japanese imperialism. In terms of healthcare, relying on new doctors would not solve such problems. New health workers must ally with Chinese medicine doctors and old intelligentsia. "Unite," he declared, "organize, criticize, educate and reform!"[31] It was a clarion call that would get harsher as the problems lingered on and the revolution unfolded.

---

[29] Zhu Hongzhao (朱鸿召) (2008). Prof. Zhu is a specialist in the social history of the Yan'an era.

[30] 'Dong Ping' and Wang Fang (2007): "Zhonggong lingxiu yu Yan'an zhongyang yiyuan wangshi (2)."

[31] Mao Zedong (1944): For an English version see Mao (1944), 235–237.

Military Medical Service: "Rescuing the Dying and Healing the Wounded"
with Limited Medical Capability

Medical services supporting the Red Army (renamed Eighth Route Army following the restoration of the United Front with the Nationalist government) were responsible for the health of army soldiers and partisans and also took on civilian patients.

A Central Military Health Commission managed military health. After the War of Resistance began in August 1937, Dr. Jiang Qixian (姜齐贤 1905–1976), a graduate of Hunan's Xiangya Medical College, who joined the Red Army in 1931 and the CCP in 1935, directed the Commission.[32] The initial vice director was Dr. Rao Zhengxi, (饶正锡 1911–1998), one of five interns at the British Methodist Universal Love Hospital in Da'ye, who joined the Red Army in 1930 (see chapter 3). Dr. Rao was also director of the health bureau of the Commission's rear service command (*zonghou qinbu* 总后勤部). This bureau oversaw two hospitals (one of which became the Norman Bethune International Peace hospital), a pharmaceutical factory, and a medical school (later China Medical University).[33] The director of the school was the highly regarded physician Dr. Li Zhi (李治 1899–1989).[34] The Commission's front line medical services became famous as a result of the work of Drs. Bethune, Kotnis and their battlefield colleagues. Its domain would in due course cover much of north China.

The military medical service faced immediate personnel and technical problems. The long marches of 1934–36 had whittled down the numbers of health workers with significant training, and medications were not easily available in the desolate Shaanganning region (map 7.1). The leaders sent representatives to Xi'an to scan incoming migrants for those with any medical expertise and do everything possible to persuade them to head for Yan'an, where they were sure to be welcomed.[35]

Another challenge facing the Eighth Route Army as it prepared for battle with the Japanese military was to develop standards of hygiene necessary to maintain the health of its troops. Most of the recruits were from Shaanganning, where popular knowledge of hygiene was virtually non-existent. The army's medical department set up a rear branch for

---

[32] Feng Caizhang and Li Baoding (1991), biography of Jiang Qixian, 80–81.
[33] Rao Zhengxi (饶正锡) (1986a), 3.
[34] http://www.hudong.com/wiki/李治％5B中国开国少将％5D, biography of Li Zhi.
[35] Yi Ming (2007). Jin relates that when he and his colleagues arrived in Yan'an, Mao, Zhu De and Zhou Enlai all turned out to greet them.

training recruits, which began operating early in 1938. Personal hygiene was stressed. Each squad was to have a hygiene orderly. Squads built their own bath and washhouses. Clothes were changed twice a week, and bathing was obligatory at least once a week. Troops underwent a daily inspection of personal appearance and cleanliness. In each room a removable earthenware jug was dug into the ground to serve as a spittoon. Large posters with arrows pointing to the spittoon were posted on the walls. Latrine pits were dug twenty-seven feet deep and provided with an outhouse. No flies or unpleasant odors hung around them. As a result of this Spartan regime, dysentery and intestinal infections dropped to 0.0042% during the dangerous summer months. Kitchens also were made fly proof by screening the windows.[36]

A report by Dr. Rao Zhengxi indicated that the medical leadership understood that effective public health depended on improving standards of living and education as well as public health. Troops were responsible for passing on knowledge about healthy living to students and country people. A health protection section provided teachers for schools and issued health protection pamphlets. In July 1939 it put on a two week medical and health exhibit in Yan'an, which attracted over 30,000 visits. The organizers distributed street posters and ran anti-fly, anti-rat and anti-spitting campaigns. Fieldwork included vaccinations, digging of hygienic latrines and cesspools, and physical examinations.[37] The army also ran courses for its medical staff. In each hospital, clinic and outpatient department two hours each day were available for organized study. The medical department printed and distributed study pamphlets and published a journal with the title National Defense Hygiene (*Guofang weisheng* 国防卫生). Weekly discussion meetings took place among more advanced practitioners.[38]

A separate review of the medical training school of the Eighth Route Army traced its evolution from Jiangxi, through the Long March to north Shaanxi, and to the Eighth Route Army headquarters after July 1937. According to this document, the school provided a special eighteen-month training course for junior medical officers. Candidates included university undergraduates and country youth knowing only a few hundred characters.

---

[36] Ma Hai-teh (Haide), "Medical Work in the Northwest Border Region," Yenan, January 21, 1940, in ABMAC, box 5.

[37] Included in Ma Haide's 1940 report. In 1939 79,500 smallpox and 13,360 typhoid vaccinations were administered in the Yan'an region.

[38] Ibid.

They began with three months of premedical education in elementary physics, chemistry and biology. During the next seven months the students were introduced to physiology, anatomy, bacteriology and parasitology, pharmacology, pathology and diagnosis. In the following eight months they explored medicine, surgery, otorhinolaryngology, urology, pediatrics, obstetrics and gynecology, skin diseases and medical administration. Students spent three and a half hours a week on political studies and three hours on English. Advanced students visited the school hospital twice a week for clinical practice.[39]

A model hospital (*mofan yiyuan* 模范医院) incorporating the former Eighth Route Army base hospital in Guaimao village (Yanchuan County) was inaugurated in May 1939. It served as a center for orthopedic surgery and for seriously wounded soldiers; it also provided a maternal health service. The surgical department had the use of twenty caves, each with six beds. The medical department occupied the facilities of the old base hospital as well as ten newly dug caves. The maternal health department could accommodate 100 patients and included a rest house for pregnant women.[40] Special caves housed operating rooms, an X-ray department, a laboratory with modern equipment, and staff quarters. It had no electric light plant for work after dark.[41]

After the arrival of Dr. Bethune (*Baiqiuen* 白求恩) in Yan'an at the end of March 1938, medical preparedness in northwest China rose to a new level. As Mao indicated in his famous eulogy, Bethune's impact would be hard to exaggerate. He combined intense personal experience in treating tuberculosis amongst the poor with unrivaled knowledge of military medicine gained through battlefield service in both World War One and the Spanish Civil War. His service in Spain gave him vital experience in battlefield blood transfusion and its capacity to save lives. Spain inspired him with a hatred of fascism; abandonment of poor people in Canada to tuberculosis (which Bethune himself contracted) led him to join the Communist party. Although eager to get to the battlefront Bethune was forced to wait a month in Yan'an, partly because CCP leaders were reluctant to

---

[39] Chang Shu-fatt, "Report on the Medical Training School of the Eighth Route Army," China Defense League Newsletter, No. 8, N.S., October 1, 1939, in ABMAC, box 5. The author was a correspondent of the Hong Kong Daily Press and English language teacher at the school.

[40] Information on the departments is from a report on hospitals in the Border Region, in CDL Newsletter, No. 8, NS, October 1, 1939, in ABMAC archive, box 5.

[41] Information from Dr. Ma's report supplemented by CDL Newsletter, No. 8 NS, October 1, 1939, in ABMAC archive, box 5.

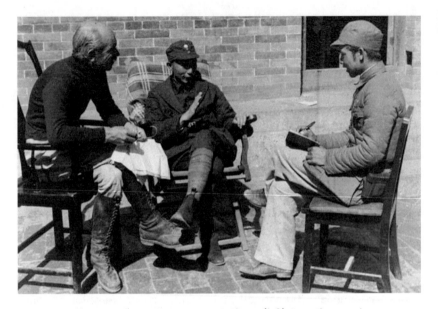

Photograph 7.1: *Dr. Norman Bethune (left) Consulting with*
General Nie Rongzhen (center)
The Canadian surgeon has become an internationally famous example of the
practice of battlefield healthcare. A Canadian Communist party member and
ardent anti-fascist, he found his true calling in his memorable and all too brief
service to soldiers of the Eighth Route Army. (*Source*: Canadian Archives)

send an aging and talented foreign friend into battle and partly so that the
medical supplies he brought from the US could catch up with him.

During the next twenty months Bethune worked at or near the front
lines in the Jinchaji military region putting his unique military medical
expertise into action on behalf of Eighth Route Army soldiers (see map
7.1). For Bethune the conditions that he found in the base hospitals were
unacceptable. Although critical and angry at what he misinterpreted as
incompetence, Bethune saw that he could make a difference. With the
aid of an interpreter he struck up a cordial relationship with General
Nie Rongzhen, the brilliant commander of the Jinchaji military district. Nie
invited him to serve as medical adviser to the Jinchaji administration with
the task of developing a medical system for regular and partisan troops
of the entire Jinchaji region. Bethune responded by launching a drive to
improve hospital organization and cleanliness, and by scheduling lectures
for medical staff, ward rounds, and weekly staff conferences.

Around this time Bethune put his blood transfusion service into operation. Using his own blood he demonstrated blood transfusion to medical

staff and villagers and persuaded the latter to organize a blood transfusion corps. At night he wrote training manuals on surgery and medicine under battlefield conditions.[42] He focused on completing a model hospital, which was unfortunately destroyed by a Japanese force only a few days after opening. Undaunted, he organized a mobile field hospital that could perform 100 operations and provide 500 dressings and 500 prescriptions. Late in November he visited the 359th Brigade and told its commander, Wang Zhen (王震), that the brigade's handling of wounded soldiers was not good enough. General Wang took the criticism seriously and sat through twenty-four hours of operations. A few days later Bethune performed 71 operations for the Brigade over a forty-hour period, during which only one patient died. From February to July 1939 Bethune's mobile medical unit in central Hebei saw action in four battles, during which it was never more than two and a half miles from the firing line and at times closer. The unit performed 315 operations in the field and on one occasion was nearly captured. It transported 1,000 wounded soldiers from central to west Hebei without losing a single one.

This front line emphasis reflected Bethune's axiom that medical staff seek the wounded (not the other way round), and that a few hours could make the difference between a successful and a failed surgical intervention.[43] The mobile medical units were now functioning as divisional field hospitals; Bethune reported that he hoped to set up seven during 1939. However he concluded that the education of medical officers and nurses should now be the main task of any foreign unit.[44] He proposed to Nie a plan to produce a whole generation of skilled doctors and nurses. This was more important, he urged, than anything that the existing mobile medical-surgical units could do.

Bethune now planned on returning to North America to generate more financial and medical aid for the Eighth Route Army, but his luck ran out.

---

[42] These included Essential Knowledge for Battlefield Rescue (Zhanchang jiuhu xuzhi); First Steps in Treating the Wounded (Chubu liaoshang); Thirteen Steps in Sterilization (Xiaodu shisan bu); Organization and Work for Field Hospitals during Divisional Mobile Warfare (Youji zhanzhong shi yezhan yiyuan de zuzhi he jishu). The latter was a 140,000-word treatise. See "Baiqiuen" in Feng and Li (1991), 616.

[43] The quote is widely reported in Bethune studies. See China Defense League (1940), 16.

[44] CDL Newsletter, No. 11, NS, 122/15/1939, in ABMAC archive Box 5. The date of Bethune's report is July 1, 1939. The same data can be found in CDL, Annual Report...1939–1940, 16–19.

He cut his finger during an emergency operation with no gloves available, contracted septicemia and died in Hebei on November 12, 1939.[45]

Bethune's death riveted attention on front line care and demonstrated what a difference it could make. In gratitude for his work the army's model rear base hospital, newly renamed the Norman Bethune International Peace Hospital, developed a song to inspire its workers. It proclaimed that:

> As soldiers commit their precious lives to resist Japan's bandit savagery,
> So we commit our precious scientific skills to safeguard their health,
> Strike down Japanese imperialism and fight for Chinese people's liberation...
> The more the difficulties we face the more we must study Baiqiuen's example,
> Overcome hardship, and provide the protection of peaceful warriors.

Bethune's work was significantly aided by Kathleen Hall (何明清), a New Zealand Anglican missionary nurse, who came to China, studied at the PUMC hospital and set up a rural mission at Songjiazhuang, a village in west central Hebei province. At considerable personal risk Hall accepted Bethune's request to visit Beijing and bring back medical equipment and supplies desperately needed for Eighth Route Army patients. She did so successfully several times by train and mules and once returned with two PUMC nurses, one of whom later married Dr. Kotnis (see below). Then the Japanese military intercepted, burned her village hospital and deported her. She escaped to Hong Kong and returned to the Eighth Route Army but contracted beriberi and had to be repatriated. She is now celebrated in China for her work on behalf of Chinese soldiers and civilians.[46]

In February 1939 a five-person team of antifascist physicians selected by the Indian Congress succeeded in arriving in Yan'an after many delays. Zhu De precipitated this initiative by writing to Jawaharlal Nehru with a request for medical aid. The team leader, Dr. M. Atal (爱德华), served as a physician in the Spanish civil war. The two youngest members, Drs. Basu

---

[45] Gordon and Allen (1952), Stewart (2002). It is clear from correspondence in the latter source that the trials of working under harsh circumstances, with only minimal supplies and only modestly trained individuals, continued to weigh heavily on Bethune right up to his last days. He also felt that supervision of medical units by staff officers was far less than what the circumstances required. He made these concerns known, especially to Ye Qingshan.

[46] Miss Hall was often accompanied by a dog given to her by General Nie Rongzhen. A scholarship in her (Chinese) name now supports nursing students from rural areas in China. Newnham (1992) and on-line sources.

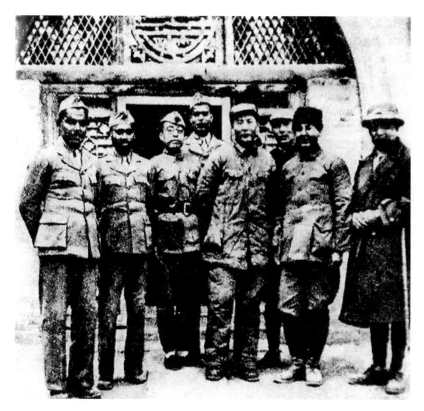

Photograph 7.2: *Indian Medical Delegation Greeted by Mao Zedong, March 15, 1939*
The Indian volunteer physicians answered a call from Zhu De to come to Yan'an
and assist the struggle against fascism. Dr. Kotnis, second from left, took that
call to heart and like Bethune gave his life assisting the Eighth Route Army's
wounded soldiers and villagers in need of medical care. Mao Zedong (fourth from
right) welcomed the delegation. (*Source*: http://www.china.com.cn/chinese/zhuanti/
kzsl/851715.htm)

(巴苏华) and Kotnis (Dwarkanath Shantaram Kotnis, known in China as
Kedihua 柯棣华), stayed longest in China; Dr. Kotnis remained until his
death in December 1942.[47] The arrival of the team added to the international medical presence in northwest China established by Drs. Bethune
and Ma Haide and added to Mao's international standing as China's anti-
fascist leader.

---

[47] The team members added 'hua' (华) to their names to indicate affiliation with China.

At first the Indian physicians worked in or around Yan'an, with Atal, Basu and Kotnis serving at the Eighth Route Army rear hospital. In early November 1939 the three of them, joined by the German Jewish physician Dr. Hans Mueller (汉斯米勒), set off for southeast Shanxi. They crossed the Yellow River and reached the Eighth Route Army Headquarters at Wuxiang on December 21. Six weeks later Dr. Atal contacted bad eczema and returned to India; the two younger physicians and Dr. Mueller joined units of the 129th division and soon learned the essentials of medical care during guerrilla warfare. Like Smedley they were struck by the contrast between the care given by Eighth Route Army medical orderlies to their wounded soldiers and the intolerable situation facing the thousands of wounded conscripts discarded by the Nationalist 17th Route Army in south Shanxi and north Henan. The latter, shivering in tattered, unlined clothes, or as corpses dead from hunger and cold, reminded Mueller of Napoleon's doomed army retreating from Moscow.[48] During a fierce battle in southeast Shanxi the Kotnis team set up an operating unit close by, and Kotnis carried out surgery for forty-six hours. After further experience of guerrilla medicine in Hebei, Basu, Kotnis and Mueller arrived in August 1940 at Gegong in west Hebei, where the medical school and a field hospital named for Dr. Bethune were then located. This was on the eve of the Hundred Regiments campaign and the radical intensification of war in north China.

The Japanese Military Onslaught in North China, and Its Effect on Army and Civilian Healthcare

The ability of north China's Communist leaders to exploit antifascism as a driving political and moral force benefited greatly from the waves of destruction of life and property unleashed by the Japanese military in north China, especially during 1940–43. The fact that the Japanese campaigns targeted both military and civilians placed a huge burden on the available health services. Often the members of those services were in great danger and not a few lost their lives. But the force of the attacks inspired them to greater efforts and reinforced the will of soldiers and health workers to achieve victory over what they regarded as a drive to reimpose colonial subservience.

---

[48] Sheng Xiangong (盛贤功) (1986), 63.

Summaries of these campaigns must suffice to explain the circumstances in which the Eighth Route Army health services operated. The Eighth Route Army's Hundred Regiments Campaign of autumn 1940 (*baituan dazhan* 百团大战) was the single most significant anti-Japanese campaign mounted by the Communist military forces in north China. The campaign had various goals, one of which was to break apart the Japanese military strategy to 'encage' the Communist armed forces. Both sides suffered heavy losses. The eruption of the Pacific War in December 1941 forced the Japanese to begin withdrawing military forces from north China before they could fully press their advantage. As a result, by 1944 the Chinese Communist forces were able to recoup lost ground and build their military strength under more favorable circumstances.

Japanese punitive counterattacks began at the end of 1940 with a two-month campaign of indiscriminate destruction in the Taiyue base area in north Shanxi. On this occasion the Japanese goal was reportedly to destroy the Eighth Route Army and its base area, kill all civilians of any age or sex, destroy their habitations, carry off or burn their grain, destroy their utensils and fill up or poison their wells.[49] This was the onset of the three year campaign known as 'three all' in English language accounts (burn all, kill all, loot all), and in Chinese as *san guang zhengce* (三光政策 three eliminations policy). Appointed Commander in Chief of the Japanese army in north China in July 1941, General Okamura Yasuji ordered the construction of ditches and walls to impede movement of Eighth Route Army patrols and restrict movement of agricultural goods. Chinese labor was commandeered to carry out this work. In August he inflicted a comprehensive, two-month *san guang* campaign on northern Shanxi. Males between the ages of 15 and 60 were targeted.[50] In November 1941 Okamura launched a second campaign in the Jinjiluyu border area (including parts of Shanxi, Hebei, Shandung and Henan).[51]

The *san guang* destruction carried on through 1942 and most of 1943. In May 1942 the Japanese military reportedly broke 128 river and lake dikes in central and western Hebei, flooding 6,752 villages and hamlets and 1.54 million *mou*, and destroying 168,900 buildings. Up to two million people

---

[49] "Sanguang Zhengce," (2011). Earlier mopping-up campaigns occurred in 1938 and 1939, but the aim of this one was to destroy the means of survival of north China soldiers and people.

[50] "Sanguang Zhengce" (2011); Bix (2000).

[51] "Sanguang Zhengce" (2011).

were affected by this devastation.[52] A text frequently cited online states that in the Spring of 1942 the Japanese military created depopulated areas in nine counties spread along either side of the Great Wall from Gubeikou to Shanhaiguan, driving off 500,000 people in the process. In May 1942 a force of 50,000 Japanese soldiers carried out a brutal mopping-up campaign in Central Hebei.[53] During a three month campaign carried out in the Jinchaji border area beginning September 1943 the Japanese military is reported to have killed 6,274 people, burned 54,779 dwellings, confiscated or burned 29 million Jin (14.67 million kg) of grain, confiscated 19,300 or more livestock, and destroyed 172,600 farming tools.[54] The overall campaign substantially reduced the size of the terrain and the numbers of people and amount of resources accessible to the Eighth Route Army. Thus from a Japanese military perspective it achieved significant immediate gains.[55]

A Chinese summary of Japanese use of chemical (gas) weapons in China states that during conflicts in 14 provinces and 77 districts, the Japanese military made use of chemical weapons on 2,091 occasions. Four hundred and twenty-three of these occasions involved conflicts with guerrilla forces in north China and resulted in over 33,000 injuries and deaths. The

---

[52] 1) //wenda.tianya.cn/wenda/thread?tid=7573bd99ad3ce8f8; 2) //zhidao.baidu.com/question/42892612. Because of the multiple existence of sites providing simultaneous wording of this atrocity, it has not been possible for the writer to determine which one is the original text and from there to assess by what means and with what level of authority the evidence was assembled. However, extraneous data dealing with the Japanese military's *sanguang* campaigns is prima facie evidence that some level of atrocity, of the sort described in these iterations, is likely to have happened. Certainly Chinese writers dealing with this topic have no doubt about it.

[53] e.g. 1) iask://sina.com.cn/b/5940327.html; 2) www.cnrand.com/jrjd/2010-10-28/1517_6.html; 3) //wenda.tianya.cn/wenda/thread?tid=4cdfb1257ca7abfc.

[54] The main source for this information has been "Sanguang Zhengce" (2011). An extended biography of Okamura is available at http://baike.baidu.com/view/14888.htm. The *sanguang* campaign is discussed in Whitson (1973), 164–165. Whitson dates it as beginning in March 1941 and continuing on for 18 months. He notes that it may have "surpassed even the Rape of Nanking in sheer brutality." That is an understatement, as a study by Himeta Mitsuyoshi on the *sanguang* 'three eliminations policy' (not seen by the writer) reportedly put the number of deaths of Chinese civilians at more than 2.7 million. That number is found in several on-line articles and reported by Bix (2000, 367). Bix maintains that the *sanguang* campaigns were "incomparably more destructive and of far longer duration than either the army's chemical or biological warfare or the 'rape of Nanking.'" Available evidence supports this judgment.

[55] According to Whitson, the Eighth Route Army lost 100,000 out of 400,000 men in 1941, and the population (and territorial scope) under Communist control was reduced by one-third by mid 1942 "from about 45 million to fewer than 30 million." Whitson (1973), 165.

Japanese military also employed gas warfare in civilian areas to contaminate wells and rivers. Overall Chinese casualties from chemical warfare are calculated to have amounted to over 100,000 military and civilian people. It is also calculated that during the War of Resistance Japan produced 7.46 million chemical shells, the majority of which were used or left on Chinese battlefields.[56]

During the last four months of 1940 the Hundred Regiments Campaign precipitated an increased use of chemical warfare as Japanese military units found themselves unexpectedly on the defensive. According to one source Japanese military forces used chemical weapons over thirty times during the later stages of this campaign, causing 21,800 Chinese casualties.[57] In the first half of 1941 the Japanese military launched a devastating mopping-up drive across the flat lands of west Shandong, central and east Hebei, and Henan. This was followed in the second half of 1941 by another major mopping-up campaign in the Jinchaji base area, characterized as 'iron wall encirclement' (铁壁合围 *tiebi hewei*). Reportedly these campaigns frequently used chemical weapons, especially on the flatlands. A Japanese chemical weapons unit, returning to one battlefield, found over 1,000 Chinese soldiers, unprotected by gas masks, lying in disarray, grievously wounded.[58] Another unit, employing Chinese puppet soldiers, gassed forty-six villagers in a schoolhouse.[59] In 1942, another bad year for the villagers of north China, a Japanese military unit released gas into a cave housing a rear base hospital, killing 192 people, and another unit gassed a tunnel in a village in Dingxian, Hebei (once the center of a great experiment in mass education and public health), eliminating over 800 people.[60]

The Chinese Communist military lacked the technical capacity to counteract chemical warfare. Thanks to the initiative of the senior political commissar Zuo Quan (左权), the Yan'an authorities organized in 1939 two six-month chemical warfare training classes, from which some

---

[56] Information is from "Kangri Zhanzheng Gei Zhongguoren Dailai Zainan You Naxie?" (2009).

[57] Wan Xuefeng (万学锋) and Wang Jihong (王季红), "Rijun dui Balujun, Xinsijun de Huaxuezhan." Senior victims included Chen Geng (陈赓), Zhou Xihan (周希汉), Chen Xilian (陈锡联), Fan Zixia (范子侠), Xie Fuzhi (谢富治), and Yin Xianbing (尹先炳).

[58] The battlefield information, cited in "Rijun dui Balujun, Xinsijun de Huaxuezhan" was sourced from a Japanese Ministry of the Interior document. The reported campaign during the first half of 1941 preceded the arrival of Okamura.

[59] Gao Xiaoyan (高晓燕) (2009).

[60] Wan Xuefeng, "Rijun dui Balujun." This incident is also reported in Yu Ge (余戈) (2009), 95–97.

sixty people graduated. Thirty were sent to divisional units to begin training in anticipating unexpected chemical warfare attacks and providing
emergency relief. To be effective, trainees would have to immediately:
1) remove all clothing of affected individuals, 2) thoroughly wash the
entire body, preferably with soap and water, or at the very least with water.
These steps would not be easy to carry out on an emergency basis, if at
all. In March 1942, when the Japanese military use of chemical warfare
was at its peak, the Chinese Communist military leadership issued further
instructions about preventive care and 1) when entering houses of villagers
in enemy-occupied areas, carry out inspections before staying overnight,
2) all food and drinking water left behind by the enemy should be examined to ensure that it was uncontaminated, 3) anything contaminated
should be burned or buried.[61] Under the circumstances these were appropriate provisions. But often such measures must have been inoperable.[62]

On the other hand the Eighth Route Army military medical services
did find ways to counteract the scorched earth *san guang* campaigns.
One way was to ensure complete maneuverability of treatment centers—
hospitals in name but often decentralized networks of huts, whose equipment could be packed and moved at half an hour's notice. During 1940–42
the Bethune International Peace Hospital in Wutaishan (northeast Shanxi)
moved twenty times, ending up in a village in west Hebei. Despite numerous staff casualties it maintained 1,500 beds, two operating theaters, and
handled an average of 100 outpatients daily.[63] The southeast Shanxi International Peace Hospital had oxcarts and mule teams to ensure "instant
departure and rapid mobility."[64]

Another way was to train health workers to be willing to risk life and
limb and to coordinate their work from company to divisional levels.
Company health workers were responsible for battlefield triage during
and after armed combat, including burial of fallen comrades. Regimental health units were responsible for providing wounded soldiers with
medical treatment within six hours (an outcome of Bethune's work). Divisional health units were responsible for field hospital care and for covert
healthcare operations, including organization of local civilian assistance.

---

[61] Wan Xuefeng and Wang Jihong, "Rijun dui Balujun . . ."
[62] Saddam Hussein's bombing of the Kurdish city of Halabja in 1988 is a reminder of
how difficult it is to guard against mustard gas.
[63] Sheng Xiangong (1986), 128.
[64] Remark by Prof. William Band of Yanjing University after visiting the hospital in
1942, cited in China Defense League (1943).

An example of devotion to duty occurred when Zhang Hanbin (张喊斌), a veteran Red Army health worker, advanced under a hail of bullets to rescue an injured comrade during one of the Japanese military *saodang* (mopping up) battles. The injured soldier's life was saved. Zhang was killed, but his heroism set an example to others and was reported by his divisional health commander.[65]

Maxims widely practiced during the exceptionally hard years of 1941–42 were "valiantly struggle" (*jianku fendou* 艰苦奋斗) and "be (totally) self-reliant" (*zili gengsheng* 自力更生). In practice this meant that units should take care of their own needs by all means possible and not rely on help from other units. If a unit was short of medications and equipment, there were two solutions, both practiced: 1) infiltrate health workers through Japanese lines to towns to buy whatever was needed (e.g. anesthetics, iodine, sulphanilamide, potassium, stethoscopes and operating knives) and find patriotic citizens to pay for them; 2) purchase materials needed to set up pharmacy plants, collect herbs with the aid of local Chinese doctors or pharmacists and produce medications, as well as make gauze, absorbent cotton, plaster bandages and soap. All this had been done in pre-long march times, but without the crushing burden of life in north China under the pressure of Japanese military *sanguang* campaigns and Japanese and Nationalist military blockades. Difficult as these tasks were, they were done on behalf of sick and wounded patients (一切为了伤病员), who whether military or civilian were treated as soldiers of the revolution.[66]

Under Dr. Kotnis' leadership the Bethune International Hospital even took steps to address the emotional trauma of seriously wounded patients and engage in heart to heart talks to treat their anxieties and regrets as well as treating their bodies. This was seen as a way of manifesting revolutionary comradeship, deepening the relations between patients and healers and strengthening the will of patients to triumph over their physical and mental adversities. It was the duty of everyone on the clinical staff to engage in this critical work, which though political in its overall goal was recognized as being part of the process of individual healing. Patients who

---

[65] Information from He Biao (贺彪) (2007). He Biao (1909–1999) was chief health officer for the 120th division, reporting directly to the division commander He Long. His report gives considerable insight into the healthcare work in the 120th division during the extended period of the Japanese *saodang* campaigns. Of Zhang Hanbin he wrote, "Even today I can never forget his fearless and devoted spirit."

[66] He Biao (2007).

were able to return to front line service would then send reports back to the hospital, allowing staff to share in their battlefield successes.[67] A pervasive will to overcome militant fascism had a lot to do with this remarkable healing of wounded fighters.

This is the point at which to mention the special services provided at the army rear hospital near Yan'an (later named after Dr. Bethune (photo 7.3)) by the Korean physician, Dr. Bang Wooyong (방우용, Chinese name Fang Yuyong 方禹镛).[68] Dr. Bang was noted for the kindness with which he treated his patients. Born in 1893 and educated in Korea and at Tokyo University, Bang worked for several years in the Nationalist military medical system before shifting his services to Yan'an. He arrived there in 1939 at the age of 46. His kindly and tireless bedside service so impressed the staff of the Norman Bethune International Peace hospital that the young nurses referred to him as "mother doctor" (*mamadaifu* 妈妈大夫). Dr. Bang believed that the attitude of medical staff had much to do with a patient's capacity to heal, and letters from grateful patients agreed with him. In 1943 the hospital celebrated his fiftieth birthday, and Mao Zedong was requested to send an inscription. Mao chose a saying from the Analects of Confucius: "After the year turns cold, one knows the pine and cypress are the last to wither."[69] This compliment reflected Mao's recognition of the value of dedicated healthcare. When Dr. Bang saw the inscription his eyes teared up. He stayed at his post till the end of the war and then returned to North Korea.[70]

Many of the army's patients were civilians targeted by the Japanese *san guang* campaigns, which raged throughout 1941 and 1942. The Chinese military units depended on local people to provide intelligence and cover and therefore could not neglect them when they became war casualties. Jiang Qixian, director of health for the Jinchaji military district, told his colleagues that no matter how bad their circumstances the local people heroically struggled to resist the enemy. "Therefore we should exert every effort to preserve their health. *This is our exalted duty* (这也是我们应有的天职)." To give two examples of how this duty played out, Dr. Qi Kairen (祁开仁), a graduate of Zhongshan Medical University and director of a surgical hospital serving the Eighth Route Army's 120th division

---

[67] Zhang Yumin (张育民) (2004).
[68] I am indebted to Prof. Jonghyun Lee for the Korean spelling.
[69] For a literary treatment of this theme see Chiu-mi Lai (2004), 131–150.
[70] Feng and Li (1991), biography of Dr. Bang, 685–686; Huang Shuze (黄树则) (1986b), 73–75.

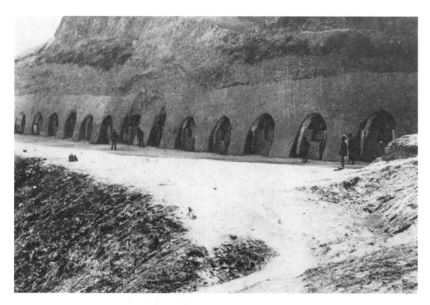

Photograph 7.3: *Upper Tier of Bethune International Peace Hospital near Yan'an*
Hospitals near Yan'an were built into caves as protection against Japanese bombers. After Dr. Bethune's death two were named in his honor. Despite the improvised accommodation and often improvised equipment, Yan'an's political leaders
demanded high standards of service. (*Source*: ABMAC Archive)

with no-cost service to civilians, took on a young female patient who for
some time showed no signs of recovery. Dr. Qi suspected an ovarian cyst,
operated, found and removed the cyst, the patient recovered and soon
gave birth to a child.[71]

Dr. Kotnis also performed heroic feats. He and his aide found a very
pregnant young woman in an abandoned hut in a village that a Japanese
military unit was approaching. He persuaded his assistant to go up the hill
and bring down a stretcher team while he prepared hot water in case her
time came. Fortunately the stretcher team arrived and they got her away
before the Japanese military unit moved in. Up in the hills Kotnis safely
delivered her baby girl. Kotnis once arrived at a village already destroyed
by the enemy, and there he treated nine badly wounded villagers between
dusk and midnight.[72]

---

[71] Feng and Li (1991), 86, 517.
[72] Sheng Xiangong (1986), 138–143, 148.

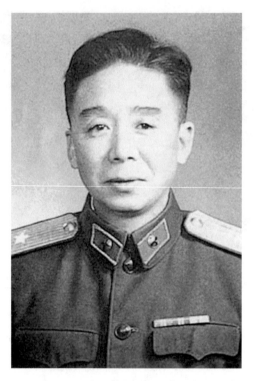

Photograph 7.4: *Dr. You Shenghua*
Trained in a short course at the Red Army Medical School near Ruijin, Dr.
You survived the Long March and became one of the Eighth Route Army field
surgeons most admired by Dr. Bethune (see chapter 3). (*Source*: China Medical
University, www.cmu.edu.cn/new/showpage.asp?pageid=345)

Such stories indicate the high level of service performed by healthcare workers, particularly during the years when the Japanese military
were most aggressive in ravaging north China's people and habitations.
The north China War of Resistance was carried out by military, partisans
and civilians, and the Eighth Route Army health services served them all.
When Kotnis (by then a Communist party member) died in the field in
December 1942 of starvation, exhaustion and epilepsy at the age of 32,
it illustrated the toll exerted by devoted front line service during the *san
guang* campaigns (see photo 7.2). At the same time it embodied revolutionary humanitarianism in action. Kotnis' life and death, like Bethune's,
proved inspirational. Zhu De said of him,

He knew the greatness of the masses and he ardently loved China's soldiers and people in the War of Resistance...he never feared danger...he did his work in the midst of battle.[73]

It was this fearlessness in the face of militant fascism and the commitment to serving wounded country people shared by Bethune and Kotnis that proved so impressive to Chinese colleagues. Both men died while serving as directors of a front line international peace hospital that Bethune founded. As director of the Health Bureau of the Jinchaji military district, Jiang Qixian urged medical workers to follow the examples of Bethune and Kotnis, "be committed to technical skill and become revolutionary medical professionals."[74] And this revolutionary resonance still matters. Looking back on the work of these two great men the historian Zhang Qi'an concluded that: "Their lofty medical ethics and practice and their spirit of self-sacrificing work will for ever inspire today's white-coated warriors."[75]

Civilian Healthcare: Confronting Superstition, Maternal-Child Mortality and Infectious Disease

The other great task of revolutionary healthcare in north and northwest China was to ameliorate disease and struggle against the influence of superstitious thinking on country people. From the perspective of China's Communist leaders—as also from the perspective of epidemiological transition—such thinking was most deeply rooted in treatment of infectious disease, childbirth and maternal and child health. Consequently these problems badly needed addressing by advocates of radical change.

Management of border area healthcare got under way late in 1937 with the establishment of a border area government and hospital and the creation of a Border Health Commission in January 1938. The hospital was originally located in Yan'an with the mission of serving party leaders and people and backing up the military healthcare system. During 1938 the management of the border government was removed from Zhang Guotao and placed under the leadership of Lin Boqu (林伯渠 also known as "old

---

[73] Zhu De (1986), 28.
[74] Feng and Li (1991), 84.
[75] Zhang Qi'an (2001). Prof. Zhang is on the faculty of Xi'an Jiaotong University. (Several websites carry this article).

Lin"), a Hunan native and one of the CCP's veteran administrators. The hospital went through several transitions of leadership and late in the fall of 1938 was relocated outside of Yan'an to be less vulnerable to Japanese bombing raids. Ouyang Jing (欧阳竞, 1914–1992), a trusted medical worker with one year of education at the Red Army healthcare school in Jiangxi and several years of front line medical work, became the hospital director. In spring 1939 a new location was excavated at Ansai (安塞, 40 km north of Yan'an) and the cave hospital began receiving patients in July.[76]

The hospital got off to a rocky start. When Dr. Bethune and Jean Ewen first arrived in Yan'an at the end of March 1938 they visited the border hospital and found no running water, sinks or flush toilets. Bethune was appalled by the primitive conditions, but Drs. Ma Haide and Jiang Qixian quietly explained the circumstances, with the result that Bethune agreed to carry out some operations.[77] Some of the hospital's difficulties were described in a report covering the period February to September 1938 by Dr. Jean Chiang (Jiang Zhaoju 姜兆菊) a Canadian-Chinese obstetrician from Montreal, who was then head of the CRCMRC's 29th mobile unit.[78] Dr. Chiang noted that the hospital had no outpatient clinic yet was handling around eighty visits a day. The patient wards were miserable and the bedding often lice-ridden. The hospital at the time had a very small supply of drugs, practically no surgical and only a very few obstetrical instruments.

Under Dr. Chiang improvements were made. The local administration helped build incinerators and latrines, and a League of Nations Epidemic Commission gave $500 to help set up a city outpatient department. The CRCMRC provided an X-ray machine and a nursing unit to assist Dr. Chiang. With the arrival of Dr. Wan Fuen (万福恩, F. E. Wan, Red Cross Medical Relief Corps 10th unit leader), the surgical service improved; old orthopedic deformities were corrected and the hospital was able to undertake major operations.[79] A tuberculosis sanitarium was also opened

---

[76] *Shaanxi Shaanganning bianqu yiyuan* (2010). This is the most comprehensive source found for an account of this hospital. Several sources state that the hospital moved to Ansai in autumn 1938, but the Shaanxi and Ansai documents are clear that the move to Ansai took place in the spring and summer of 1939.

[77] Jean Ewen (1981), 89–90.

[78] Information on Dr. Chiang comes from a note by Dr. Norman Bethune, transcribed in Larry Hannant (1998), 205. Dr. Chiang's father had been head of the Department of Chinese Studies at McGill University, Montreal. Her work for the New Fourth Army is reported in both Smedley (1943) and Ewen (1980).

[79] Dr. Jean Chiang, "Report of the 29th Unit at Yenan, February to September 1938" (received January 6, 1939), in ABMAC, box 5.

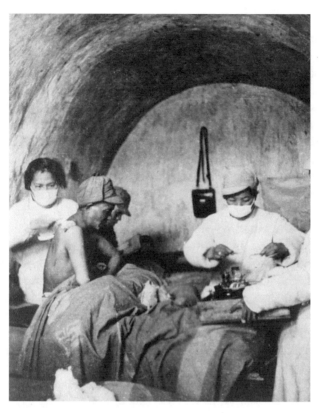

Photograph 7.5: *Two Women Medical Specialists at Work in Eighth Route Army Cave Hospital* (see photo 7.3)
As this photo comes from the ABMAC archive it probably documents the work of a Red Cross Medical Relief Corps team that visited Yan'an. One such team was led by the Chinese Canadian obstetrician Dr. Jean Chiang (Jiang Zhaoju). The photograph may well have accompanied her report to Dr. Lin Kesheng late in 1938. (*Source*: ABMAC Archive)

because, as Dr. Chiang reported, the disease was rife in the Northwest. The sanitarium was located 12 miles outside Yan'an.[80] By June 1939 it had departments of internal medicine, surgery, obstetrics and pediatrics.[81]

---

[80] Information from Chiang report, see note 79.

[81] Information on this hospital from "Ba Xiandai Yixue Daijin Shaanbei," (2006), first section inside article entitled Shandan Huakai (山丹花开, the theme of a Northern Shaanxi revolutionary song). Another source more broadly states that before or after 1940 the Border area hospital, the Yan'an central hospital, and the Bethune International Peace hospital successively added departments of pediatrics. He Zhaoxiong (1988), 263.

Earlier in 1939 the Health Commission held a conference, which identi-fied priorities for the work of local health agencies. They included raising people's health knowledge, emphasizing public health and maternal child health, setting up pharmacies, training health cadres, attacking superstitions and campaigning against witch doctors and sorcerers. The health services were constantly short of funds and materials, especially western medical drugs, thus they had to depend all the more on training cadres and emphasizing preventive health strategies.[82] At a parallel conference in Yan'an Mao urged participants not to let material and financial difficulties get in the way of applying the essence of public health work in the course of popular revolution (*fayang minzu geming zhong weisheng gongzuo de jingshen*).[83]

This was the broad agenda that Shaanganning border officials were expected to address. In twenty-three counties they developed two cooperative systems: a health preservation pharmaceutical cooperative which combined drug sellers and manufacturers under local government leadership and mandates, and a clinical services cooperative which combined Chinese and Western clinics and human and veterinarian, also under local government leadership, to provide clinical services to country people. These cooperatives registered commercial operations, coordinated local health services and mobilized health workers and campaigns.[84] Among their noted workers was a Chinese medical practitioner who was a leader of the health cooperative, by name Li Changchun (李常春). He was willing to see patients at all hours and in all conditions at very low cost; in the first four months of 1944 he saw over 1,600 patients and became known as a model practitioner. Another model physician, Dr. Xu Genzhu (徐根竹), was famous for studying and successfully treating an outbreak of enteritis with yellow water discharge in northern Shaanxi province in or around 1941. He was killed in 1947 during the civil war. Another health-care worker, Dr. Bai Lang (白浪), donated blood ten times for patients in need. In December 1944 she received a certificate of merit from Mao Zedong naming her a model worker.[85]

---

[82] Zhang Qi'an (2001), 58.

[83] Zhang Qi'an, op. cit.

[84] See Zhang Wenjun (张文军) (2008). This system of cooperatives is now being reviewed as a forerunner for rural collective health services in China today.

[85] Zhang Qi'an (2001). Mao's certificate for Bai Lang is also mentioned in www.yapop .gov.cn.

Rural Health: Addressing the Drastic Problems of
Maternal and Child Health in Northwest China

As the introduction to this chapter indicated, maternal child health in Shaanxi and Gansu provinces was a catastrophe calling for political leaders with skills of modern medical science and sensitivity to the needs of the poor as well as to traditional Chinese values and practices around childbirth. An investigation around Yan'an in 1937 found that in one village 67 deliveries had occurred in 1935, of which only 22 children were still living two years later, two of them with deformities.[86] A recently published essay on maternal and child health notes that border government data for Ansai county reported that 50 children were born in April and May 1939, of whom only 10 were still living by July 1940. Undated data for Baoan district reported that 188 women had given birth to 1,028 children, of whom 645 had died. Most children died from tetanus, diphtheria, influenza, or pneumonia and dysentery. Most of the mothers succumbed to miscarriage or post partum hemorrhage.[87]

A variety of factors could be held responsible for these conditions, among them the "three great calamities" (三大害) of illiteracy, superstition and unhygienic practices. Xu Teli told Edgar Snow, "This is culturally one of the darkest places on earth. People . . . believe that water is harmful to them . . . they hate to wash their feet, hands or faces, or cut their nails or their hair."[88] Smedley reported that the people were "always on the verge of starvation." She saw foot-bound women, disheveled and dirty, with dirty babies.[89] When women had their periods they bled into their pants or stuffed in a rag or piece of sheepskin. At time of childbirth they depended on charms and witch doctors.[90]

Traditional birthing procedures were dangerous. Traditional midwives could not be counted on to wash their hands before delivering a child. They used such unsanitary materials as a broken tile or millet stalk to cut the umbilical cord. In one particularly gruesome case, reported by Liberation Daily, delivery started with the presentation of an arm. The midwife tugged at the arm and it came off. According to incomplete statistics in an

---

[86] "Ba Xiandai Yixue Daijin Shaanbei," (2006), also available at cpc.people.com.cn/GB/64093/67507/4934112.html.

[87] Information on this topic, unless otherwise noted, is drawn from Liu Juanzhi (刘娟芝) (2010).

[88] Snow, (1961), 234. Liu Juanzhi drew on this passage.

[89] Smedley (1938), 9, 216.

[90] Liu Juanzhi, (2010).

East Gansu (*Longdong*) branch district, out of 104 births fifty-five infants died.[91] Another district in East Gansu reported a comparable rate of infant deaths.

Early marriage was another liability. In an area of Yan'an, sixty-three out of seventy-six women had not yet reached the age of eighteen sui (eighteenth year, i.e. seventeen) at the time of marriage. Twenty-three of them had not yet menstruated, and the rest were all young children (*wawa*). In three villages belonging to Zizhou district (130 km northeast of Yan'an) almost fifty percent of women were only 12–15 sui at the time of marriage, and over eighty percent were only 12–17 sui.[92] Health complications for teenage girls resulting from premature marriage are many and dangerous. Often the teenage girl was married to an older, sexually active male whose family wanted a child right away, thus there was little or no chance for the girl to negotiate consensual sexual intercourse. The pelvis of a teenage girl was often too small to deliver an infant. The consequences of delivery under these circumstances, especially for girls under the age of fifteen, were likely to be obstructed labor, followed (in the absence of c-section) by death for the neonate or the mother, and very often at least obstetric fistulas for the mother. The latter would cause prolonged leakage of urine, feces, and blood. Other medical consequences for girls driven into premature marriage include increased risk for sexually transmitted disease and cervical cancer, along with delivery of infants with low birth weight, inadequate nutrition and anemia. Social consequences could include domestic violence, social stigmatization, deprival of education, and isolation.[93] Given such appalling circumstances, the least a writer on this subject can do is, in Liu Juanzhi's words, "cast a brick to attract jade." All we can do here is to note the seriousness of the problem, describe responses and acknowledge their limitations.

Mao Zedong took a step in the right direction by calling for protection of women workers, lying-in women and children.[94] Early help came with

---

[91] Liu Juanzhi (2010).

[92] Liu Juanzhi, ibid.

[93] Information from 1) Ana Lita (2008), and 2) International Women's Health Program (2009). According to the latter source, countries where the majority of girls are still married before the age of 18 include Niger (76%), Democratic Republic of Congo (74%), Nepal (60%), Afghanistan (54%), and India (50%).

[94] Liu Juanzhi (2010). Given Mao's view, expressed in his study of the peasant movement in Hunan, that male domination was one of the four thick feudal ropes binding the Chinese people, the development of protections for women and children was a logical outcome of this perspective.

the arrival of the Red Cross Medical Relief Corps 29th unit in Yan'an in or around March 1938. During eight month's work it supervised one hundred deliveries, during which only one mother and three infants died.[95] In April 1939 a party resolution covering the whole Shaanganning border region set the minimum age for marriage at twenty sui for men and eighteen sui for women. A Shaanganning government resolution of November 1939 urged education of lying-in women on protection of infants, decreasing the risk of death due to lack of hygiene, and protection against infectious diseases. Another resolution sought education on how to maintain health during menstruation and requested doctors in health centers to help women manage their health. A resolution of September 1940 called on obstetricians, pediatricians, nurses, and women party members to follow through on the work of protecting mothers and children.

All this was part of a broader drive by the Shaanganning border area government to elevate the social position of women and achieve greater gender equality, through marriage regulations, banning of foot binding and protection of rights of female infants. Acknowledging that up to 1940 the border area infant mortality rate was still at around sixty percent, the Shaanganning government instituted classes in modern midwifery training and health for infants and passed a regulation permitting pregnant women one month's time off before delivery and two weeks afterwards.[96] In January 1942 the Shaanganning government resolved that all administrative agencies down to the rural (*xiang*) level should appoint a child care worker to oversee the health and registration of pregnant and lying-in women and children.[97] Such policy-making was ahead of many worldwide attitudes and policies even today towards protection of women's health.

To promote these ideas Communist Party leaders decided to work through educational propaganda that would enable the masses themselves to struggle against old thinking. As of 1940 mobile exhibitions taught that during delivery the fetus should enter the birth canal head first, not in any other position. Children are not a gift from *"Lao Tian Ye"* (老天爷 the Daoist Jade Emperor) but are born like so (illustrated)! For the 1945 Women's Day Festival the Women's Commission organized a woman's health exhibit, dealing with knowledge about pregnancy, delivery and birthing.

---

[95] Information on Red Cross unit from report by Dr. Jean Chiang in ABMAC, box 5 (see note 79).

[96] Li Jinlong (李金龙) and Zhang Juan (张娟) (2008).

[97] Wang Yuanzhou (王元周) (2009), part two, on beginning of border area large-scale mass health work; Li Jinyong and Zhang Juan (2008).

It featured physicians such as the Chinese medicine physician Dr. Bi Guangdou (毕光斗) and the model woman physician Dr. Ruan Xuehua (阮雪华), who specialized in treating women and children.[98]

Another strategy was to utilize temple fairs, of which there were many in the Shaanganning border region, as a venue for advocacy. On or around the fifteenth day of the New Year festival was the time to make noise with 'red fire.' This was a time when women would leave their habitations to go out into the community and enjoy the fireworks. Many temples held fairs on the eighth day of the third and fourth lunar months. These events would attract women from far away. Medical teams used these occasions to talk about new methods of delivery and maternal child health. Qingyang County (also known as Longdong 陇东, i.e. east Gansu) was especially favored because of its tradition of dance theater (*yangge* 秧歌). The border area government organized small teams of women cadres to mix among the women audiences to talk about hygiene and child rearing. In another district teams performed skits about child rearing and handed out 'umbilical cord packs' containing antiseptic cloths and gauze. They advocated for better food hygiene and against reliance on witch doctors. Winter provided a further opportunity to reach some women, as did publication of articles in journals such as *Jiefang Ribao* (解放日报, *Liberation Daily*).

Upgrading the training of midwives was more difficult. An article in *Jiefang Ribao*, dated May 5, 1944, included remarks on the subject by Dr. Fu Lianzhang. Fu argued that to remold old style midwives and mobilize women's health cadres to become involved in mass health work, they should recruit women from amongst the masses and provide them with basic knowledge about practicing midwifery. A conference convened by the Central Department of Health proposed to mobilize women cadres to engage in mass public health work and teach women the essentials of public health knowledge.[99] In October 1944 a formal class in midwifery

---

[98] Liu Juanzhi (2010). Dr. Bi Guangdou (1879–1970), a native of Yan'an, received the first degree under the old imperial examination system, but at the age of 30 turned to the study of Chinese medicine. An ethicist, he treated rich and poor without regard to ability to pay. His patients included Zhang Hao, Lin Biao, and Xu Fanting. He also received Mao Zedong many times. In 1940 he advocated the establishment at Yan'an of a Chinese medicine research organization. Later he worked at the Yan'an Health station. He was committed to the transmission of medical skills and training of human talent. Unfortunately he was struggled against during the Cultural Revolution and his case-work and essays were burned. From www.hudong.com/wiki/毕光斗.

[99] Wang Yuanzhou (2009), section 3.

opened up with eighty students. The class graduated in July 1945, and thirty-five students were sent out to various localities. In November 1944 The Shaanganning border government held a conference that reviewed training of midwives. For the next two years midwifery classes were held in sixty-four rural localities remolding the work of 826 old-style midwives. As a result, new methods of delivery were made available in seventy-three percent of the rural areas.[100] Also in November a border area conference decided that preventive health should take precedence over curative. In 1945 the Jinchaji military district sent a representative to help with border area women's federation training of midwives.[101] Guanzhong and Long-dong regions and Ganqing and Xinning counties opened up local midwifery training programs, each with around thirty students and continuing for three months. In November 1945 a women's professional school opened with fifty students (later sixty) providing special training of maternal child health cadres. Meanwhile the Central Hospital's department of Obstetrics set up a newborn clinic in 1940.[102] In the first eleven months of 1943 the department delivered 470 infants weighing eight pounds or more. Only three percent of deliveries weighed five pounds or less. The normal infant weight was 6.76 pounds in the first half of the year and 6.9 pounds in the latter half. The infant death rate was only 2.4 percent.[103]

Clearly the authorities found it useful to bring information about maternal child health directly to rural women and not simply channel it through 'old-style' midwives who did not belong to a registered medical profession. According to Dr. Liu Ruiheng, (Director of the Nationalist Government's National Health Administration in Nanjing during the 1930s), a new provincial midwifery school had been set up in the Gansu provincial capital, Lanzhou, which admitted its first regular class in 1935. About forty 'old-style' midwives had undergone "new" training. Xi'an had also established a provincial midwifery school in 1935 as a result of reorganization of a private school. It had an attached maternity home with forty beds. In addition three rural maternal child health centers had been started.[104] These efforts, while laudable, were drops in the sea in which old-style midwifery prevailed.[105] The reluctance of the all-male traditional

---

[100] Information in last three sentences from Wang Yuanzhou, op. cit.
[101] Wang Yuanzhou, op. cit.
[102] Information for newborn clinic from He Zhaoxiong (1988), 263.
[103] Liu Juanzhi (2010).
[104] Wong and Wu (1936), 754–755.
[105] Estimates of the numbers of old-style midwives in China, along with hand-wringing comments by missionary and western trained Chinese physicians, can be found in Lamson

medical profession to interfere with childbirth practices reflected gender barriers and also the epistemological barriers between a world of practice designed to maintain harmony and balance and another fraught with inexplicable dangers and emotional tension, in which appeals to gods was not infrequent.

Despite these drawbacks the Communist reformers in northwest China took on a centuries old social challenge by instituting legal and public health policies to upgrade the status of women. Introduction of maternal child healthcare and retraining of old-style midwives were key steps to save lives by bringing preventive health knowledge to bear on childbirth and early childhood care. Documentation indicates that this policy was actively pursued in Shaanganning from 1940 on. Certainly the results "significantly" reduced death rates; but broad conclusions on how far this social revolution went depend on greater access to numerical data than is currently available.[106] It should also be noted that a flurry of activity to improve maternal child health training took place in Shaanganning between the decline of Japanese military activity in north China in late 1944 and the resumption of the civil war in 1946.

Fighting Epidemic Disease

Epidemic disease was another major problem confronting the Communist reformers in north China. Cholera, typhoid, malaria, typhus, tuberculosis, relapsing fever, and measles were all active, especially in areas dislocated by Japanese occupation and military repression. Detailed figures for epidemics in wartime China are still being uncovered, but there are tabulations for specific regions, districts, towns and villages, which give an idea of the incidence of diseases and their affect on families and communities.

For example, during 1938 Dr. Erich Landauer of the League of Nations Epidemic Commission unit in north China reported a cholera epidemic along the Pinghan railway line and around Zhengzhou.[107] In July 1939,

---

(1935). See index, 'midwifery', in Lamson's book for information, much of it drawn from articles in the *National Medical Journal of China*.

[106] Since individual workers were tasked to collect numerical data, it should be available in border government, county or party history records.

[107] Memorandum of November 1938 in China Defense League folder, ABMAC, box 5. Dr. Landauer reported that his appeals for help to local missionary agencies in establishing vaccine stations were unsuccessful. See next section on bacterial warfare for a pos-

the China Defense League sent 5,000 ampules of neosalvarsan to Xi'an to counter an outbreak of relapsing fever in northwest China, and sent another 5,000 by land.[108] In 1939 typhoid fever was reported in Linxian and Pingshun districts in northern Henan and southeast Shanxi. In 1940 it spread north to Licheng and Zuoquan districts, and in 1943 it was present throughout the southeast Shanxi border area. Newsletters of the China Defense League reported epidemics of typhus and relapsing fever raging in south Shanxi and in the Shuangshipu (Fengxian) region of southwest Shanxi in early 1941.[109] During a two-month period in 1943 relapsing fever and malaria struck 302 people out of 2,156 in an area of Lingshou County (west Hebei). During the same year in Lingqiu County in northeast Shanxi, sixty-seven percent of the population of one area had malaria, 7.5 percent had relapsing fever and six percent had influenza.[110]

Inevitably children were more vulnerable than adults. During the first five months of 1944 over two thousand people, representing a little over three percent of the population of Yan'an, are reported to have died of infectious diseases; but because of poor public understanding of childbirth and child rearing, the infant death rate reached sixty percent. Quite apart from ignorance of hygiene, lack of basic needs, including quilts, rendered

---

sible connection between this epidemic and Japanese military bacteria warfare carried out along railways at that time. Zhengzhou is the site of a major railway junction in north central Henan.

[108] China Defense League (1940), 8. Neosalvarsan was the trade name for neoarsphenamine, originally developed by Paul Ehrlich and colleagues for treatment of syphilis but indicated in the 1940 Merck manual as treatment for relapsing fever.

[109] CDL Newsletter #35, August-September 1941, in ABMAC, box 5. The epidemic in south Shanxi was originally reported by Kathleen Hall in CDL Newsletter #27 [dated March 15, not seen]. Hall wrote, "I don't think I had ever before seen such misery. In my village half of the people had died... Many orphans had been left behind." The epidemic around Shuangshipu was reported by George Hogg, an employee of the Chinese Industrial Cooperatives (INDUSCO) in CDL Newsletter #30 [dated May 1, not seen]. He wrote, "Where there was a chance to make anything like a detailed survey, it was found that more than half of the total population had recently been seriously ill" (with either typhoid, typhus, relapsing fever or influenza). He also wrote that: "from one third to one half of the total population had died of sickness within the past four months." The scope of these epidemics is not clear from the data seen. Both should be examined for possible connection to the activities of the Japanese military's Taiyuan bacterial warfare laboratory (see below). Unfortunately efforts by CDL to send large supplies of fish liver oil, vitamins and sulfanilamide contributed by the American Red Cross, ABMAC and other agencies for relief in the northwest were delayed and blocked by Nationalist government authorities outside Guiyang and in Chongqing, on the grounds that the supplies might be used to support Eighth Route Army activities. (Note: sulpha drugs were the main antibacterial treatment available before the discovery of penicillin and were widely used during World War II.)

[110] This is a sampling of data provided by Wang Yuanzhou (2009). Data in this section on epidemic disease is from this source unless otherwise indicated.

children especially vulnerable, as did the necessity of flight from villages attacked and destroyed by the Japanese military mopping-up (*saodang* 扫荡) campaigns.

Sexually transmitted diseases were also war-related infections. In the twentieth century civilians were fair game to be bombed, gassed, bayoneted and raped. Rape is also a strategy for terrorizing an occupied population. Data found by Prof. Wang Yuanzhou in the Henan provincial archives indicate that during the eight year War of Resistance Japanese soldiers campaigning in the Jinjiluyu border region raped 360,000 Chinese women, of whom 122,000 were infected with sexually transmitted disease. Obviously these figures are estimates, but they are not out of line with other estimates of disease and death in China during the War of Resistance.[111] Here we are concerned with the factor of sexually transmitted disease among a population already exposed to drought, famine, malaria, cholera, typhoid, and serious malnutrition, and for several years into the war lacking basic health knowledge or access to emergency health services. Thus it is difficult to avoid the conclusion that sexual disease transmitted by rape (and the killing of uncounted numbers of women after they had been raped) played a major role in contributing to the overall death and sickness that confronted Communist leaders in northwest and north China during 1937–1945.[112]

During 1936 while their survival was still on the line in northwest China, the Chinese Communist Party leaders were in little position to do anything about either rape or epidemic diseases. However, in December 1939 the Shaanganning border government began to educate the civilian public on hygiene and sanitation. As a result of an epidemic in May 1940 the Yan'an government set up a preventive health commission and a month later the Shaanganning government organized a Department of Health.[113] Each county (*xian*) was to have a health section, each sub-district

---

[111] Wang Yuanzhou calculates that during the eight-year war with Japan the Jinjiluyu base area alone lost 860,000 deaths to infectious disease out of a total population of 2.8 million.

[112] "Kangri zhanzheng shengli 50 zhounianji…" (2009) notes that the Japanese military compelled over 200,000 Chinese women to serve as 'comfort women.' Particularly during the *san guang* campaigns the number of women killed by rape was "exceedingly high" (*feichang da* 非常大). The writer cites the historian Wu Tianwei (吴天威) to the effect that there were five million or more Japanese soldiers at war in China, and that they raped at least one million Chinese women. See http://blog.sina.com.cn/s/blog_4dae258b0100eus9.html.

[113] This initiative began at much the same time as the National Health Administration's local health service system.

(*qu*) a health worker and each rural community (*xiang*) a health committee. To promote health propaganda work, the border government organized a Health Education Commission. It improved its health education newspaper, and printed various booklets on essentials of preventive health. In April 1942 it set up a Preventive Health Commission, and in May it organized a preventive health reporting system. Under this system bubonic plague, cholera and smallpox, once diagnosed, were to be reported by telephone within twenty-four hours. Less contagious and deadly diseases, such as typhoid, paratyphoid, dysentery, typhus, relapsing fever, and scarlet fever, were to be reported on a weekly basis. The Commission could adopt appropriate measures in cooperation with the county in question.[114] The region also provided some limited health care services, but the main responsibility for that work devolved on, and was accepted by, the military health services.

In due course public opinion built momentum for preventive health work. An editorial in the *New China Newspaper* published on April 7, 1939, drew a direct connection between the people's health and the capacity to wage war. Another article written a year later pointed out that a healthy people and a strong country go together. But it was Dr. Fu Lianzhang (傅连暲) who laid out the order of priorities. "In mass health work," he wrote, "the first priority is maternal child health. Next comes preventive health work, and after that treatment of ill health." "We lack grandchildren," he pointed out in another article. A new democratic society, he said, should build a system that protected people's health. Today's health was the basis for the future. Others pointed out that the spread of epidemic disease, as happened in the Jinchaji border area in spring 1944, directly lessened labor and productive power. As a result, the border area government had to turn its attention from production to health work.[115]

The conversion of an obvious need into a health campaign took time. One mechanism for action arose out of a "Double Support" (*shuang yong* 双拥) set of movements that took shape during the first two months of the 1943 agricultural calendar. The double support consisted of a movement of civilians to "support the army and favor its dependents" and another movement for the army to "support the government and cherish the people." The latter movement included ten principles; of which the

---

[114] Information on the Regional Commission from "Shandan huakai [xia]" (山丹花开 [下]) (2006).
[115] Original texts in Wang Yuanzhou (2009), section 2.

eighth was "help the people advance the movement for sanitation and hygiene (*qingjie weisheng* 清洁卫生)."On February 1, *Liberation Daily* carried an article by the military leader He Long (贺龙) supporting the movement assigned to the army. The initiative was put to work in the Shaanganning border area. Late in February 1943, 5,000 people attended a conference in Nanniwan (around 50 km southeast of Yan'an) on how to make it happen.[116]

By October 1943 Mao Zedong indicated that as of the Spring Festival in 1944 the movement should extend in very specific ways throughout the base areas.[117] Here are some examples of how that happened. In the summer of 1944 the public health plan of Heshui County in East Gansu called for every household to clean up its main entrance, make toilets and rubbish pits in suitable places, clean out wells, and clean up rubbish around the town gates. In Yan'an's Qingliang mountain locality, the ravines once full of sick people became a model public health area, thanks to the initiative of Dr. Ruan Xuehua (阮雪华) and the local area director. In a conference in November 1944 the Shaanganning border area was ready to adopt the policy of 'preventive health first, curative second' and thus emphasize public health education and the sanitation and hygiene movement.[118]

The Jinchaji border area was already emphasizing health advocacy from 1943 to 1944. Methods included campaigns against smallpox, pneumonia and measles, and publication of handbooks, wall newspapers and posters to get ideas across to the public. The Jinjiluyu border area (south Shanxi and Hebei and parts of Shandong and Henan) pushed for coordination of disease prevention strategies through such campaigns as the "four cleans" (house and yard; hands, face and clothes; wok, table and bowl; and refuse pits and streets). Beginning in January 1943 the Shandong military district set out to help villages set up medical and herbal cooperative societies and train militiamen as health workers. It declared April 12–May 12 to be the "Health Movement Month" for the entire army. Beginning March 1945 the Shandong army's Medical Affairs Journal put together a column on propagating health knowledge and teaching the masses to pay attention to hygiene, for publication in *The People's Daily* (*Dazhong Ribao*).[119]

---

[116] Shuangyong Yundong (2004).

[117] Ibid.

[118] Information on Heshui, Qinliang, and November conference from Wang Yuanzhou (2009), section 3.

[119] Shandongsheng weisheng dashiji (2007).

Recognizing the extent to which infectious diseases flourished in areas dominated by witch doctors, illiteracy, and superstition (the "three great scourges" of the border areas), north China border administrations launched drives against witch doctors, in which certain physicians who specialized in rural and military health care played an active part.[120] In Shaanganning border area administrative officials initiated a drive in 1939; in 1944 another drive was named for the Chinese physician Dr. Cui Yuerui (崔岳瑞), who had vigorously opposed witch doctors and superstition from an early age. Winter classes were designed to arouse the masses to the dangers of relying on witch doctors to control infectious disease. But following an epidemic of measles in early 1945 in the Jinchaji border area, an investigator found during a twenty day survey of eleven villages that superstitions were still embedded in the minds of the villagers that actually facilitated the spread of disease. In any case, there were not nearly enough "modern" (现代) or Chinese medicine doctors around for the villagers to consult.[121]

Efforts to unite Chinese medicine and modern style physicians in promoting public health and restoring China's strength proved more successful. In part this was due to pressure from Mao Zedong at a Shaanganning border area conference of educational and cultural workers in October 1944. Mao reminded his listeners once again that two-thirds of the people of Shanganning were still illiterate and harboring enemies inside their minds. It was often more difficult to combat mental enemies, he noted, than to fight Japanese imperialism. "We must call on the masses to struggle against their own illiteracy, superstitions and unhygienic habits. For this struggle a broad united front is indispensable."[122] Mao urged "new doctors" to collaborate with Chinese medicine doctors, warning that if they didn't it was tantamount to condoning witch doctors and high mortality rates among the masses.

First steps in this direction began in 1941, but it took the onslaught of the Japanese military campaigns of 1941–43 to demonstrate the urgency

---

[120] They included Drs Ruan Xuehua (阮雪华), Bai Lang (白浪), and Wang Ququin (王区寝). For 'three great scourges' (三大害) see Huigu: wunian he bashinian er (回顾五年和八十年 二 Review: five years and eighty years), http://www.china.com.cn/xxsb/txt/2007-08/content_8760511.htm.

[121] Wang Yuanzhou (2009), section 5.

[122] Mao Zedong (1944) contrasts "new medicine, new physicians" (新医) with "old medicine, old physicians" (旧医), referring specifically to the 1,000 or more Chinese medicine practitioners in the Shaanganning Border Area.

of unity, as well as forceful statements by Mao and Li Fuchun in October and November 1944, to get the biomedical physicians on board. Drs.
Ren Zuotian (任作田), a specialist in acupuncture and moxibustion, and
Lu Zhijun (鲁之俊), director of the Yan'an Bethune International Peace
Hospital and a surgeon who studied acupuncture with Dr. Ren, actively
responded to Mao's call and helped create in Yan'an in March 1945 a
Chinese Western Medical Research Agency combining two previously
separate agencies. Subsequently Chinese-Western medical teams went
into the countryside, and more Chinese Western medical teams started
to collaborate.[123]

One thing lacking in north China was adequate access to vaccines. Dr.
Ma Haide reported that between 1937–1939 79,490 smallpox and 13,360
typhoid vaccinations were administered in the Yan'an region.[124] During
1939, the CRCMRC personnel reportedly administered cholera inoculations to 492,898 individuals.[125] But in 1940 the Nationalist army blockade
began, and after the Wannan incident in January 1941 Red Cross units
were unable to provide further service in areas where Communist military
forces were active. Meanwhile Japanese military forces had blockades in
the east and southeast.

Local manufacture of smallpox vaccine began in 1941, along with production of a variety of medications, including novocain, glucose, ephed-
rine and quinine.[126] But for the most part control of infectious diseases in
north and northwest China depended on public health propaganda. That
meant that progress in reducing sickness and death would be slow.

Impact of Bacterial Warfare on Public Health in North China

Efforts to combat epidemic disease in north China were impeded not only
by ignorance and superstition, but also by bacterial warfare carried out by
the Japanese military under conditions of great secrecy. Typhoid, cholera,
and plague were among the organisms employed by the Japanese military.
Because of the secrecy of the campaigns and their activation during warm
summer months when epidemics could be anticipated, country people

---

[123] Zhu Hongzhao (2010), Wang Yuanzhou (2009), section 5. The idea was in part to
"scientize" Chinese medical practice and "sinify" Western medical practice.

[124] Ma Haide 1940 report.

[125] China Defense League (1940), 69.

[126] China Defense League (1943), 31–32.

assumed that they were forms of warm weather pestilence set off by the deity Lao Tian Ye (老天爷). Thus the Japanese military were able to carry out bacterial warfare in north China and elsewhere, with few people realizing their provenance.[127]

The bacterial warfare program was set up under Dr. Ishii Shiro (四郎石井) at Unit 731 in northeast China (Manchukuo). After the outbreak of war in July 1937 a number of bacterial warfare units were established in north China. In Beijing the Japanese military took over the Chinese government's preventive medicine offices and laboratories in Tiantan Park, and later the PUMC Hospital, to set up Unit 1855.[128] This unit became the primary bacterial warfare facility in north China. It was officially known as the "Tiantan Central Epidemic Prevention Bureau,"[129] (the name of the buildings under China's National Health Administration). A Chinese author has called it the "North China Death Factory." Its job was to research and manufacture bacterial weapons and supervise bacterial warfare in north China.[130]

Unit 1855 had two branch centers, one in Taiyuan, capital of Shanxi province, the other in Jinan, capital of Shandong. The Taiyuan unit was founded in May 1938. It had departments for bacterial warfare education, inspection and manufacture of cultures, dissection, special testing, and disinfection. From August 1942 to early 1944 Ishii took on responsibility for its operation. In view of Ishii's strong belief in the cost effectiveness of bacterial weapons,[131] it is inconceivable that he did not intend to put the

---

[127] This account of bacterial warfare in China mainly relies on Xie Zhonghou (谢忠厚) (2008). Mr. Xie works at the Institute of History at the Henan Provincial Academy of Social Sciences. See also Daniel Barenblatt (2004). Several other English language studies are listed in the Wikipedia article on Japanese military bacterial warfare.

[128] The properties of the PUMC were seized by the Japanese army in February 1942, since when the hospital was used officially as a Japanese military hospital. See Notes on CMB Inc. for a Brief Outline of Western Assistance to China during 1943–1944 in the Field of Medicine and Health. China Medical Board Archive, box 22, folder 157.

[129] Yuki Tanaka (1998), 143. According to Tanaka, a document put out by Unit 1855 and captured in the southwest Pacific provided information on how to develop cholera, typhoid, dysentery and other pathogens used for bacterial warfare.

[130] Xie Zhonghou (谢忠厚) (2002) describes the work of the unit 1855 departments in some detail.

[131] Examples of Ishii's thinking are in the articles by Xie Zhonghou and are also in other publications on this subject. While there is no clear trail of Ishii's activity while directing the Taiyuan unit, a hint can be found in a memoir by the Japanese Army medical doctor Yuasa Ken (湯浅 謙). Yuasa arrived in a city hospital in southern Shanxi in January 1942. He soon discovered that his work required him to carry out practice operations on Chinese prisoners. Some of these operations were done under anesthetic; others, such as removal of bullets, were not. Yuasa reported that: "Dr. Ishii Shiro came to our hospital many times

work of the Taiyuan unit into active support of Japanese military campaigns in north China, of which there were many.[132] This implies that incidences of epidemic disease anywhere in Shanxi and more broadly the Jinchaji and Jinjiluyu military regions during the period of the Taiyuan unit's operation must be examined for the possibility that they were activated by bacterial warfare. That would include the epidemic diseases occurring in the Jinchaji base area in spring 1944, as noted in the previous section.[133]

There were also mobile bacterial warfare units attached to Japanese divisions and regiments. An example is given by Xie Zhonghou (谢忠厚) of a unit attached to the 59th division in Shandong, set up in April 1942. It had four people in leadership positions and 25 to 30 subordinates. A surviving Chinese prisoner of war reported in 1954 that its activities were confined to preparation for bacterial warfare.[134]

The largest bacterial warfare campaign in north China took place between late August and October 1943. After an unexpectedly heavy rainfall, the attack was launched in west Shandong along the banks of the Wei River. The Wei runs along the border with Hebei province and leads into the Grand Canal, which takes water traffic up to Tianjin and Beijing. Soldiers from the Japanese 12th army deposited cholera organisms in the water supplies of various towns and villages. They reportedly left infected food bundles in places where hungry local people could collect and eat the contents. After the disease had taken hold, Japanese troops broke the Wei and Zhang river embankments, forcing local inhabitants to flee, carrying the disease with them. The epidemic spread into twenty-four districts in southern Hebei and further into Shandong and northern Henan; it reached as far as Beijing and Tianjin. Barenblatt, writing in 2004, estimated the number of deaths to be 200,000. The Shandong historians Cui Weizhi and Tang Xiu'e, based on over ten years of documentary research

---

for education." In the next sentence Yuasa declares: "If the only way to win a war against America is bacterial warfare, I am ready, I will do anything. This is war." Evidently Ishii came not only to observe lethal operations but also to propagandize. See Haruko Taya Cook and Theodore F. Cook, (1992), 145–151.

[132] The Taiyuan unit did at one point send a team to study frostbite and cholera in the Yuncheng region of southwest Shanxi, and in May 1945 it sent a team to northwest Henan to assist a military unit with water supplies. Information from Xie Zhonghou (2002).

[133] The writer shifted a discussion of two outbreaks of cholera from the section in this chapter dealing with epidemic disease after realizing that they occurred during the time, and near the epicenter, of the Japanese military cholera campaign in west Shandong and south Hebei from August to October 1943.

[134] Xie Zhonghou (2008).

and extensive interviewing of survivors, put the number of deaths at 427,500. They point out that the cholera organisms took root in the region and continued to exact a toll in later years.[135]

Several episodes in north China indicate that Eighth Route Army leaders knew they were dealing with bacterial warfare. On March 29, 1938, Zhu De and Peng Dehuai sent out a telegram stating that the Japanese military were planning to release bacteria with the aim of killing people in northern Shaanxi and regions in Shanxi, Hebei and Shandong. The generals called on the entire country and people across the world to protest so as to prevent the campaign from happening. In September 1938, the *Xinmin News* reported that the Japanese military retaliated to surprise attacks by spreading typhoid and cholera cultures along major roads and railroads in north China and infecting wells; as a result some 40–50,000 people are believed to have died.[136] On October 11, 1938, Zhu De and Peng Dehuai sent a telegram to Wuhan stating that the Japanese military were indiscriminately releasing cholera and malaria organisms in certain districts in northern Henan. In March 1942 the Nationalist government's preventive medicine office issued a report stating that bubonic plague had appeared in Suiyuan, Ningxia, Shaanxi and Shanxi with fatalities already rising into the hundreds. Other such episodes are now known to have happened that could not at the time be attributed to bacterial warfare.[137]

We are again left with the realization that saving lives is far more arduous than killing them. Lives of injured or sick people are saved one by one, whereas they can be destroyed en masse. The Japanese military use of bacterial warfare in China was successful in reducing the numbers of Chinese people with whom the Japanese military were in conflict. Its negative effect on the Chinese wartime economy has not yet been authoritatively assessed, partly because much of what we need to know about this warfare is still being uncovered. Whereas knowledge of the Holocaust and the atomic bombs has been with us since 1945, information about Japanese

---

[135] Daniel Barenblatt (2004), 170–172. Cui Weizhi (崔维志) and Tang Xiu'e (唐秀娥), a married team, have published three books on Shandong history in the 1940s, including *Luxi Xijun Zhan Da Tusha Jiemi* (鲁西细菌战大屠杀揭秘 Unveiling the Great Massacre of the West Shandong Bacterial War) published in July 2003. The account of their findings in this paragraph draws from "Jiemi Shijie Zuida de Luxi Xijun Dusha 42 Wan Guoren Yu'nan" (揭秘世界最大的鲁西细菌屠杀 42 万国人遇难 Unveiling the World's Greatest Bacterial Warfare Massacre in West Shandong Killing 420,000 of our People) (2005).

[136] This is the episode that correlates with the League of Nations cholera report discussed in the previous section of this chapter.

[137] These episodes are enumerated in Xie Zhonghou (2002).

military bacterial warfare in China still lurks behind a screen of misinformation and ignorance. More study of this phenomenon and its effect on Chinese lives is needed.

Conclusion: Results Obtained from Mao's Ideas on Health

Despite their destructiveness, the Japanese military campaigns in north China were unable to inflict lasting damage on the Communist military and civilian institutions. Even with the loss of several million people and uncounted numbers of medical workers, the idea prevailed that the lives of poor people mattered. This was such a fundamental plank of Mao Zedong's ideology in those days that it is hardly surprising to find it reflected in the work of Communist party military and civilian health workers. Even more significant is Mao's insistence on the strategic role of modern biomedicine in undermining the traditional world of superstition.

Thus it is impressive to see the extent to which health workers went during the Yan'an era to save lives and educate the people about science and hygiene. This was the revolutionary change in public health policy that dedicated healthcare workers sought to contribute to the revival of north China. The campaigns to improve maternal child health and reduce mortality from infectious diseases and childbirth made some progress despite having to wrestle with deeply embedded social traditions, extreme poverty and relentless enemy assaults. Yet at war's end infectious diseases were still active, and the lives of young women, infants and small children were still endangered. Due to Mao Zedong's recognition of healthcare's strategic potential, the epidemiological transition needed to get beyond these problems in north China had begun. But by 1945 that transition was still in its early stages.

CHAPTER EIGHT

SAVING LIVES IN WARTIME CHINA: WHY IT MATTERED

Oh, the pain and misery of China.
—Ai Qing, 1937[1]

The 1930s and 40s represent a watershed era in Chinese history, between the gradual withering away of the chaotic warlord era and the establishment of the People's Republic. Politically the rise and fall of the Nationalist government, and the success of the Communist forces in gaining control throughout China delineate this era. More to the point of this study, it was a time of massive amounts of premature death due to fecal-borne diseases, tuberculosis, smallpox, malaria, typhus, childbirth complications, other infectious and parasitic diseases, opium, starvation, drowning, and military and civil oppression, amounting to tens of millions of uncounted and uncountable fatalities. All that pain and misery is summed up in an unforgettable poem by Ai Qing.

Yet this era saw both Nationalists and Communists paying attention to saving military and civilian lives under some of the most difficult circumstances imaginable. What have we learned from their efforts?

The modern health movement in early to mid twentieth century China rose up in response to the widespread evidence of premature mortality and its association with scientific and national incapacity. As we have seen, the healthcare reformers recognized that a strategy focused on curative medicine would not suffice to bring the vast population of rural China into the modern era, let alone dig them out of misery, nor could it be afforded. Preventive health care was the only way to go. Preventive healthcare meant hygiene and sanitation on the one hand and prophylactic strategies to combat epidemic disease on the other. We have observed district nurses visiting families to initiate sanitary methods to control trachoma, and Red Cross and army medical teams using oil drums and other

---

[1] From Ai Qing (艾青), "Snow Falls on China's Land" (雪落在中国的土地上), written in 1937 following the outbreak of the War of Resistance, translated by Marilyn Chin, and published in Joseph S. M. Lau and Howard Goldblatt (1995). The original text is 中国的痛苦与灾难, 像这雪夜一样广阔而又漫长呀. Oh, the pain and misery of China, as long and vast as this snowy night!

improvised materials to set up delousing, bathing and scabies stations to bring typhus and scabies under control. We have also seen national health, provincial health and Red Cross units delivering hundreds of thousands of prophylactic inoculations and vaccinations to control cholera and smallpox in infected regions, and issuing millions of quinine pills to mitigate malaria. They engaged in propaganda drives to visit schools and teach rural and urban children and their families the basics of hygiene and sanitation. This focus on public hygiene was a new phenomenon in the history of modern China.

Efforts were also launched to train modern midwives in registered schools of midwifery, to set up child health centers, to undertake ante- and postnatal examinations, and to make birthing available in hygienic settings. In epidemiological transition theory, however, this puts China in the 1930s and 1940s in a primary phase still dominated by acute infectious diseases and severe maternal child mortality. In demographic transition theory China was still in a high fertility and high mortality stage. Those were the civilian challenges to lifesaving. What made those challenges so lethal was the ignorance of both the educated and uneducated population as to their dangers, in consequence of which healthcare reformers too often found themselves working in an atmosphere of suspicion and noncooperation.

It should be added that while the healthcare initiatives can be explained to a certain extent through epidemiological and demographic analysis, such analysis did not motivate them. However, greater attention to epidemiological transition theory would help to explain the problems and transitions going on in China at this time and provide an explanatory alternative to dependence on political and military factors to explain historical development.

A third area of lifesaving health care, which has received somewhat more attention in the public record, has to do with front line rescue of wounded soldiers. Dr. Norman Bethune is the most publicized advocate of this approach, and Communist Eighth Route Army soldiers were the fortunate beneficiaries of his work. Clearly the Red Cross Medical Relief Corps and the work of the Nationalist Army's medical reformers must also be credited for tens of thousands of saved lives that would otherwise have been lost due to gangrene and hemorrhagic shock. Here, as with maternal childcare, we have marveled at the work of key medical reformers, who were motivated by patriotism to engage in this ill-paid, dirty, and dangerous work. One outstanding example of this concern for human life is Dr. Lin Kesheng, who gave up an internationally respected career as a physiologist to take on the task of organizing an emergency relief system for wounded soldiers. Although reared in Singapore and Scotland Dr. Lin had on several occasions expressed a pro-Chinese patriotism, and like Dr. Bethune he knew a good deal about military medical care. His charisma and leadership drew in colleagues and medical students from both within China and the Chinese Diaspora, who felt a strong patriotic calling to serve their ancestral country. A similarly strong patriotic motivation drew thousands of young people to Mao's side in Yan'an. Despite the blood, the stench of gangrene and human waste, the cries and groans, the lack of medical supplies and painkillers, these patriots realized that compassionate and scientifically trained intelligentsia were needed and could truly save lives of poor people.

Those who went into healthcare during this wartime era realized that war could no longer be the burden solely of disposable peasants used as cannon fodder. We have seen rural people working as bearers, dressers, nursing aides, scouts, cooks, hosts, providers of food, collectors of herbs, and even as organizers of paramilitary forces supporting the formal divisions and armies. Collectively they played a huge part in aiding China in its time of need.

Because of their experience in World War One and Spain, medical leaders such as Dr. Lin and Dr. Bethune were able to bring parts of Chinese military health care much closer to international norms than their civilian colleagues were able to do in the arena of public health. Dr. Lin was able to use the war to train young, patriotic and well-educated physicians to grasp the new norms of military health care. Drs. Bethune and Kotnis were able to do the same in the smaller context of Eighth Route Army health care. Chinese Communist leaders welcomed Bethune, Kotnis and other international healthcare workers; they knew well that they could not survive without the active engagement of poor country people in the war effort.

The Nationalist military leadership, by contrast, was not as attuned to the importance of rank and file soldiers. They believed they could discount battlefield losses by maintaining a hugely inefficient and often life-threatening system of conscription. They also evaded the need for developing effective services of supply—particularly supply of nutritious food—by leaving soldiers to depend on age-old practices of forage and pillage.

Healthcare education constituted another major wartime activity focused on life saving. Before the Japanese war China's modern medical colleges were primarily in the business of capacity building. Faculty at colleges, such as the Peking Union Medical College, with activist departments of public health, helped to found medical colleges specifically to promote State Medicine, that is, to make certain preventive health services available to China's predominantly rural population. Others, such as the Xiangya Medical College, had a strong sense of loyalty to their home provinces. The Red Army healthcare schools produced health workers to serve in the Red Army; the Emergency Medical Service Training Schools produced a large range of health workers to support soldiers primarily enrolled in pro-Nationalist armies. If pushed, all the medical colleges would say that life saving through clinical training was a central mission.

What is undeniable is that none of the formal colleges, including the Army Medical College, were equipped to withstand the pressure on military healthcare created by the massive Japanese military invasion of China in 1937. The Chinese soldiers who faced the Japanese armies in 1937 had virtually nowhere to go for help. At first they died on the battlefield, or under bushes, or in miserable hovels masquerading as field hospitals. But once improvised medical relief services were developed by the Red Cross Medical Relief Corps and by the Red Army, the civilian medical colleges played a vital role in educating physicians and nurses to serve in those medical relief agencies.

The Red Army leaders, in particular, had no choice but to mobilize human energy to turn life saving into a central goal. Much smaller in size than the Nationalist armies, they had to save lives to preserve their mission from destruction. Even so, it is instructive to recall how Mao Zedong and Zhu De went about this task. After the collapse of the 1927 uprisings Zhu De enlisted the services and hospital facilities of Dr. Fu Lianzhang to treat his wounded soldiers. After the collapse of the 1930 uprisings Mao Zedong enlisted the services and skills of Dr. Dai Jimin. In both cases they stumbled on remarkable individuals who were motivated by the Christian missionary ideal of serving others. As a graduate of St. John's Medical College in Shanghai, Dr. Dai could have opted for a lucrative urban practice. But he preferred to work in a country town in Jiangxi province, and he was a devout Christian. He listened to Mao and accepted the challenge that Mao presented. Revolutionary humanitarianism was the idea that brought Mao Zedong and Dr. Dai together. A natural mobilizer of others, Dr. Dai and his colleagues succeeded in getting seven hundred wounded soldiers back on their feet in short order. It was the idea that motivated several other great healthcare leaders during the time of the Communist government in Jiangxi. Mao's Eighth Route Army had young trained healthcare workers willing to give their lives on the front lines following the examples of front line service set by Drs. Bethune and Kotnis, examples that still resonate in China today.

For the idealists serving in the much more diffuse world of Nationalist army medical service, a great deal depended on Dr. Lin Kesheng's ability to attract young people to his side and mobilize the resources needed to make the Red Cross Medical Relief Corps effective across large distances. As the data in chapter 4 reveals, Dr. Lin pulled a significant number of medical relief teams together. He was also able to mobilize a very large transportation system and obtain a considerable supply of materials suitable for both front line relief and long term care. Through his overseas Chinese, British and American connections, Dr. Lin was also able to organize long term overseas financial, human and material aid. No one else had the breadth of international connections as well as managerial drive and military medical and scientific skills that he had to make all this aid available to China's military forces. Dr. Lin received strong backing from senior Guomindang leaders such as Song Ziwen and Mme. Chiang.

But as we have seen, that was not enough to save him from being sucked into a vortex of criticism and hostility from conservative military leaders, opponents within the Chinese Red Cross, and indignant American civilian representatives, who thought that his work was getting too big a share of American relief aid. Because of his willingness to serve both nationalist and communist military forces in the United Front he was harassed by Chiang Kaishek, He Yingqin and the Red Cross leaders. His ability to operate was effectively cut short for almost eighteen months, and during that time the Red Cross Medical Relief Corps languished. His close associate and PUMC colleague Dr. Lu Zhide also ended up frustrated by Guomindang politics and resigned from his position as Army Surgeon General. It was not until the tide turned with the development of the Alpha Plan in late 1944 that these two gifted and honorable men were able to return to positions of influence within the Nationalist government's military medical orbit.

In the War of Resistance to Japan we witnessed a combination of savagery towards civilian enemies and disregard of the lives of powerless people that raises uncomfortable questions. Why, for example, did the Japanese military engage in bacterial warfare? Why were the leaders of such warfare allowed to escape examination in postwar trials (other than in the Soviet Union)? But the era also provides us with examples of savagery by Chinese people towards other Chinese people, as well as gross indifference to the human consequences of taking such drastic strategic

steps as breaching huge river dikes. These examples are part of the context
in which commitments to life saving took place. The modern history of
East Asia needs to put such questions onto center stage, as that is where
questions of life and death belong.

Beyond such intentional destruction of human life, we have encountered four other types of activity destructive of human life that occurred
during these times: 1) rigorous exaction of rents and taxes during times of
near famine that precipitated famine, such as what occurred in Henan in
1942–1943; 2) customs permitting 'marriage' of early teenage girls unready
for birthing to sexually active men, ensuring dangerous and often deadly
consequences for mothers and children; 3) Indifference to the lives and
welfare of conscripted soldiers manifested in the wretched conscript
medical services of the time; 4) habits of mind among empowered people
that concluded that military medical care was not all that important, and
neither were the lives of rural people.

Finally we should pay attention to the epidemic and contagious diseases
that assailed the Chinese people on a virtually year-round basis. Among
these diseases tuberculosis, smallpox, malaria, dysentery and cholera
were probably the most widespread and fatal, but there were others such
as plague, typhoid fever, typhus, relapsing fever, hookworm, diphtheria,
measles, scarlet fever, tetanus, and venereal diseases, that took a heavy
toll on the population. The most pervasive disease of all was malnutrition,
a state of near starvation that dominated the countryside and country
people in times of stress, such as characterized the era on which this study
is focused. And what kept these evils flourishing, apart from crop failure
and oppressive government, was a near complete absence of any popular
understanding (including among traditionally 'educated' people such as
scholar-officials) of basic hygiene and sanitation.

One might think that under such circumstances governments would
pay very close attention to the health of the public, on whose wellbeing
their present and future depended. The Nationalist government leaders
did pay lip service to the importance of public health and did attract
some very capable people to serve the public through the field of civilian
healthcare. But the record demonstrates that for the senior political and
military leaders, including Chiang Kaishek as overall leader, public health
was never a top priority. China had survived for millennia without modern public health, and it would continue to do so. Mme. Chiang was one
of the few top Nationalist leaders whose thinking was not constrained by
such blinders. Although lacking medical training and getting in the way of

those who had it, she saw that healthcare mattered. She helped thousands of orphans, and she tried to help Dr. Lin. She supported various organizations that made efforts to ameliorate the health of soldiers.

The early years of the War of Resistance to Japan mark the time when the reformers had the best chance to utilize waves of pro-Chinese patriotism to put their ideas into action. This patriotism helped materially to fuel lifesaving healthcare reform during these few precious years (1937–40), before renewed Japanese military aggression, hyperinflation and general war weariness set in. Even then, the energy in civilian public health and health education did not peter out until 1944, while the Nationalist military healthcare reformers obtained a renewed but last ditch boost of energy thanks to support from the burgeoning American military and medical presence in Southwest China.

This tells us that there were Chinese leaders who devoted themselves to the public interest by committing in a variety of ways to save lives, putting that interest above professional career, economic benefit or personal security. They did this at a time when plenty of other people thought that such idealism was a waste of time and money, or worse—a way of getting into bed with Communists. We should not underestimate the degree of human trauma and fear in wartime China that played its part in corrupting the judgment of individuals who might otherwise have remained above reproach. But it is precisely in those circumstances that moral commitment makes a difference. It was by all accounts hard to survive in wartime China. That is what makes the work of the people who cared about rescuing human lives all the more meaningful.

Was all the death mitigated by the lives saved? Could one at least commemorate the lives of refugees gunned down by Japanese bombers or farmers drowned as a result of ambitious but futile Chinese maneuvers to stop the Japanese military advance into central China? The answer to that is obviously yes. Dr. Bethune's work is rightly celebrated in the grand new museum adorning the central space of the city of Yan'an. But those who worked very hard to save the lives of drowning peasants, newborn children or Nationalist conscripts and soldiers do not get the same publicity. For that to happen, historical perspective will have to take account of both epidemiology and ethics. It must make the case that in any feasible development policy science and ethics receive equal attention. How fortunate it was that in wartime China so many healthcare patriots lived up to that challenge.

BIBLIOGRAPHY

Archives Consulted

American Board of Commissioners for Foreign Missions, Shaowu archive, volume II, Harvard University Houghton Library.

American Bureau for Medical Aid to China (now Advancement in China), Columbia University, Rare Books Library. This archive is a major source for ABMAC's relations with the Chinese Red Cross Medical Relief Corps, the wartime National Health Administration, and China's wartime medical and nursing schools. It contains a large photographic collection; prime examples of its wartime photographs are accessible through the digital library of Indiana University-Purdue University Indianopolis at http://www.ulib.iupui.edu/digitalscholarship/collections/WMIC.

American Red Cross Archive, Washington, D.C. National Archive.

China Medical Board and Rockefeller Foundation Archives, Pocantico Hills, N.Y.

Jiangsu Provincial Archives, Nanjing.

Shanghai Municipal Archive.

Stanford University Chen Cheng archive (in microfilm at Harvard Yenching Library).

Western Language Sources

CDL   China Defense League
CMJ   Chinese Medical Journal
NMJC   National Medical Journal of China

"ABMAC's Chinese Blood Bank" (1944): *CMJ*, 62/2, April–June 1944, 218, 304.

Leonard P. Adams (1972): "China: the Historical Setting of Asia's Profitable Plague," Appendix to Alfred W. McCoy et al., *The Politics of Heroin in Southeast Asia*, New York, Harper and Row.

Emmanuel S. Akinboye and Oladapo Bakare (2011): "Biological Activities of Emetine," The Open Natural Products Journal, 4, 8–15 and note 27.

Alitto, Guy S. (1986): The Last Confucian, 2nd ed., Berkeley, CA, University of California Press.

American Journal of Public Health (October 1926): "A Welcome Publication," 16/10, 1030.

Armfield, Blanche B. (ed.) (1963): *Medical Department, United States Army, in World War II: Organization and Administration*, Washington, D.C., Office of the Surgeon General, Department of the Army.

Arnold, David (1993): *Colonizing the Body: State Medicine and Epidemic Disease in Nineteenth-Century India*, Berkeley: University of California Press.

Auden, W. H. and Christopher Isherwood (1939): Journey to a War, London: Faber and Faber.

Balinksa, M. A. "La Pologne: du Choléra au Typhus, 1831–1950," (accepted 1999): www.pathexo.fr/documents/articles-bull/T92-5-1962.pdf.

Balme, Harold (April 8, 1939): "The Medical Emergency in China," Lancet, 1, 836–839.

Barenblatt, Daniel (2004): *A Plague Upon Humanity: The Secret Genocide of Axis Japan's Germ Warfare Operation*, New York, HarperCollins, 2004.

Belden, Jack (1944): Still Time to Die, New York and London: Harper.

Benton, Gregor (1992): Mountain Fires: the Red Army's Three-Year War in South China, 1934–1938, Berkeley, CA, University of California Press.

Bix, Herbert (2000): Hirohito and the Making of Modern Japan, New York, HarperCollins.

Boorman, Howard L. (1967): Biographical Dictionary of Republican China, New York: Columbia University Press.

Bowers, John Z. (1972): Western Medicine in a Chinese Palace, New York, Macy Foundation.

Brauer, Max, E. Briand-Clausen and Dr. A. Stampar (January 1934): Report of Survey of Certain Localities in Kiangsi, [Nanjing], National Economic Council.

Bu, Liping (2009): "Social Darwinism, Public Health and Modernization in China, 1895–1925," in Iris Borowy, ed., Uneasy Encounters: The Politics of Medicine and Health in China, 1900–1937, Frankfort am Main, Peter Lang, 93–124.

Bullock, Mary Brown (1980): An American Transplant, Berkeley, CA, University of California Press.

Calame, Louis (November 1938): "La Misère dans la Nord de la Chine," Revue Internationale de la Croix-Rouge, 967–1016.

Carlson, Evans Fordyce (1940a): The Chinese Army: Its Organization and Military Efficiency, New York, Institute of Pacific Relations.

—— (1940b): Twin Stars of China, New York, Dodd, Mead, 1940.

Central Field Health Station (1934): The First Report of the Central Field Health Station, April 1931–December 1933, Shanghai: Kelly and Walsh.

—— (1936): Report for 1935, Nanking.

Chang, K. and H. T. Ch'in (January 1943): "An Evaluation of Pickled Vegetables in the Dissemination of Ascaris Lumbricoides," CMJ, 61A/2, 63–69.

Chang, P. Y. (1923): "A General Review of the Treatment of Tuberculosis," NMJC, 9/4, 297–304.

Chen, C. C. (1933): "A Practical Survey of Rural Health," CMJ, 47/7, 680–688.

—— (1989): Medicine in Rural China: a Personal Account, Berkeley, University of California Press.

Chen, S. P. (Chen Sibang 陈祀邦) (June 1916): "Medical Education in China." NMJC, 2/2, 4–19.

Chia K'uei (Jia Kui) (1925): "A Sanitary Survey of Tsunhwa (Zunhua)." NMJC, 11/5, 313–323.

Chiang, May-ling Soong (1940): China shall Rise Again, New York, Harper.

China Defense League (1940): Annual Report and Survey of Projects, 1939–1940. Hong Kong: Central Committee, China Defense League.

—— (1943): In Guerrilla China.

China Weekly Review (1936): Who's Who in China, 5th ed., Shanghai, China Weekly Review.

Chinese Medical Directory (1941): Shanghai, Chinese Medical Association.

Chinese Ministry of Information

—— (1943): China Handbook, 1937–1943, New York, Macmillan.

—— (1944): China Handbook, 1937–1944, Chungking, Chinese Ministry of Information.

—— (1947): China Handbook, 1937–1945, New York, Macmillan.

—— (1950): China Handbook, 1950, New York, Rockfort Press.

Chun, J. W. H. (陈永汉 John Wing-hon Chun/Chen Yonghan) (1919): "Influenza including its Infection Among Pigs." NMJC, 5/1, 34–44.

"Control of Epidemics: the Epidemic Commission of the League," (August 1938): CMJ, 54/2, 182–189.

Cook, Haruko Taya and Theodore F. Cook (1992); Japan at War: An Oral History, New York, The New Press.

Correspondence (1929): NMJC, 15, 520–524.

Crozier, Ralph C. (1968): Traditional Medicine in Modern China, Cambridge, MA, Harvard University Press.

Davenport. Horace W. (1980): Biographical Memoirs, 51 Biography of Robert K. S. Lim, Washington D.C., National Academy of Sciences.

Day, Clarence Burton (1969): Chinese Peasant Cults, 2nd ed., Taipei, Ch'eng Wen Publishing Co.

De Groot, J. J. M. (1972): *The Religious Systems of China*, 6 volumes, reprint, Taipei, Ch'eng Wen Publishing Co.

Department of Health (May 1991): Malaria Eradication in Taiwan, Taipei, DOH.

Dictionary of Traditional Chinese Medicine (1984): Taipei, Southern Materials Center.

Dikotter, Frank (2010): *Mao's Great Famine: The History of China's most Devastating Catastrophe*, New York, Walker, 2010.

Dixon, Norman (1994): *On the Psychology of Military Incompetence*, London, Random House (Pimlico Edition).

Dreyer, Edward L. (1995): China at War: 1901–1049, New York, Longman.

Dyer, Brian R. (Chinese name Daiya 戴雅) (January 1936): "Methods Developed at the Central Field Health Station for the Training of Sanitation Personnel," *CMJ*, 50, 76–81.

Eastman, Lloyd (1991): "Nationalist China during the Nanking Decade, 1927–1937," in Eastman et al., The Nationalist Era in China, 1927–1949, New York, Cambridge University Press, 29.

Editorials:

—— (March 1918): "The Recent Plague Epidemic," *NMJC*, 4/2, 37–39.

—— (September 1918): "Pneumonic Plague," *NMJC*, 4/3, 88–94.

—— (March 1921): *NJMC*, 7/1, 2–4.

—— (June 1921): "Progress of Medical Science in China," *NMJC*, 7/2, 38.

—— (1923): "The Relation between the Mission Hospitals and Public Health Work in China," *The Caduceus*, 2/3, 154–157.

—— (1926): "A Challenge to Posterity," *NMJC*, 12/3, 253–257.

—— (1929): "Financing Public Health in China," *NMJC*, 15/1, 49–52.

Eiler, Keith E. (1987): *Wedemeyer on War and Peace*, Stanford, CA, Hoover Institution Press.

Epstein, Israel (1947): *The Unfinished Revolution in China,* Boston, Little, Brown.

Ewen, Jean (1981): Canadian Nurse in China, Halifax, NS, Goodread Biographies.

Fan, J. H. (1945): "Communicable Diseases during Recent Years," United Nations Relief and Rehabilitation Administration, *Epidemiological Information Bulletin*, 1/12, 495–536.

Faust, Drew Gilpin (2008): *This Republic of Suffering: Death and the American Civil War*, New York, Knopf.

Fee, Elizabeth (1987): Disease and Discovery: A History of the Johns Hopkins School of Hygiene and Public Health, 1916–1936, Baltimore, The Johns Hopkins Press.

Field, Mark G. (1967): *Soviet Socialized Medicine*, New York: Free Press.

Field Service Hygiene Notes 1945, Calcutta: Government of India Press, 1945.

Flood Relief, (1932): *CMJ*, 46/2, February 1932, 233.

Flowers, W.S. (1946): *A Surgeon in China: Extracts from Letters from Dr. W. S. Flowers*, London, Carey Press.

Gachelin, Gabriel and Annick Opinel (April/June 2011): "Malaria Epidemics in Europe after the First World War: the Early Stages of an International Approach to the Control of the Disease," *História, Ciências, Saúde-Manguinhos*, 18/2. Available online.

Gordon, Sydney and Ted Allan (1952): *The Scalpel, the Sword: The Story of Doctor Norman Bethune*, New York, Monthly Review Press. Revised 1971, 1973.

Graham, David Crockett (1961): *Folk Religion in Southwest China,* Washington, D.C., Smithsonian Press.

Grant, John B. (1928): "State Medicine—A Logical Policy for China," *NMJC*, 14/2, 65–80.

—— Oral History, Columbia University Oral History Archive.

Grant, John B. and T. M. Peng (彭达谋) (October 1934): "Survey of Urban Public Health Practice in China," *CMJ*, 48/10, 1074–1079.

Hannant, Larry (1998): The Politics of Persuasion: Norman Bethune's Writing and Art, Toronto, University of Toronto Press.

Harrison, Mark (2004): *Disease and the Modern World*, Cambridge, UK, Polity Press.

Hayford, Charles W. (1990): *To the People: James Yen and Village China*, New York, Columbia University Press.

"Health Work in Kiangsi," (1934): *CMJ*, 48/11, 1173.

"Health Work in Kiangsi," (1937): *CMJ*, 51/1, 102–104.

"Health Work in the Central China Flood" (January 1933): *CMJ*, 47/1, 75–76.

Heaton, Leonard D. (1968): *Medical Supply in World War II*, Washington, D.C. Office of the Surgeon General, Department of the Army.

Hensman, Bertha, (1967): "The Kilburn Family…" Canadian Medical Association Journal, 97, August 12, 1967, 471–483.

Hinton, David (2008): *Classical Chinese Poetry*, New York, Farrar, Strauss and Giraux.

Hochschild, Adam (2012): *To End All Wars: A Story of Loyalty and Rebellion, 1914–1918*, Boston: Houghton Mifflin.

Honda Katsuichi (1999): The Nanjing Massacre, Armonk, N. Y., M. E. Sharpe.

Hsu, Francis K. L. (1983): Exorcising the Troublemakers: Magic, Science and Culture, Westport, CT, Greenwood Press.

Hsu Long-hsuen and Chang Ming-kai (1971): *History of the Sino-Japanese War (1937–1945)*, Taipei, Chung Wu Publishing.

Huang, H. H., M. D. and T. H. Wang M. D., (王祖祥) (1936): Survey of the Maternity and Child Health Work in Nanking," *CMJ*, 50, 554–561.

Huang, J. L. (1984): Memoirs of J. L. Huang, Taipei, Yingzhong Chubanshe. Institute of Social Sciences, Demographic Research Center (1974): The Population of Yugoslavia, Belgrade. Available online.

Huang, Tsefang F. (1927): "Public Health in China: A Proposed Program," National Epidemic Prevention Bureau, Special Bulletin No. 3, (Beijing, 1927), reported in Herbert Day Lamson (1935).

Institute of Social Sciences, Demographic Research Center (1974): *The Population of Yugoslavia*, (Belgrade). Available on line.

International Women's Health Program (2009): "'Til Death Do Us Part: Understanding the Sexual and Reproductive Health Risks of Early Marriage," iwhp.sogc.org/index .php?page=early-marriage&hl=en_US.

Ishikawa Tatsuzo (2003): Soldiers Alive, translated and with introduction by Zeljko Cipris, Honolulu, University of Hawai'i Press.

Japan International Cooperation Agency (2005): *Japan's Experiences in Public Health and Medical Systems*, jica-ri.jica.go.jp/IFIC_and_JBICI-Studies/english/publications/reports/ study/topical/health/pdf/health_01.pdf.

Jefferys, W. Hamilton and J. L. Maxwell, (1910, 1929): *The Diseases of China Including Formosa and Korea, 1*st ed., Philadelphia, Blakiston's Son and Co., 2nd ed., Shanghai, A.B.C. Press.

Jettmar, H. M. (1932): "Plague in Shansi and Shensi," *CMJ*, 46/4 (April 1932), 429–435.

Jha, Prabhat (2012): "Counting the Dead is one of the World's best Investments to Reduce Premature Mortality," *Hypothesis*, 10/1. doi:10.5779/hypothesis.v10i1.254.

Johnson, Steven (2006): *The Ghost Map: The Story of London's Most Terrifying Epidemic— and how it Changed Science, Cities and the Modern World*, New York, Riverhead Books.

Johnson, Tina Phillips (2011): *Childbirth in Republican China*, Lanham, MD, Rowman and Littlefield.

Keen, William Williams (1917): The Treatment of War Wounds, Philadelphia, W. B. Saunders.

Keeper, Frank R. (1918): A Textbook of Elementary Military Hygiene and Sanitation, Philadelphia and London, W. B. Saunders.

King, P. Z. (金宝善 Jin Baoshan) (1940): "The Chinese National Health Administration During the Sino-Japanese Hostilities," in May-ling Soong Chiang (1940), 198–228.

—— (January–March 1943): "Epidemic Prevention and Control in China," *CMJ* 61/1, 47–54.

—— (1946): "Thirty Years of Public Health Work in China," *CMJ* 64 (January–February 1946), 3–16.

Koenig, William J. (1972): Over the Hump: Airlift to China, New York, Ballantine Books Inc.

Kwok, D. W. Y. (1965): *Scientism in Chinese Thought, 1900–1950*, New Haven, Yale University Press.

Lai, Chiu-mi (2004): "Reinvention of the 'Late Season' motif in the Wen Xuan," Early Medieval China 10/11.1 131–150.

Lai, Daniel G. (Lai Douyan 赖斗岩) and C. M. Chu (Zhu Jiming 朱既明) (May 1941): "The Kutsung (Yunnan) Health Demonstration Centre—a Review for 1939–40," *CMJ* 59/5, 468–475.

Lamley, "Harry J. (May 1965): "Liang Shu-ming, Rural Reconstruction, and the Rural Work Discussion Society, 1933–1935," Chongji Xuebao (崇基学报), 8/2, 50–61. Available online.

Lamson, Herbert Day (1935): *Social Pathology in China*, Shanghai: Commercial Press.

Lary, Diana and Stephen MacKinnon, (2001): *Scars of War: The Impact of Warfare on Modern China*, Vancouver: UBC Press.

Lary, Diana (1985): Warlord Soldiers: Chinese Common Soldiers, 1911–37, Cambridge, Cambridge University Press.

—— (2010): *The Chinese People at War: Human Suffering and Social Transformation, 1937–1945*, Cambridge, Cambridge University Press.

Lasnet, A., (1939): "Dix Mois de Mission Sanitaire dans le Sud de la Chine," Bulletin de L'Academie de Medecine, 121, March 7, 1939, 300–317.

Tony Latter, (2004): "Hong Kong's Exchange Rate Regimes in the Twentieth Century: the Story of Three Regime Changes," Hong Kong Institute for Monetary Research, Working Paper No. 17. Available online.

Lau, Joseph S. M. and Howard Goldblatt (1995): *The Columbia Anthology of Modern Chinese Literature*, New York, Columbia University Press.

"Law and Legislation: Ministry of Health Organizational Regulations," (February 1929): *NMJC*, 15/1, 75–76.

League of Nations Health Organization (1930): *Proposals of the National Government of the Republic of China for Collaboration with the League of Nations on Health Matters*, February 12, 1930.

—— (1937a): Intergovernmental Conference of Far Eastern Countries on Rural Hygiene: Report of China, Geneva.

—— (1937b): Intergovernmental Conference of Far Eastern Countries on Rural Hygiene: Report of Japan, Geneva.

Lee Shu-fan, FRCS, (李树芬 Li Shufen) (1926): "The Duties and Responsibilities of the Present-day Chinese Physician." *NMJC*, 15/1, 57–61.

—— (1964): *Hong Kong Surgeon*, New York, E. P. Dutton.

Lemley, Kevin V. and Linus S. Pauling (1994): Thomas Addis, 1881–1949, Washington, D.C.: National Academy of Sciences, 1994.

Li Kuang-hsun (Guangxun) (1923): "Public Health in Soochow (Suzhou)," *NMJC*, 9/2, 122–131.

Li, Lillian (2007): *Fighting Famine in North China: State, Market, and Environmental Decline, 1690s–1990s*, Stanford, CA: Stanford University Press.

Li Ting-an (李廷安) (October 1925): "A Public Health Report on Canton, China," *NMJC*, 11/5, 324–375.

—— (1934): "Summary Report on Rural Public Health Practice in China," *CMJ* 48/10, 1086–1090.

Li, Virginia C. (2003): From One Root Many Flowers, New York, Prometheus Books.

Lie Chen Ie (2003): "China Ambulance" (Huaqiao Kangri Jiushengdui 华侨抗日救生队). CHC Bulletin, 2, September 2003, 28–31.

Lin Chia-swee and H. M. Jettmar, (1925): "The Scarlet Fever Problem in the Far East," *NMJC*, 11/6, 399–412.

Lin Jia-swee (林家瑞) and Wu Lien-teh (February 1927): "Report of a Preliminary Health Survey of Pinchiang (Chinese City of Harbin) January-June, 1926," *NMJC*, 13/1, 24–82.

Ling, W. P. (林文秉 Lin Wenbing) (February 1924): "A Plea for the Conservation of Vision in China," *NMJC*, 10/1, 20–24.

Lita, Ana (2008): "Obstetric fistula: a dire consequence of child marriage," International Humanist and Ethical Union, http://iheu.org/story/obstetric-fistula-dire-consequence-child-marriage.

Liu, J. Heng (刘瑞恒) (1929): "The Chinese Ministry of Health," *NMJC*, 15/2, 135–148.

—— (1930): "Nursing Problems in China," in Liu Sijin (1989), 313–315.

—— (1932): "The Chinese Medical Association: First General Conference Address," *Chinese Medical Journal*, 46, 1125–1127, reprinted in Liu Siqin (1989), 303–306.

Liu, Yungmao (2008): "Reflections on Lin Kesheng during the Eight-year War of Resistance Against Japan," in John R. Watt, ed., (2008): *Health Care and National Development in Taiwan*, 1950–2000, New York, The ABMAC Foundation, 18–20. (Chinese text in Chinese bibliography).

Lucas, AnElissa (1982): *Chinese Medical Modernization*, New York, Praeger.

Machiavelli, Niccolo (1950): *The Prince and the* Discourses, New York, Random House, Modern Library.

MacKinnon, Janice R. and Stephen R. (1988): *Agnes Smedley: The Life and Times of an American Radical*, Bderkeley, CA, University of California Press.

MacKinnon, Stephen R. (2008): *Wuhan, 1938,* Berkeley, CA, University of California Press.

Mallory, Walter H. (1926): *China: Land of Famine*, New York, American Geographical Society.

Malone, Thomas (1942): "Hospital Work in China under War Conditions," Hospital Progress, 23, August 1942, 256–260.

Mao Zedong (1927): "Report on an Investigation of the Peasant Movement in Hunan, March 1927," *Selected Works of Mao Tse-tung*, vol. I, Peking, Foreign Languages Press. 1965, 23–59.

—— (1934): "Be Concerned with the Wellbeing of the Masses, Pay Attention to Methods of Work," vol. I, 147–152.

—— (1935): "On Tactics against Japanese Imperialism," vol. I, 153–178.

—— (1936): "Problems of Strategy in China's Revolutionary War," vol. I, 179–254.

—— (1944): "The United Front in Cultural Work," Selected Works, vol. III, 235–237.

McClure, Robert Baird (November 1941): "Medical Aspects of the China War," *Public Health Nursing* 33, 640–645.

McCord, Edward A. (2001): "Burn, Kill, Rape and Rob: Military Atrocities, Warlordism, and Anti-Warlordism in Republican China," in Diana Lary and Stephen MacKinnon, (2001), 18–47.

McLynn, Frank (2011): *The Burma* Campaign, London, Vintage Books.

McNeill, William H. (1976): *Plagues and Peoples*, Garden City, New York: Doubleday.

"Medical Help for China," (1939): Lancet, 1 (March 11, 1939): 616.

Mote, F. W. (2010): *China and the Vocation of History in the Twentieth* Century, Princeton, East Asian Library Journal.

"National Board of Health Conference,"(1929): *NMJC*, 15, 203–204.

National Flood Relief Commission, (1933): "Health Work in the Central China Flood," *CMJ*, 47/1, 75–76.

"National Health Administration," (1943): report dated December 1942, *CMJ*, 61/1, 75–84.

Newnham, Tom (1992): He Mingqing: The Life of Kathleen Hall, Auckland, NZ, Graphic Publications.

Osterhammel, Jurgen (1979): "'Technical Cooperation' between the League of Nations and China," Modern Asian Studies, 13/4, 661–680.

"Pneumonic Plague" (September 1918): *NMJC*, 4/3, 88–94.

Peiping Branch, National Medical Association (1929): *NMJC*, 15, 469–470.

Peking United International Famine Relief Committee (1922): The North China Famine of 1920–21, Peking.

Peter, W. W. (1920): "The Work of the Council on Health Education," *NMJC*, 6/4, 234–236.

Porter, Edgar A. (1997): The People's Doctor: George Hatem and China's Revolution, Honolulu, University of Hawai'i Press.

Powell, Lyle Stephenson (1946): A Surgeon in Wartime China, Lawrence, KA, University of Kansas Press.

Rajchman, L. (1927): "Report to the League of Nations." *NMJC*, 13/3, 288–292.

Ramsay, Alex. (1922): *The Peking Who's Who 1922*, Beijing, Tientsin Press.

Reeves, Caroline Beth (1998): The Power of Mercy: The Chinese Red Cross Society, 1900–1937, Cambridge, MA, Harvard University Dissertation.

"Review of Journals," (1926): *The Caduceus*, 5/1, 58–60.

Robertson, R. Cecil (1940): "Malaria in Western Yunnan with reference to the China-Burma Highway," *CMJ* 57/1, 57–73.

Rogaski, Ruth (2004): *Hygienic Modernity: Meanings of Health and Disease in Treaty Port China*, Berkeley: University of California Press.

Romanus, Charles F. and Riley Sutherland (1959): *Time Runs Out in* CBI, Washington, D.C., Department of the Army, 1959. Available online.

Rue, John E. (1966): *Mao Tse-tung in Opposition, 1927–1935*, Stanford CA, Stanford University Press.

Rumsey, Henry Wyldbore (1856): *Essays on State Medicine*, London: John Churchill.

Scott, Munroe (1977): McClure: The China Years, Markham, ONT, Penguin Books.

Sevareid, Eric (1978): Not so Wild a Dream, New York, Atheneum.

Sheng Xiangong (盛贤功) (1986): An Indian Freedom Fighter in China (柯棣华大夫 Kedihua Daifu), Beijing, Foreign Languages Press.

Slack, Edward R. Jr, (2001): Opium, State and Society: China's Narco-Economy and the Guomindang, 1924–1937, Honolulu, University of Hawai'i Press.

Smedley, Agnes (1934): *China's Red Army Marches*, New York, Vanguard Press.

—— (1938): *China Fights Back: An American Woman with the Eighth Route Army*, New York, Vanguard Press.

—— (November 1938): "The Wounded in China," *CMJ* 54/5, 475–6, originally published in Manchester Guardian Weekly (August 26, 1938), 176.

—— (1943): *Battle Hymn of China*, New York, Knopf.

—— (1956): The Great Road: The Life and Times of Chu Teh, New York, Monthly Review Press.

Snow, Edgar (1961): Red Star Over China, New York, Grove Press.

Stampar, Andrija, (June 1937): "A Health Program for Fukien, April 1936" *CMJ*, 51/6, 1091–1101.

—— (1938a): "Observations of a Rural Health Worker," *New England Journal of Medicine*, 218/24, 991–997.

—— (1938b): Public Health in Jugoslavia, London, School of Slavonic and East European Studies.

—— (August 2006): "On Health Politics," American Journal of Public Health, 96/8, 1382–1385.

Stewart, Roderick (2002): *The Mind of Norman Bethune*, Markham, Ont., Fitzhenry and Whiteside.

Stowman, Knud (1945a): "Cholera," UNRRA, Epidemiological Information Bulletin, I/13 (August 15, 1945).

—— (1945b): "Progress Report of Health Division," UNRRA, Epidemiological Information Bulletin, I/16 (September 30, 1945).

Su Kai-ming (1985): Modern China: a Topical History, Beijing, New World Press.

Sun, Shuyun (2006): *The Long March*, London, HarperPress.

Tanaka, Yuki (1998): Hidden Horrors, Boulder, CO, Westview Press.

Tanaka, Yuki (1988): "Hidden Horrors: Japanese War Crimes in World War II," Boulder, CO, Westview Press.

The China Lantern (US armed forces newspaper) (May 4, 1945): 3/13. Available online.

"*The Cholera Epidemic*" (September 1919): *NMJC*, 5/3, 141–142.

Tawney, R. H. (1964): Land and Labor in China, New York, Octagon Books.

Thomson, James C. Jr., (1969): While China Faced West: American Reformers in Nationalist China, 1928–1937, Cambridge, MA: Harvard University Press.

Tian Xiang Yue and nine other authors (2005): "Surface Modelling of Human Distribution Population in China," Ecological Modelling 181, 461–478, online at www.igsnrr.cas.cn/xwzx/jxlwtj/200711/W020090715580896042625.pdf.

Tirman, John (2011): The Deaths of Others: The Fate of Civilians in America's Wars, New York, Oxford University Press.

Tregear, T. R. (1965): A Geography of China, London, University of London Press.

Tuchman, Barbara (1970): Stilwell and the American Experience in China, New York, Macmillan.

Tyau, E. S. (刁信德, born 刁庆湘, Edward Sintak Tiao/Diao Xinde) (November 1915): "The Demand of Modern Medicine on the Profession, the College and the Government." NMJC, 1, 11–6.

Tyau, Min-ch'ien T. Z., (刁敏谦, 字德仁 Diao Minqian) (1930): Two Years of Nationalist China, Shanghai, Kelly and Walsh.

Unschuld, Paul U. (1986): Medicine in China: A History of Pharmaceutics, Berkeley, CA, University of California Press.

Utley, Freda (1939): China at War, London, Faber and Faber.

Wampler, Ernest M. (1945): China Suffers, Elgin, IL: Brethren Publishing House.

Wang Zheng (1999): Women in the Chinese Enlightenment, Berkeley, CA: University of California Press.

Watt, John R. (1989): "J. Heng Liu and ABMAC," in Liu Sijin (1989), 188–205.

—— (2004): "Breaking into Public Service: The Development of Nursing in Modern China, 1870–1949," Nursing History Review, 12, 67–96.

—— (2008): Health Care and National Development in Taiwan, 1950–2000, New York, The ABMAC Foundation.

—— (2012): Public Medicine in Wartime China: Biomedicine, State Medicine, and the Rise of China's National Medical Colleges, 1931–1945, Boston, Suffolk University, Rosenberg Institute for East Asian Studies.

White, Theodore H. and Annalee Jacoby (1946): Thunder out of China, New York, William Sloane, 1946.

Whitson, William W. (1973): The Chinese High Command: A History of Communist Military Politics, 1927–71, London MacMillan.

Wilbur, C. Martin (1983): The Nationalist Revolution in China, 1923–1928, Cambridge, Cambridge University Press.

Williamsen, Marvin (1992): "The Military Dimension, 1937–41," in James C. Hsiung and Steven I. Levine ed., China's Bitter Victory: The War with Japan, 1937–1945, Armonk, N.Y., M. E. Sharpe Inc., 147–153.

Winfield, Gerald F. (1948): China, the Land and the People, New York, William Sloane.

Wong, I. K. (1925): "Dr. Sun Yat-sen." NMJC, 11/3, 193–195.

Wong, K. Chimin and Wu Lien-teh (1936): History of Chinese Medicine, Shanghai: National Quarantine Service.

Wou, Odoric Y. K. (1994): Mobilizing the Masses: Building Revolution in Henan, Stanford, Stanford University Press.

Wu Lien-teh and J.W. H. Chun (December 1919): "The Recent Cholera Epidemic in China," NMJC, 5/4, 182–198.

—— (1920): "The Management of the 1919 Cholera Epidemic in Harbin," NMJC, 6/1, 4–16.

Wu Lien-teh (1915): "Awakening the Sanitary Conscience of China," CMJ 29/4, 222–229.

—— (1918): "North Manchuria Plague Prevention Service: Summary of Sixth Annual General Report, 1918," NMJC, 4/4, 132–139.

—— (1920): "The Management of the 1919 Cholera Epidemic in Harbin," NMJC, 6/1, 4–16.

—— (1922): "The Future of Medical Research in the Orient," NMJC, 8/4, 286–290.

—— (1923): "A Survey of Public Health Activities in China Since the Republic," NMJC, 9/1, 1–6.

—— (1924): Editorial on preventive medicine, *CMJ* (January 1924), 44, 45, cited in Lamson (1935), 455.

—— (1959): Plague Fighter: The Autobiography of a Modern Chinese Physician, Cambridge, Heffer.

Wu, S. M. (胡宣明 Hu Xuanming), (1924): "The Problem of School Hygiene in China," *NMJC,* 10/2, 98–100.

—— (January 1924): Editorial on preventive medicine, *China Medical Journal,* 44, 45.

Yang Daqing, (2001): "Atrocities in Nanjing: Searching for Explanations," in Lary and MacKinnon (2001), 76–96.

Yang Hsien-yi and Gladys Yang (1972): *Selected Stories of Lu Hsun,* Peking: Foreign Languages Press.

Yang Jisheng (2012): *Tombstone: The Great Chinese Famine 1958–1962.* New York: Farrar, Straus and Giroux.

Yang, Marian (杨崇瑞) (1934): "First Report of the Peiping Committee on Maternal Health," *CMJ,* 48/8, 786–791.

Yang Ting-kuang and W. H. Shih (1924): "Scarlet Fever in China," *NMJC,* 10/3, 153–170. Lin Chia-swee and H. M. Jettmar, "The Scarlet Fever Problem in the Far East." *NMJC,* 11, 6, (December 1925): 399–412.

Yao Hsun-yuan, (姚寻源 H. Y. Yao) (1938): "The Provincial Health Administration: A Brief Report on its Activities since its Establishment, July 1, 1936, to December 31, 1937," *CMJ,* 53, 577–583.

—— (1939): "Plan for Malaria Control in Yunnan," *CMJ,* 56/1, 63–68.

Yao, Y. T., L. C. Ling, and K. R. Liu (1936): "Studies on the So-called Chang-ch'i," Part I in *CMJ* 50, 726–738; Part II in *CMJ* 50, 1815–1828.

Ye Shaojun (1995): "A Posthumous Son," in Lau, Joseph S. M. and Howard Goldblatt, *The Columbia Anthology of Modern Chinese Literature,* New York: Columbia University Press.

Yip, Ka-che (1995): *Health and Reconstruction in Nationalist China,* Ann Arbor, Association of Asian Studies.

Young, Arthur N. (1963): *China and the Helping Hand, 1937–1945,* Cambridge, MA, Harvard University Press.

Yue, M. K. (1928): "The Epidemic of Cholera in Hinghwa City Fukien, 1–25 September 1927," *CMJ* 42/3, 151–153.

Yung, W. W., M. D. (1936): "Child Health Work in Peiping First Health Area," *CMJ,* 50, 562–572.

Zhang Chunhou (2007): *World Perspectives on 100 Poems and Ci of Mao Zedong in English and Chinese: A Comprehensive Political, Social and Historical Research,* Hong Kong, Wenwei Publishing.

Zinsser, Hans (1935): *Rats, Lice and History,* Boston: Little Brown.

Chinese Language Sources

Many of the sources listed here have been found on the Chinese internet. There are certain problems in dealing with such sources. 1) The urls are not permanent, so it may be necessary to check by author and/or title to find the document. 2) Online documents vary in quality. Some are texts already published in journals, some have been published by well-established agencies. Others rely heavily on copying texts published elsewhere or provide little if any back-up documentation for the data presented. 3) Many such documents lack author attribution. 4) Documents originally accessible through google are now mostly accessible through baidu; a few are still accessible through google, a few are not accessible through baidu, and one or two are now not accessible at all. 5) It is generally possible to sort out stylistically which accessible documents are usable.

NMJC: National Medical Journal of China.

"Ba Xiandai Yixue Daijin Shaanbei," (2006): (把现代医学带进陕北 Bringing modern medicine to northern Shaanxi), first section inside article entitled Shandan Huakai (山丹花开—the theme of a Northern Shaanxi revolutionary song). From Beijing Ribao. url: //news.sohu.com/20061019/n245878718.shtml.

"Changzheng lushang zoulai de hongse yisheng yaolan" (长征路上走来的红色医生摇篮 Cradle of Red Physicians: Walking the Road of the Long March) (2009): at http://wenku .baidu.com/view/20f0572bb4daa58da0114ad2.html.

Chen Tao (陈韬) (1987): "Lingdao Zhanshi Jiuhu zhi Lin Kesheng Xiansheng" (领导战时 救护之林可胜先生 Dr. Lin Kesheng: Leader of Emergency Relief), in Zhang Dehua (1987), 191–198.

Chen Wenda (陈闻达) (1928): "Jinhou suo Xiwang yu Xuexiao Dangju, Xuexiao Xiaoyi, ji Xuexiao Xueshengzhe" (今后所希望於学校当局学校校医及学校学生者 Henceforth what one hopes for from school authorities, medical people and students), NMJC, 14/2, 105–107.

Cui Yueli (催月犁) et al. (1987): Zhongguo Dangdai Yixuejia Huicui (中国当代医学家 荟萃 Anthology of Contemporary Chinese Physicians), Changchun, Jilin Kexuejishu chubanshe.

'Dong Ping' (东平) and Wang Fan (王凡) (2007): "Zhonggong Lingxiu yu Yan'an Zhongyang Yiyuan Wangshi" (3) (中共领袖与延安中央医院往事, Chinese Communist Leaders and Recollections of the Yan'an Central Hospital), at Zhongguo gongchandang Xinwen 中国共产党新闻, http://cpc.people.com.cn/GB/64162/64172/85037/85039/60 40385.html.

Fan Pu (樊圃) (general ed.) (1988): Zhongguo Yixue Shi (中国医学史 History of Chinese Medicine), Guizhou, Renmin Chubanshe.

Fenxi Guomin Zhengfu Shiqi Gongyi Zhidu Fazhan de Sange Jieduan (2011): (分析国民 政府时期公医制度发展的三个阶段 Analysis of the three stage development of the public healthcare system during the time of the Nationalist Government), at www.lw61 .com/html/mianfeifanwen/wenkelunwen/2011/0421/15853.html.

Feng Caizhang (冯彩章) and Li Baoding (李葆定) (1991): Hong Jun Jiangling (红军将领 Red Army Generals), Beijing, Kexue Jishu Chuban She.

Feng Zhongen (鄷仲恩) (1928): "Saochu Feijiehebing zhi Yijia Fuwu," (扫除肺结核病之 医家服务 What physicians should do to get rid of pulmonary tuberculosis), NMJC, 14/3, 149–153.

Fu Hui (傅惠) and Deng Zongyu (邓宗禹) (1989): "Jiu Weishengbu zuzhi de bianqian (旧卫生部组织的变迁 Changes in the Organization of the Old Ministry of Health), in Wenshi Ziliao Xuanbian (文史资料选编 Anthology of Literary and Historical Materials), #37, Beijing, Beijing Chubanshe, 253–277.

Fu Weikang (傅维康) (1989): Zhongguo Yixueshi (中国医学史 History of Chinese Medicine), Shanghai, Zhongyi Xueyuan Chubanshe.

Gao Hang (高航), ed. (2005): "Hongjun Jinxing di Sici Fan 'Weijiao' Douzheng," (红军进行 第四次反围剿斗争 Red Army Launches the Fourth Counter Encirclement and Suppression Campaign); on line at various urls, e.g. news.xinhuanet.com/mil/2005–07/28/ content_3278934.htm.

Gao Wei (高维) (1926): "Shehui Yixue," (社会医学 Social Medicine), NMJC, 12/6, 563–568.

Gao Xiaoyan (高晓燕) (2009): "Rijun zai Shanxi de Duqizhan," (日军在陕西的毒气战 Japanese military gas warfare in Shanxi), at www.tydao.com/2009/90901/ws90901duqi .htm.

"Gonggong weisheng shiye de fajan: xiangcun weisheng" (公共卫生事业的发展: 二乡 村卫生 Development of Public Health: 2, Village Health), in Zhongyi Lishi (中医历 史 History of Chinese Medicine), at www.cintcm.com/lanmu/zhongyi_lishi/jindaijuan/ xiyi/mulu/diliuzhang3.htm.

"Gonggong weisheng shiye de fazhan: fuyou weisheng" (妇幼卫生 Maternal Child Health). (Same url as previous entry).

"Gonggong weisheng shiye de fazhan: 1. chengshi weisheng gongzuo"(城市卫生工作 Urban Health Work). (Same url as previous two entries).

Gu Xinwei (顾鑫伟) and Liu Shanjiu (刘善玖), "Shilun Zhongyang Suqu Yiliao Weisheng Guanli Tizhi Jianli yu Wanshan," (试论中央苏区医疗卫生管理体制建立与完善 On the Establishment and Realization of the Central Soviet Medical and Healthcare System), Journal of Gannan Medical University, 26, 5 (October 2006): 807–808, at http://www.doc88.com/p-19254437705.html.

"Guanyu Zhonghua Minguo Zhengfu de Weisheng Jigou" (关于中华民国政府的卫生机构 Health Organizations of China's Nationalist Government) (2011): http://blog.sina.com.cn/s/blog_676014580100vsrm.html.

"Guo Gong Neizhan Zhandou Liebiao" (国共内战战斗列表 Chart of Nationalist and Communist Civil War Battles), http://zh.wikipedia.org/wiki/國共內戰戰鬥列表.

"Guomin zhengfu shiqi gongyi zhidu shouxiao shenwei yuanyin tanxi," (国民政府时期公医制度收效甚微原因探析 Why Public Medicine had very little Impact during the time of the Nationalist Government) (2011): at www.lw61.com/html/mianfeifanwen/wenkelunwen/2011/0421/15854.html.

Guo Shaoxing (郭绍兴) (1987): "Huiyi Kangzhan Shiqi Dang zai Zhongguo Hongshizihui Jiuhu Zongdui de Gongzuo," (回忆抗战时期党在中国红十字会救护总队的工作 Remembering the Party's Work in the Chinese Red Cross Medical Relief Corps during the time of the War of Resistance), in Zhang Dehua (1987), 3–8.

Guo Zuyuan (1987): "Feng Yuxiang Jiangjun Guancha Guiyang Honghui Jiuhu Zongduibu," (冯玉祥 将军观察贵阳红会救护总队部 General Feng Yuxiang Surveys the Guiyang Red Cross Medical Relief Corps), in Zhang Dehue (1987), 9–10.

He Biao (贺彪) (2007): "120 shi de yiliao weisheng gongzuo,"(120 师的医疗卫生工作 120th division medical health work), at www.crt.com.cn/news2007/news/YYSC/11330132557DCBOHKH9K75BH26BD500.html.

He Tao (何涛) (1987): "Honghui Jiuhu Gongzuo Shiyi,"(红会救护工作拾遗 Anecdotes from Red Cross Medical Relief Work) in Zhang Dehua (章德华) ed., (1987).

He Zhaoxiong (何兆雄) (ed.) (1988): Zhongguo Yide Shi (中国医德史 History of Medical Ethics in China), Shanghai: Shanghai Medical University.

"Hongse Fangmianjun zai Jingyuan Qiangdu Huanghe," (红色方面军在靖远强渡黄河 The Red Front Army Crossing of the Yellow River at Jingyuan), (March 18, 2010): http://61.178.146.167/jfq/shownews.asp?nid=639.

Hsiung Ping-chen (熊秉真) (1991): Yang Wenda Xiansheng Fangwen Jilu (扬文达先生访问记录), Taipei, Academia Sinica, Institute of Modern History.

Huang Jiasi(黄家驷) (ed.) (1985): Zhongguo Xiandai Yixuejia Zhuan (中国现代医学家传 Biographies of China's Modern Physicians), Hunan Kexue Jishu Chubanshe.

Huang Shuze (黄树则) (1986a): "Lingxiu de Jiaohui" 领袖的教诲 ([our] leaders' instructions), in Rao Zhengxi (1986), 6–12.

—— (1986b): "Sui han ran hou zhi song bai zhi hou diao," (岁寒然后知松柏之后凋 After the year turns cold one knows the pine and cypress are the last to wither) Rao Zhengxi (1986), 73–75.

Huashuo Lao Xiehe (话说老协和 Recollections of PUMC) (1987): Beijing, Zhongguo Wenshi Chubanshi.

Jiangning gang: minzhong shiqi de mofan shiyan xian (江宁网: 民中时期的模范实验县 a Model Experimental County during the Nationalist era, [section 3 on medicine and health 医疗卫生]) (no date): at www.jnmh.net/index.php3?file=detail.php3&kdir=2182553&nowdir=2160967&id=807894&detail=1.

"Jiemi Shijie Zuida de Luxi Xijun Dusha 42 Wan Guoren Yu'nan" (揭秘世界最大的鲁西细菌屠杀42万国人遇难 Unveiling the World's Greatest Bacterial Warfare Massacre Killing 420,000 of our People in West Shandong province) (2005): at http://hi.baidu.com/gslh8/blog/item/c5814c8d9a625513b31bbafd.html. The review originally appeared in *Lishi fengyun* 历史风云, July 4, 2005.

Jin Baoshan (金宝善) (1926): "Beijing zhi Gonggong Weisheng," (北京之公共卫生 Public Health in Beijing), *NMJC*, 12/3, 253–261.

"Jinggangshan Hongjun Yiyuan Yiwen" (井冈山红军医院轶闻 Jingangshan Red Army Hospital Anecdote[s]) (2008); from Zhongguo Ji'an web, at http://ja.jxcn.cn/247/250/270/html/20080228/20080228151113.htm. A more detailed account with the same title is at http://www.jgsdaily.com/247/250/270/html/20080228/20080228151113.htm.

Jiuhu Shouce (救护手册 First Aid Manual) (1937): Beijing: Chinese Red Cross, Beijing Branch.

"Kangri Zhanzheng Gei Zhongguoren Dailai Zainan You Naxie?" (抗日战争给中国人带来灾难有哪些, What Calamities did the War of Resistance bring about for the Chinese People?) (2009): http://wenda.tianya.cn/wenda/thread?tid=7573bd99ad3ce8f.

Kangri zhanzheng shengli 50 zhounianji de diaocha tongji shuzi (Examination of statistics on the occasion of the fiftieth anniversary of the victory of the War of Resistance (dated 2009 on blog.sina): at http://wenda.tianya.cn/wenda/thread?tid=7573bd99ad3ce8f8 (or http://wenda.tianya.cn/question/7573bd99ad3ce8f8 http://wenda.tianya.cn/question/7573bd99ad3ce8f8), also available as a separate document at http://blog.sina.com.cn/s/blog_4dae258b0100eus9.html.

Li Haiwen (李海文) (2006): Changzheng zhong Weisheng Jiaoyu he Yiliao Gongzuo, (长征中卫生教育和医疗工作 Health Education and Medical Work during the Long March). This source is available on several websites, e.g. http://vip.book.sina.com.cn/book/chapter_40933_25324.html.

Li Ji (李吉) (2002): "Hongjun Dongzheng" (红军东征) at www.tydao.com/suwu/2002/1223-3.htm. Li Ji (李吉) (2002): "Hongjun Dongzheng" (红军东征) at www.tydao.com/suwu/2002/1223-3.htm.

Li Jinlong (李金龙) and Zhang Juan (张娟) (2008): "Guanyu Kangzhan shiqi Shaanganning bianqu liangxing hexie jianshe de lishi yanjiu" (关于抗战时期陕甘宁边区两性和谐建设的历史研究 Historical Research on the Establishment of Gender Harmony in the Shaanganning Border Area during the War of Resistance). *Yan'an Daxue Xuebao*, 30/2 (April 2008), 50–53.

Li Lixia (李丽霞) (December 2006): "1928–1930 Nian Nianjin Shaanxi Zaihuang Yimin Wenti." (1928–1930 年年馑陕西灾荒移民问题 Analysis of Shaanxi Migrants during the Famine of 1928–1930), Journal of Institute of Disaster-Prevention Science and Technology (Fangzai Keji Xueyuan Xuebao 防灾科技学院学报), 8/4, online e.g. at http://d.wanfangdata.com.cn/periodical_fzjsgdkxxxb200604007.aspx.

Li Qingying (李庆英), "Hongjun Xilujun Lishi Zhenxiang Chengqing Shimo (红军西路军历史真相澄清始末 The Real Facts of the History of the Red Army's Western Route Army Clarified from Beginning to End)" (online date 2005): Article originally published in Dangshi Wenyuan; available online e.g. at //news.xinhuanet.com/newmedia/2005-10/24/content_3675981.htm.

Li Tingan (李廷安) (1935): Zhongguo Xiangcun Weisheng Wenti (中国乡村卫生问题 China's Rural Healthcare Problems), Shanghai, Commercial Press.

Li Xiangming (李向明) et al. (ed.) (1984): Zhongguo Xiandai Yixuejia Zhuanlue, (中国现代医学家传略 Brief Biographies of China's Modern Physicians), Beijing, Kexue Jishu Wenxian Chubanshe, 280–286.

Liao Haoping (廖皓平) (2009): "Mao Zedong zai Jinfeng Dashan, (毛泽东在金丰大山 Mao Zedong at Jinfeng Mountain), at http://www.baomi.org/bmyw_info.php?optionid=62&auto_id=375.

Lin Jingcheng (林竞成) (1987): "Canjia Honghui Jiuhu Zongduibu Gongzuo de Huiyi," (参加红会救护总队部工作的回忆 Memories of Taking Part in the Work of the Red Cross Medical Relief Corps), Zhang Dehua (1987), 64–75.

Liu Juanzhi (刘娟芝) (2010): "Kangzhan Shiqi Shaangangning Bianqu de Fuyou Baojian," (抗战时期陕甘宁边区的妇幼保健 Maternal-Child Health in the Shaanganning Border Area during the War of Resistance), at lsx.ldxy.edu.cn/message/biyelunwen/ljz.doc.

Liu Sijin (刘似锦) (1989): Liu Ruiheng Boshi yu Zhongguo Yiyao ji Weisheng Shiye (刘瑞恒博士与中国医药及卫生事业, Dr. J. Heng Liu and Medical and Health Development in China), Taipei, Commercial Press.

Liu Yongmao (刘永懋) (1970): "Kangzhan Banian Zhuisui Lin Kesheng Xiansheng Huiyi," (抗战八年追随林可胜先生回忆 Recollections of Following Dr. Lin Kesheng during the Eight year War of Resistance), Zhuanji Wenxue (传记文学) 16/1, 95–98.

Lü Yunming (吕运明) (1987): "Lin Kesheng Jiaoshou Zai Kangri Zhanzheng Qijian de Zhuoyue Gongji," (林可胜教授在抗日战争期间的卓越功绩 Professor Lin's outstanding Contributions during the War of Resistance against Japan), Zhang Dehua (1987), 187–190.

Mao Zedong (1944): "Wenhua gongzuo zhong de tongyi zhanxian," 文化工作中的统一战线 The United Front in Cultural Work), see www.people.com.cn.

Qiu Yunhong (仇云红) (2011): "Mao Zedong yiliao weisheng sixiang dui dangdai xinxing nongcun yiliao weisheng shiye de qishi (毛泽东医疗卫生思想对当代新型农村医疗卫生事业的启示 Light thrown by Mao Zedong's Medical and Health Thinking on the Present-day Style of Village Medical and Health Practice), at http://www.chinareform.org.cn/Economy/Agriculture/Practice/201109/t20110921_122194.htm.

Rao Zhengxi (绕正锡) (ed.) (1986): Yan'an Bai Qiuen Guoji Heping Yiyuan (白求恩 国际和平医院 Bethune International Peace Hospital), Beijing, Jiefangjun Chubanshe.

—— (1986a): "Junwei lingdao tongzhi dui Yan'an Baiqiuen guoji heping yiyuan de guanhuai" (军委领导同志对延安白求恩国际和平医院的关怀, Solicitude of military commission leader comrades towards the Bethune International Peace Hospital), in Rao, ed. Yan'an Baiqiuen guoji heping yiyuan, 3–5.

"Sanguang Zhengce," (三光政策 Three Eliminations Policy) (2011): baike.baidu.com/view/71188.htm.

Shaanxi Shaanganning bianqu yiyuan (2010): ([宁晋]第四节陕西陕甘宁边区医院 Section 4: Shaanxi Shaanganning Border Hospital), at http://www.sxsdq.cn/dqzlk/sxsz/weisz/201004/t20100416_245491.htm, also at www.qxdyxx.com/njdsyy/news11035.html.

Shaanxi Zhongyi Xueyuan, (1988): Zhongguo Yixueshi (中国医学史 History of Chinese Medicine), Guizhou Renmin Chubanshe.

"Shandan huakai [xia]" (山丹花开[下]) (2006): section headed "Ba Xiandai Yixue Daijin Shaanbei," (把现代医学带进陕北 Bringing modern medicine to northern Shaanxi), at http://news.sohu.com/20061019/n245878718.shtml.

Shandongsheng weisheng dashiji (山东省卫生大事记 Shandong Provincial Health Record of Major Events) (2007): at http://www.shdma.com/show.aspx?id=304&cid=63.

Shi Zhengxin (施正信) (1987): "Huiyi Tuyun'guan,"(回忆图云关 Remembering Tuyun'guan) in Zhang Dehua (1987), 81.

Shi Yuquan (史玉泉) and He Liangjia (何亮家) (1985): "Shen Kefei," (沈克非) in Huang Jiasi (黄家驷) ed., Zhongguo Xiandai Yixuejia Zhuan (中国现代医学家传 Biographies of Modern Chinese Physicians), Changsha, Hunan Kexue Jishu, 115–116.

Shuangyong Yundong (双拥运动 'double support' movement) (2004): at http://news.xinhuanet.com/ziliao/2004-07/20/content_1618426.htm.

Tian Gang (田刚) (2009): Zhongguo Gongchangdang Lingdao de Suqu Weisheng Fangyi Yundong (中国工厂党领导的苏区卫生防疫运动 Soviet Area Health Prevention Movement of the Leadership of the Chinese Communist Party), published on-line by Zhongguo Gongchangdang Xinwen (News of the Communist Party of China) at http://cpc.people.com.cn/GB/64162/64172/85037/85039/6040454.html.

Wan Xuefeng (万学锋) and Wang Jihong (王季红), "Rijun dui Balujun, Xinsijun de Huaxuezhan," (日军对八路军新四军的化学战 Japanese Military Chemical Warfare against the Eighth Route and New Fourth Armies), at http://richsp.com/userlist/731/newshow-18130.html. [This url is no longer freely available, but a book by these authors with this title is at 731部队罪行国际学术研讨会论文选编祸移中国东北—侵华日军第七三…at www.731museum.org.cn/jy/pagelist.asp?id=112].

Wang Chunjing (王春菁) (1987): "Canjia Zhongguo Hongshizihui Gongzuo de Huiyi," (参加中国红十字会工作的回忆 Memories of Participating in Chinese Red Cross Work), in Zhang Dehua (1987), 114–121.

Wang Congyan (王从炎) (1987): "Jiuhu Zongduibu Yiliaodui Gongzuo Jianjie," (护总队部医疗队工作简介 Brief Introduction to the work of the MRC Healthcare Units), in Zhang Dehua (1987), 131–133.

Wang Tianjiang 王天将 (September 1990): *Henan Jindai Dashiji 1840–1949* (河南近代大事记 Record of Major Events in the Modern History of Henan 1840–1949), Henan Renmin Chubanshe 河南人民出版社, at http://new.ssreader.com/ebook/detail.jhtml? id=11713635.

Wang Xiuying (1987): "Wode muxiao—Xiehe huxiao," (我的母校协和护校 My Mother School—PUMC School of Nursing), in Huashuo Lao Xiehe (话说老协和), Beijing, Zhongguo Wenshu chuban she, 224–230, also reproduced (in large part) in Liu Sijin, op. cit., 33–37.

Wang Xueli (王学礼), Yin Xing (尹醒) (1986): "Qinqie de Jiaohui, Juda de Guwu" (亲切的教诲巨大的鼓舞, Attentive teaching, great inspiration), in Rao Zhengxi (1986), 13–15.

Wang Youchun (汪犹春), (1987a): "Zai Honghui Jiuhu Zongduibu de Huiyi," (在红会救护总队部的回忆 Recollections of Being with the Red Cross Medical Relief Corps), in Zhang Dehua, (1987), 101–106, 113.

—— (1987b): "Nanwang de Suiyue—Ji Zhongguo Hongshizihui Guiyang Yiliaodui zai Miandian," (难忘的岁月—记中国红十字会贵阳医疗队在缅甸 Unforgettable Times: Remembering the CRC Guiyang Healthcare Units in Burma), in Zhang Dehua, (1987), 177–186.

Wang Yuanzhou (王元周) (2009): "Kangzhan Shiqi Genjudi de Yibing Liuxing yu Qunzhong Yiliao Weisheng Gongzuo de Fazhan," (抗战时期根据地的疫病流行与群众医疗卫生工作的发展 Epidemic Disease in Base Areas during the War of Resistance, and Development of Medical and Public Health Work among the Masses). Kangri Zhanzheng Yanjiu (抗日战争研究 Journal of Studies of China's Resistance War against Japan), 2009, 1, 59–76.

Wei Hongyun (魏宏运) (1986): *Zhongguo xiandai shigao* (中国现代史稿 Draft Modern History of China), Heilongjiang, Renmin Chubanshe.

Wu Hongzi (吴宏子) (1987): "Ji liushisi yiliaodui (记六十四医疗队 Remembering the 64th Medical Care Unit), in Zhang Dehua (1987), 145–148, 141.

"Xiangjiang Zhanyi" (湘江战役 Xiang River Battle), www.baike.com/wiki/湘江战役.

Xie Benshu (谢本书) (November 2010): "Riben zai Dianxi de Xijunzhan" (日本在滇西的细菌战, Japan's Bacterial War in Western Yunnan), at www.balujun.org/qhrj/xjz/5420.html.

Xie Zhonghou (谢忠厚) (2002): "Huabei Jia di 1855 Xijunzhan Budui ji Yanjiu" (华北甲第一八五五细菌战部队之研究 Research into North China's top bacterial warfare Unit #1855). This is a book chapter, accessible at http://www.balujun.org/qhrj/xjz/5426.html, or at http://www.lw23.com/pdf_547043de_92ad-44ae-8f2d-6f07559c96f1/lunwen.pdf.

—— (2008): "Jiekai bei Yangai de Lishi Zhenshi—Huabei de '731'—Rijun (jia) 1855 Xijun Budui Jiemi," (揭开被掩盖的历史真实: 华北的"731": 日军[甲] 1855 细菌部队揭秘 Uncovering a Concealed Historical Truth: North China's 'Number 731': The Secret of The Japanese Military's Top 1855 Bacterial Unit), at http://bbs.1931-9-18.org/redirect.php?tid=238605&goto=lastpost.

Xin Zhongguo Yufang Yixue Lishi Jingyan (新中国预防医学历史经验 Historical Experience of Preventive Medicine in New China) (1988): volume 3, Beijing: Renmin Weisheng Chubanshe.

Xu Shusheng (徐书生) (2008): "Peizhi Gongyi Rencai de Guoli Zhongzheng Yixueyuan (培植公医人材的国立忠正医学院 The National Zhongzheng Medical College for Training Physicians to Serve State Medicine) (no date accessible): at http://www.ncsjx.cn/?artid=13593&F=view.html, also http://blog.sina.com.cn/s/blog_569c4ca30100cbl5.html.

Xu Zhi (徐植) (1987): "Wo zai honghui jiuhu zongdui de jingli" (我在红会救护总队的经历 My Experience with the Red Cross Medical Relief Corps), Zhang Dehua (1987), 149–153.

Xue Qingyu (薛庆煜) (1987): "Zai Guiyang Tuyun'guan de Honghui Jiuhu Zongdui." (在贵阳图云关的红会救护总队 The Chinese Red Cross Medical Relief Corps in Tuyun'guan, Guiyang), Zhang Dehua (1987), 38–55.

Yan Fuqing, (1927): "Guomin Zhengfu Ying She Zhongyang Weishengbu zhi Jianyi," (国民政府应设中央卫生部之建议 Proposal to the Nationalist Government to Establish a Central Ministry of Health), *NMJC*, 13/4, 229–240.

Yan Yiwei (颜宜葳) and Zhang Daqing (张大庆) (2006): "Wo guo di yizuo xueku de jianli zhanzheng huanjingxia yixiang yixue xinjishu de zhuanrang, jieshou ji yingxiang," (我国第一座血库的建立战争环境下一项医学新技术的转让接受及影响 The First Blood Bank in China: Transfer, Incorporation and Consequence of a New Medical Technique in Wartime), *Kexue wenhua pinglun* (Science and Culture Review), 3/1. Available online.

Yanan Baiqiuen guoji heping yiyuan (1986): (延安白求恩国际和平医院 Yan'an Bethune International Peace Hospital), Beijing, Jiefangjun chubanshe.

Yang Lifu (杨立夫), ed., (1988): Fenghuo Xiaoyan zhong de Baiyi Zhanshi (烽火硝烟中的白衣战士 White-coated Warriors Amid the Fire and Brimstone), Beijing, Military District Logistics Department, Office for Collection of Party Historical Materials.

Yang Wenda (杨文达) (1989a): "Liu Ruiheng Boshi Qi Ren Qi Shi," (刘瑞恒博士其人其事, Dr. Liu Ruiheng: the Man and his Work), in Liu Sijin (刘似锦) (1989), 65–69.

—— (1989b): "Yishi Jiaoyu yu Xunlian (医事教育与训练 Medical Education and Training)," in Liu Sijin, Liu Ruiheng Boshi, 123–127.

Yang Xishou (杨锡寿) (1987): "Huiyi Guiyang Lujun Yiyuan," (回忆贵阳陆军医院, Recalling Guiyang's Army Hospital), in Zhang Dehua (1987), 167–176.

Yijiuerqi 1927 nian dageming shibai hou de da tusha he zhanshou (2011): (1927 年大革命失败后的大屠杀和斩首 (massacres and decapitations following the failure of the great revolution in 1927), www.360doc.com/content/11/1108/22/1241083_162918954.shtml.

Yi Ming (佚名) (2007): "Jin Maoyue xiansheng fangtan lu," (金茂岳先生访谈录 Record of conversation with Dr. Jin Maoyue), http://www.eywedo.com/huizuyanjiu/hzyj20070206.html.

Yinni Huayi Mingyi Ke Quanshou [san] (2010): (印尼华裔名医柯全寿 [三] The Indonesian of Chinese descent and famous doctor Ke Quanshou [three]), http://blog.sina.com.cn/s/blog_614c191d0100jj7l.html.

Yu Ge (余戈) (2009): "Rijun Fangduju yu Dui Hua Duqizhan," (日军防毒具与对华毒气战 Japanese military gas protection equipment and gas warfare against China), Shijie Junshi 世界军事, 2009:8, 95–97, at http://pdlishi.dhsvr.net/pdlishi/Article/wzfl/200907/450.html.

Yu Shifa (余世法) (1987): "Honghui Jiuhu Zongduibu de Yixie Qingkuang" (红会救护总队部的一些情况 Some factors regarding the Red Cross Medical Relief Corps), in Zhang Dehua (1987), 111–113.

Zhang Dehua ed. (章德华) (1987): Honghui Jiuhu Zongdui, (红会救护总队 Red Cross Medical Relief Corps), Guiyang, Guiyang Wenshi Ziliao Xuanji.

Zhang Jian (张建) (1984): Guofang Yixueyuan Yuan-shi (国防医学院院史 History of the National Defense Medical Center), Taipei, National Defense Medical Center.

Zhang Li'an (张丽安) (2000): *Zhang Jian yu Junyi Xuexiao* (张建与军医学校 Zhang Jian and the Army Medical School), Hong Kong, Cosmos Books Ltd.

Zhang Pengyuan (张朋园 Chang Peng-yuan) (1992): Zhou Meiyu Xiansheng Fangwen jilu (周美玉先生访问记录 Oral Memoir of Ms. Zhou Meiyu), Taipei, Nankang, Academia Sinica, 27–28.

Zhang Qi'an (张启安) (2001): "Shaanganning Bianqu de Yiliao Weisheng Gongzuo he Yide Jianshe," (陕甘宁边区的医疗卫生工作和医德建设 Shaanganning Border Area Medical Health Work and Formation of Medical Ethics), Zhongguo Yixue Lunlixue, March 2001, 77, at http://journal.shouxi.net/upload/pdf/145/2619/1370280_6323.pdf.

Zhang Ruguang, Guo Fangfu, He Manqiu (1989): Zhongguo Gong Nong Hong Jun Weisheng Gongzuo Shilue (中国工农红军卫生工作史略 History of Healthcare Work of China's Worker-Peasant Red Army), Beijing, Jiefangjun Chubanshe.

Zhang Taishan 张泰山 (2008): *Chuanranbing yu Shehui* (传染病与社会, Infection and Society in the Republic of China), Beijing: Shehui Kexue Wenxian Chubanshe.

Zhao En-yuan (赵恩源) (c. 1933): "Guo-li Beijing diyi Zhuchan Xuexiao Lueying" (国立北京第一助产学校掠影 A Glimpse of National Beijing Number One Midwifery School), in Liu Sijin (1989), 170–173.

Zhao Shifa (赵士法), (February 1925): Weisheng Jiaoxuefa" (卫生教学法 Methods of Health Education), *NMJC* 11/1, 4–17.

Zhang Wenjun (张文军) (2008): "Shaanganning bianqu de baojian yaoshe he weisheng hezuoshe" (陕甘宁边区的保健药设和卫生合作社 Shaanganning border area pharmaceutical and health service cooperatives), MA dissertation, Shanxi Zhongyi Xueyuan, online at www.doc88.com/p-470422266067.html.

Zhang Yumin (张育民) (2004): "Kangzhan shiqi heping yiyuan de jixiang gongzuo zhidu," (抗战时期和平医院的几项工作制度 Aspects of Peace Hospital work during the War of Resistance), 4: shangbingyuan sixiang zhengzhi gongzuo zhidu (伤病员思想政治工作制度 System of ideological political work with sick and wounded soldiers), http://www.peacehospital.com/jianjie/book_1/chuanren_5.htm.

Zhongguo Hongshizi Hui (中国红十字会 Chinese Red Cross Society) (1947): Shanghai, Executive Yuan News Bureau, in Shanghai Municipal Archive.

Zhongguo Hongshizihui Bainian (中国红十字会拜年, Centenary of the Red Cross Society of China) (2004): Beijing, Red Cross Society of China.

Zhongguo Hongshizihui Huabei Jiuhu Weiyuanhui Baogao (中国红十字会华北救护委员会报告 Report of Chinese Red Cross North China Relief Commission) (c. 1934): in Shanghai Municipal Archive.

Zhongyang Suqu (中央苏区 Central Soviet), http://www.fj.xinhuanet.com/zb/2007-09/07/content_14798071.htm.

Zhonghua Renmin Gongheguo Guofangbu (2009): Zhongyang Suqu Diwuci Fan Weijiao" (中央苏区第五次反围剿 Central Soviet Area Fifth Counter Encirclement and Suppression) (2009): http://www.mod.gov.cn/hist/2009-07/22/content_4005819.htm.

Zhou Meiyu (1936): "Dingxian Xiangcun Gonggong Weisheng Hushi Shishi Fangfa," (定县乡村公共卫生护士实施方法 Practical Methods of Public Health Nursing in Dingxian Townships and Villages), in Liu Sijin (刘似锦) (1989), 23–26.

Zhu Baotian (朱宝钿) (c.1930): "Liu Ruiheng Boshi dui huli zhi changdao" (刘瑞恒博士对护理之倡导 Dr. Liu Ruiheng's Proposals for Nursing), in Liu Sijin (1989), 115–117.

Zhu Chao, (ed.) (1988): Zhongwai yixue Jiaoyushi (中外医学教育史 History of Chinese and Foreign Medical Education), Shanghai, Shanghai Yike Daxue.

Zhu De (1986): "Jinian Kedihua Daifu," (纪念柯棣华大夫, Remembering Dr. Kotnis), in Rao Zhengxi, (ed.), Baiqiuen Guoji Heping Yiyuan, 28–29.

Zhu Hongzhao (朱鸿召) (2008): Yanan Zhongyang Yiyuan, Yanan shiqi zuihao de yiyuan (延安中央医院延安时期最好的医院, Ya'nan Central Hospital—the best Hospital in the Yan'an Period), www.djbkw.com/Html/wenhua/5452628215.hstml. (djbkw stands for dajia baokan wang 大家报刊网). The date of entry is January 4, 2008.

—— (2010): "Yan'an 'Zhong-Xi Yi Hezuo' yundong shimo" (延安中西医合作运动始末 The Movement in Chinese-Western Medical Cooperation in Yan'an from Start to End), at wenku.baidu.com/view/bacb03c708a1284ac8504318.html.

INDEX OF NAMES

INDEX OF SUBJECTS

Printed in the United States
By Bookmasters